THE ART OF
EKG INTERPRETATION
A Self-Instructional Text

Third Edition

With Special Sections on

ANTIARRHYTHMIC AND THROMBOLYTIC DRUG THERAPY
HEMODYNAMIC MONITORING
PEDIATRIC EKG INTERPRETATION
PACEMAKER BASICS

Karen S. Ehrat, Ph.D.

KENDALL/HUNT PUBLISHING COMPANY
2460 Kerper Boulevard P.O. Box 539 Dubuque, Iowa 52004-0539

Front cover photography by Memories In Time, Doug Duncan, Mt. Clemens, Michigan: Shadow box design by Bing Veryser.

THIS BOOK IS DEDICATED
TO MEMBERS OF
THE HEALTHCARE COMMUNITY
... PROFESSIONALS and STUDENTS ...
WHO ARE STRIVING TO LEARN THE
COMPLEXITIES of EKG INTERPRETATION
AS PAINLESSLY AS POSSIBLE!

CONTRIBUTING AUTHORS

DEANNA M. CULBERSON, B.S.N., R.N.

MIKE LUCEY, Pharm. D.

DELORES D. SCHULTZ, B.S.N., R.N.

JANE D. WERTH, M.S., R.N.

Acknowledgments

Every writer struggles with *meaningfully* recognizing all those individuals who support or assist with a publication effort. This author is no different! Clearly, any published work is the end product of multi-faceted ideas and labor.

I especially want to recognize and thank past learners who have generated numerous questions. Those questions served as the foundation for this publication.

Tucson Medical Center, Tucson, Arizona, deserves special credit for supporting the genesis of this work. The *cactus belt* contributed creative talents and scholarly insight. Thank you to all those special people, too many to name personally!

Special recognition goes to the staff of 31 West, ICU/CCU and PAR at St. Joseph's Mercy Hospital, Mt. Clemens, Michigan, who have *arduously* watched for, and collected, unique monitor tracings.

Deanna Culberson, Mike Lucey, Jane Werth, and Delores Schultz win best supporting author awards for their contributions to this text. Their efforts speak for themselves.

Last, though certainly not least, I must thank Deborah Smith, Terri Cory, Tracey Toth, and Peggy Reihner for their typing and editorial support. Without their able assistance, this text would be a mere collection of EKG strips and meaningless diagrams! A warm hug goes out to Bing Veryser, the best shadow box builder "UP NORTH".

For the many supporting individuals I have not named, I trust a sincere *thank you* will be accepted!

A Long-winded Introduction
Still Worth Reading

(From the first edition of this book)

Traditionally, educators have cautioned students NOT TO JUDGE A BOOK BY ITS COVER, though I assume you have picked up this book because it stands out amidst the more conservatively bound books. If that is the case, you should know a bit about the book and a bit about the author.

It has been my experience that, in order to grasp the complexities of EKG interpretation, one must have (out of necessity) a mind for abstractions, the ability to make conceptual leaps, and an unrestricted book budget. In many regards, those expectations are unrealistic for either the practicing professional or the student.

So . . . this book has been designed to eliminate those difficulties by drawing together the relevant theory pertaining to rhythm anomalies—and do it in a systematic way that allows for PAINLESS learning!

Educators (from the "Humor Has No Place In The Classroom" vintage) may look critically at my illustrations and analogies. My theory, however, is that learners tend to remember analogies . . . or stated another way, association aids learning. Beyond that, I believe learning should be fun and completely non-threatening . . . particularly when dealing with a technical subject!

As for me, I suppose I am one of those nontraditional educators who enjoys the lighter side of learning. I trust THE ART OF EKG INTERPRETATION will meet your expectations. I have built in enough structure to prevent even the novice from floundering. My expectation is that when you have completed the book, you will be *comfortable* describing the various dysrhythmias and know when action is warranted. I do not expect EKG interpretation to become the focal point of your existence, nor do I expect you to suffer any physical or psychosomatic symptoms from your study!

There are several things you should be aware of before you start through the book. People working around monitoring equipment (and cardiac patients) have a tendency to use a lot of "jargon" terminology . . . "aberrantly conducted premature junctional beats interposed on a sinus rhythm with periods of rate related right bundle branch block" . . . much like the scientist who complained that a Canis familiaris upset the structural design of his Tupi petyn—he can't just tell you that a dog dug up his petunias! It's the same reason that surgeons wear green, ICU nurses wear stethoscopes around their necks, surgical nurses clip a Kelly clamp to their pockets, and firemen have dalmations. It's simply a form of identity in a complex world!

My theory is, if confusing terminology is addressed secondarily, with a primary focus on descriptive analysis, EKG interpretation is actually quite simple. Rest assured, the terminology will follow as a natural consequence! The important thing to remember when dealing with any abnormality in rhythm is this: There are only a few treatments available—regardless of the dysrhythmia name. So, it is pointless to become overly focused on *inconsistent* naming jargon.

To illustrate what I mean—following are the available dysrhythmia treatments:

- speed up the heart rate
- slow down the heart rate
- administer drugs to control ectopic or irritable beating
- introduce a pacemaker to initiate or control a rhythm
- administer electric shock
- or, simply do nothing!

So, in essence, arrhythmia interpretation deals with determining whether:

- the heart rate is too slow
- the heart rate is too fast
- there is irritable or ectopic activity
- there is no activity (you'll usually have a clue—the patient will be coding!)
- the heart rate is normal, or of no physiologic consequence to the patient

SOUNDS SIMPLE . . . RIGHT?

This book has been structured to allow you to learn at your own pace. In the event that you have difficulty pacing yourself, the book has been divided into major sections, each section becoming slightly more challenging. So, take each section as it comes!

You are probably familiar with self-instructional material. You will be provided with information and encouragement under headings labeled INPUT. Practice exercises follow the input sections. Last, but not least, practice exercise answers are provided under FEEDBACK headings.

Contents

(Participant Objectives Precede Each Section)

LEADing Into Section I

Welcome to this book! You're probably wondering who I am . . . Right? Well, this is me.

Actually, this is the back of my head. If you think it would be difficult to recognize me in a crowd . . . I'll help you out by showing you my best side. . . .

(Cute, huh?)

If you're still uncertain about what I look like . . . you can look at me from any angle that you choose.

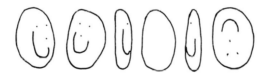

Sometimes if one has a common face, it's necessary to look closely to know who that someone is!

The same thing holds true when looking at monitors or electrocardiograms! Sometimes all those "peculiar" waves and bumps are *almost* **impossible** to identify. . . .

But, by looking at them from different views or angles, identity becomes more clear.

Before you start through this book, there are several things you should know. For instance, all cell membranes in the body are charged . . .

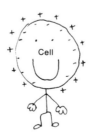

. . . and *CHARGED* means that the cell membranes have *ELECTRICAL POTENTIALS*.

When cells are in a RESTING or POLARIZED state, the cell membrane carries a net positive charge.

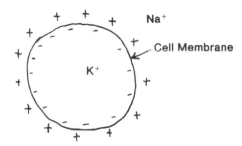

This charge or electrical potential results from the difference of intra and extracellular electrolyte concentrations. Technically speaking, the development of energy or electrical potential is dependent upon the dissipation or restitution of the ionic gradient across the cell membrane! Because of this charge, electrical potentials can be measured (like on EKG's)!

When the cell is electrically stimulated, the cells depolarize and contract. The cell membrane which is usually only slightly permeable to sodium (Na^+), allows Na^+ ions to rush into the cell while potassium (K^+) moves out of the cell.

This shift in electrolyte concentrations reverses the charge on the cell membrane and is known as DEPOLARIZATION.

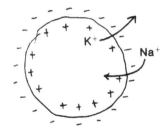

Once depolarization occurs, the cell activity transports Na^+ back to the cell membrane surface, and K^+ diffuses back into the cell.

That brings us back to where we started from. The returning to the resting state is called REPOLARIZATION.

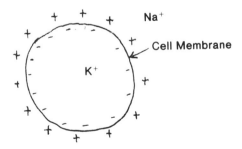

It is this process of DEPOLARIZATION and REPOLARIZATION of the myocardial cells that produces the various wave forms seen on the EKG. The EKG measures electrical potential . . . it tells one nothing about muscle contraction.

It is perhaps worth remembering that electrical depolarization occurs *before* cardiac muscle contraction . . . and that electrical repolarization follows cardiac muscle contraction!

Rather than tackling the history of electrical potential measurement, we will just accept the fact that the standard EKG machine has the capability of measuring electrical potential using a 12 lead system.

If you think of leads as simply providing different views or angles from which to view the heart's electrical activity, the subject is less frightening.

The standard 12 lead EKG system has 5 electrodes. One electrode is placed on each extremity, while the 5th electrode is used as a FLOATING ELECTRODE . . . or used for recording from the chest wall.

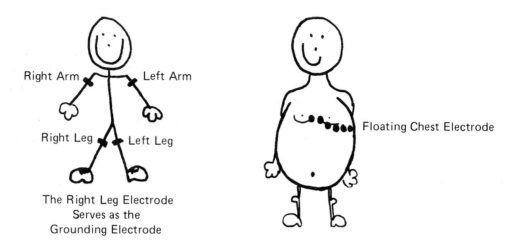

Right Arm   Left Arm

Right Leg   Left Leg

The Right Leg Electrode
Serves as the
Grounding Electrode

Floating Chest Electrode

There are actually three different kinds of leads . . . standard limb leads, augmented leads, and precordial or chest leads. Each lead is made up of a negative (−) and a positive (+) electrode. These electrodes sense both the magnitude and the direction of the electrical forces and also record surface information from the heart borders. Whew!

That sounds confusing, so let's talk about each kind of lead separately.

Lets make certain though, that we understand the important points before we tackle the various leads.

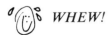 Though these points will be discussed later in the book, they will assist you in understanding the EKG picture associated with the various leads.

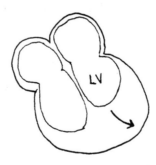

LV

FIRST, the major direction of ventricular activation is leftward, through the free wall of the left ventricle (see arrow).

SECONDLY, ventricular depolarization or activation is recorded on the EKG as a QRS complex. QRS complexes are either positive (upright) or negative (directed downward) depending upon the placement of the electrodes and the movement of depolarization toward or away from those electrodes.

WHEW!

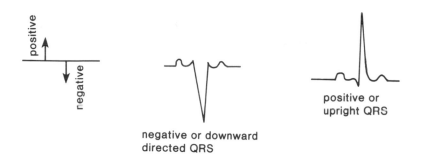

negative or downward
directed QRS

positive or
upright QRS

Remember . . . the QRS represents ventricular depolarization or activation.
NOW . . . *the good stuff.* . . .

When the major force or direction of depolarization spreads through the heart muscle toward a positive (+) electrode, the QRS deflection on the EKG will appear upright or positive.

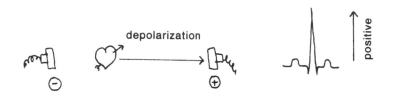

depolarization

positive

If the major force or direction of depolarization spreads through the heart muscle away from a positive (+) electrode or toward a negative (−) electrode, the QRS deflection will appear negative or directed downward.

depolarization

negative

Sounds *fairly simple* . . . right?!

You will notice as we move forward that various electrodes change their *polarity* . . . in other words, sometimes a given electrode is positive (+), and sometimes that same electrode is negative (−). *NOT TO WORRY!* The EKG recording machine is programmed to change the polarity when the various lead channels are selected. *WHEW!*

Now . . . more about the 12 leads. . . .

The Standard Limb Leads

The STANDARD LIMB LEADS are leads I, II, and III and they record frontal plane activity. These leads are *bipolar leads* . . . which means that each of these leads has two electrodes which record the electrical potential of the heart flowing toward two extremities. In other words, each lead records the difference of electrical potential between two selected electrode sites.

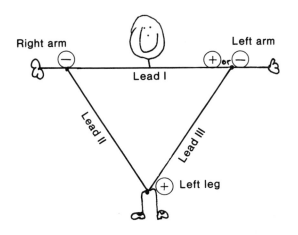

Leads I, II, are III are all electrically equidistant from the myocardial activity. The right arm is always the negative (−) pole, while the left leg is always the positive (+) pole. The left arm electrode is positive in Lead I and negative in Lead III.

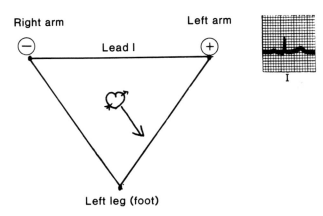

Lead I records the difference of potential between the left arm and the right arm. Specifically, in Lead I, the positive electrode is on the left arm and the negative electrode is on the right arm. The important thing to observe is that the direction of depolarization (see arrow) moves generally toward the positive (+) electrode. Thus, the QRS (which represents ventricular depolarization) is predominantly positive or upright in Lead I.

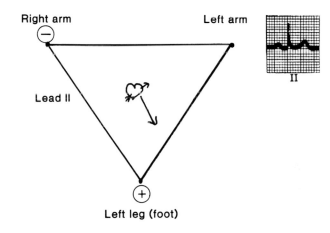

Lead II records the difference of potential between the left leg and the right arm. In Lead II, the left leg electrode is positive and the right arm electrode is negative. Notice the direction of depolarization (see arrow) moves generally toward the positive (+) electrode. Therefore, the QRS in Lead II is positive or upright.

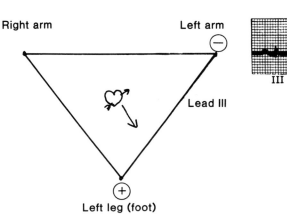

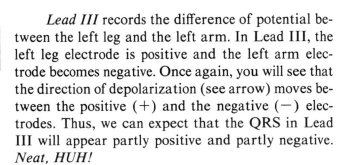

Lead III records the difference of potential between the left leg and the left arm. In Lead III, the left leg electrode is positive and the left arm electrode becomes negative. Once again, you will see that the direction of depolarization (see arrow) moves between the positive (+) and the negative (−) electrodes. Thus, we can expect that the QRS in Lead III will appear partly positive and partly negative. *Neat, HUH!*

The Augmented Leads

The AUGMENTED LEADS, leads aVR, aVL, and aVF are designed to increase the amplitude of the deflections by 50% over those recorded by the standard limb leads. The augmented leads are unipolar in nature (one electrode on the body) and record electrical potential from both the right and left arms and the left leg.

> P.S. aVR stands for augmented voltage right arm
> aVL stands for augmented voltage left arm
> aVF stands for augmented voltage foot

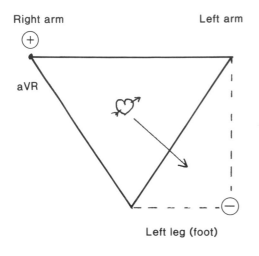

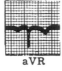

Lead aVR faces the heart from the right shoulder and is oriented to the cavity of the heart. In lead aVR, the right arm electrode extends in an imaginary direction between the left arm and left leg electrodes. The *important* thing to notice is that the direction of depolarization (see arrow) moves toward the negative (−) electrode. Thus, the QRS is directed negatively in lead aVR.

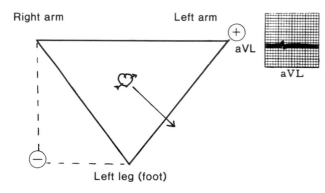

Lead aVL faces the heart from the left shoulder and is oriented to the left ventricle. In lead aVL, the left arm electrode is positive. The negative electrode extends in an imaginary direction between the right arm and left leg electrodes. The *important* thing to notice is that the direction of depolarization (see arrow) moves more or less perpendicular to the positive and negative electrodes. Thus, the QRS complex viewed from lead aVL is neither extremely positive nor negative.

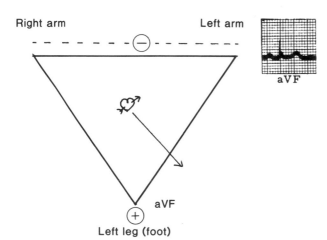

Lead aVF faces the heart from the hip and is oriented to the inferior surface of the left ventricle. In lead aVF, the left leg electrode is positive. The negative electrode extends in an imaginary direction between the right arm and left arm electrodes. The *important* point to notice is that the direction of depolarization (see arrow) moves principally toward the positive (+) electrode. Thus, the QRS complex viewed from lead aVF is positive.

Precordial Leads

There are *six CHEST* or *PRECORDIAL LEADS* that are identified by the letters V-V_1, V_2, V_3, V_4, V_5, and V_6. The V leads record electrical potential in the *horizontal plane* and provide six views of the heart's activity! 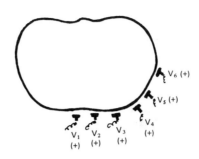 There is a single positive electrode which is moved to all six positions on the chest wall.

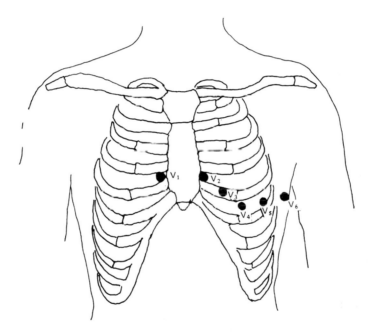

Lead V_1 is located over the 4th intercostal space to the right of the sternal border.
Lead V_2 is located over the 4th intercostal space to the left of the sternal border.
Lead V_3 is located between V_2 and V_4.
Lead V_4 is located at the 5th intercostal space on the mid-clavicular line.
Lead V_5 is located at the 5th intercostal space on the anterior axillary line.
Lead V_6 is located at the 5th intercostal space on the midaxillary line.

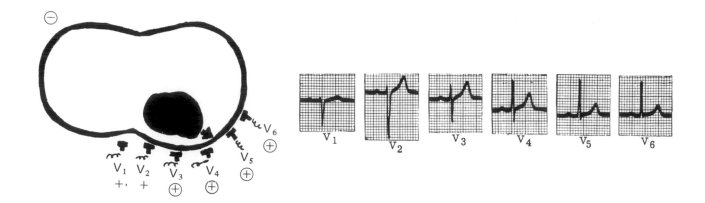

You are probably wondering where the negative electrodes are if the V leads are all positive! (You will remember that each lead is made up of both a positive (+) and a negative (−) electrode . . . remember? Well, in the precordial leads (V leads), the negative electrode extends backwards or posteriorly toward an imaginary point created by the limb leads.

Normally the *major* forces of depolarization move from *right to left*. Thus, the QRS deflections in the right precordial leads (V_1 and V_2) are mostly negative (moving away from the positive chest electrode). As the chest electrode is moved further left, the QRS deflections become positive (the wave of depolarization is moving toward the positive electrode).

Now that you are no doubt THOROUGHLY perplexed, let me reinforce the important points to remember about leads. . . .

When the major force or wave of depolarization (electrical activity) spreads through the heart muscle toward a positive pole (electrode), the QRS deflection on the EKG will appear upright or positive.

depolarization

positive

When the major force or wave of depolarization (electrical activity) spreads through the heart muscle away from a positive pole (electrode) or toward a negative pole (electrode), the deflections will be inverted or negative.

depolarization

negative

IMPORTANT

If there is no electrical activity occurring, there will be no recorded wave forms. . . .

. . . In other words, there will be a straight line _____ called an ISOELECTRIC LINE. So here's an isoelectric line.

P.S. We'll review this depolarization nonsense again near the end of this book.

Whew!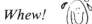

If you think all this is confusing, you're right! . . . It also means that you're progressing in a *normal* fashion. HONEST!

Probably the most important thing to remember is that the 12 leads allow one to look at the various surfaces of the left ventricle . . . or simply look at the electrical activity from different views or angles.

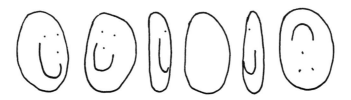

Since the left ventricle (*THE PUMP*) is the most important heart chamber, the various leads are designed to look at its surfaces!

LEFT VENTRICLE

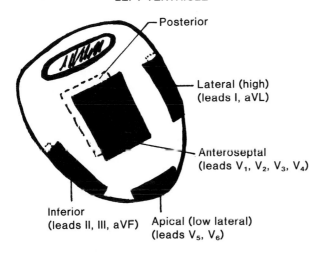

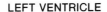

Leads I and aVL look at the lateral surface of the left ventricle (high lateral).

Leads II, III, and aVF look at the inferior surface of the left ventricle.

Leads V_1, V_2, V_3, and V_4 look at the anteroseptal surface of the left ventricle.

Leads V_5 and V_6 look at the apical surface of the left ventricle (low lateral).

There are no leads that view the posterior region of the left ventricle directly.

So, with that under your belt, you can proceed to Section I.

P.S. If you don't have it under your belt yet . . . *don't worry!* "LEADing Into Section I" only comes at the beginning because history and tradition so dictates! It makes much more sense if you reread this section at the end of the book! So progress ahead without a care!

Bedside Monitoring

Because all this business about leads is somewhat confusing in the beginning, it may be useful to talk briefly about bedside monitoring. Most bedside monitoring systems use a three lead system made up of a positive (+) electrode, a negative (−) electrode, and a ground (G) electrode. Depending upon how those three electrodes are arranged on the chest surface, the resulting monitor picture will closely resemble the standard limb leads I, II, or III. (You will remember that the standard limb leads are bipolar leads. The following examples also use a bipolar lead system.)

In each of these diagrams, notice the electrode placement.

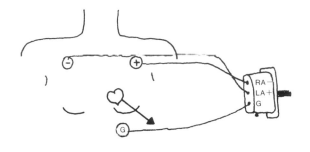

Lead I

In the bedside version of lead I, the general direction of ventricular depolarization (see arrow) is toward the positive (+) electrode. So . . . the QRS in lead I will be positively deflected.

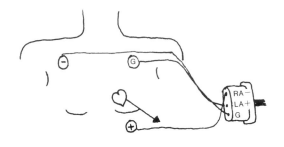

Lead II

In the bedside version of lead II, the direction of ventricular depolarization (see arrow) is toward the positive (+) electrode. Thus, the QRS in lead II is positively deflected.

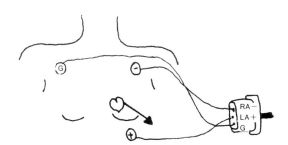

Lead III

In the bedside version of lead III, the direction of ventricular depolarization (see arrow) is between the positive (+) and negative (−) electrodes. Thus, the QRS observed in lead III is partly positive and partly negative.

Makes sense . . .

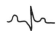

It is also possible to arrange the three electrodes to mimic certain precordial leads, specifically leads V_1 and V_6. However, since the precordial leads are unipolar in nature (they use a positive electrode on the chest wall; the negative electrode is imaginary ⊙), and our bedside monitoring system is bipolar, certain modifications must be made. Thus, these leads are referred to as modified chest leads!

Lead MCL₁ (modified V₁)

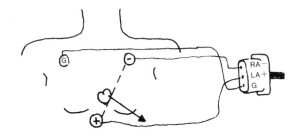

The positive (+) electrode is positioned as V_1 at the 4th intercostal space to the right of the sternum (see page 7).

REMEMBER . . . V_1 is a right chest lead . . . so, MCL_1 is a modified right chest lead.

Because the direction of depolarization (see arrow) moves between the positive (+) and negative (−) electrodes, the QRS in lead MCL_1 will be partly positive and partly negative.

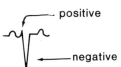
positive

negative

Lead MCL₆ (modified V₆)

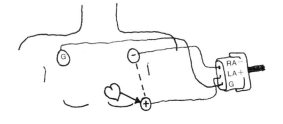

The positive (+) electrode is positioned as V_6 at the 5th intercostal space on the mid-axillary line (see page 7).

REMEMBER . . . V_6 is a left chest lead . . . so, MCL_6 is a modified left chest lead.

You will notice that the direction of depolarization (see arrow) is toward the positive (+) electrode. Thus, the QRS observed in lead MCL_6 will be positive or upright.

In the above modified systems (MCL_1 and MCL_6), the left arm electrode is the negative (−) electrode. The positive electrode is placed in the appropriate V lead position. If you need review, please turn back to page seven.

Just a trivial thought . . . MCL stands for "modified chest—left arm" lead. Fascinating . . . right?

Let me REASSURE you once again! If you are uncertain or confused, please understand that this is a NORMAL state. It will all begin to fall into place as we move along. TRUST ME!

11

Section I
The Conduction System and Related Matters

OBJECTIVES

When you have completed Section I, you will be able to describe or identify

1. normal electric impulse transmission across the myocardium
2. P, Q, R, S, T cardiac cycle
3. calculating heart rate
4. paper time
5. sinus rhythm
6. the conduction system
7. the method utilized for interpreting dysrhythmias

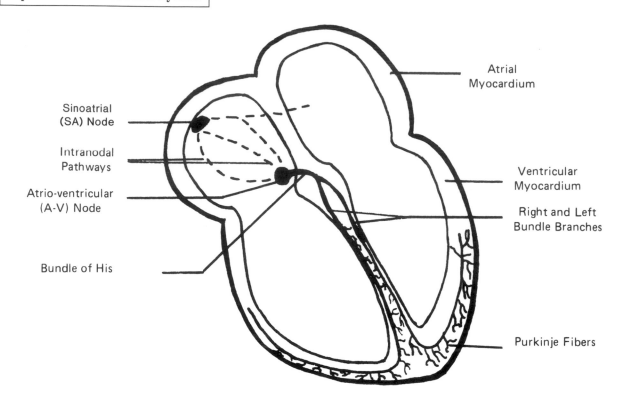

Sinoatrial (SA) Node

Intranodal Pathways

Atrio-ventricular (A-V) Node

Bundle of His

Atrial Myocardium

Ventricular Myocardium

Right and Left Bundle Branches

Purkinje Fibers

Each normal heart beat is the result of an electrical impulse that originates in the sinoatrial (SA) node. The SA node lies at the junction of the superior vena cava and the right atrium. *The SA node is the normal heart's physiologic pacemaker, firing between 60–100 times per minute. From the SA node the impulse travels across intranodal pathways activating the atria. The intranodal pathways connect the SA node and the AV (atrio-ventricular) node. Current physiologic evidence cites that activation of the atria occurs through these preferential or semi-specialized pathways that are concentrations of normal myocardial cells and Purkinje cells. (The tissues between these cells consist mainly of collagen and fat which have high electrical resistance.) The AV node lies on the floor of the right atrium. Conduction through the intranodal pathway is rapid; conduction is then slowed in the AV node itself. The AV node serves only to transmit the impulse. Impulse conduction speeds up as it leaves the AV node passing to the bundle of His. From the bundle of His, the impulse passes rapidly down the right and left bundle branches to the terminal Purkinje fibers. Ventricular depolarization or activation then occurs, producing the QRS complex on EKG. After depolarization, the muscle rests (repolarizes) while the ventricles fill with blood. The next impulse arrives when filling is completed and ventricular depolarization again occurs. *Each cardiac cycle consists of depolarization and recovery (repolarization).*

IMPORTANT NOTE:
*The SA node is the normal pacemaker of the heart because it has the *fastest* rate of impulse formation and discharge. The SA impulse reaches slower potential pacemakers and discharges their immature impulses before they have the opportunity to discharge spontaneously. Sounds complicated, right? The important thing to remember is that the *fastest* pacemaker always controls the heart . . . just like the *fastest* runner controls the race! It's also helpful to know that the SA node is influenced by both the sympathetic and parasympathetic nervous systems . . . thus, the sinus rate of discharge fluxuates with nervous stimulation.

Practice Exercise 1

Now it's your turn.

The electrical impulse normally originates in the sinoatrial node and travels across the heart to initiate myocardial muscle depolarization. Trace and label the parts of the conduction system on this diagram.

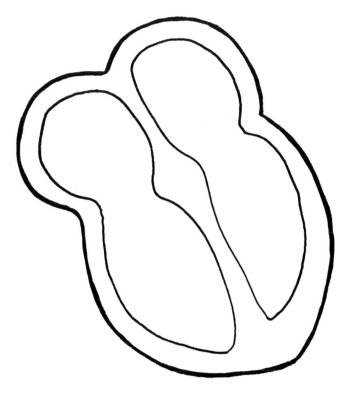

The activation phase of the cardiac cycle is known as _____ .

The recovery phase of the cardiac cycle is known as _____ .

Normally, the SA (sinoatrial) node fires _____ to _____ times per minute.

For **Feedback 1,** refer to page 35.

Input 2: The P Wave and P-R Interval

All electrical activity can be recorded. As the impulse travels across the myocardium, a monitoring device will show various wave forms.

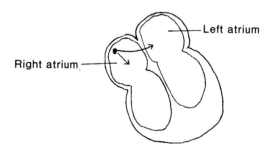

Atrial excitation begins at the SA node and spreads through the right and left atria. The monitor will show a wave form that usually looks like this.

For reasons unknown to me, this is called a P wave! Owing to the direction of electrical activation, P Waves are *normally upright* in leads I, II, aVF, and V_3-V_6. P waves are normally inverted in leads aVR and may be inverted in leads V_1 and V_2. P waves may be upright, flat, diphasic, or inverted in leads III and aVL.

The P wave represents depolarization of both the right and left atria. Remember, muscle contraction follows electrical depolarization.

So, whenever a P wave is observed, the monitor watcher will know that depolarization of the atria has occurred.

Since the impulse originates in the sinoatrial node and since the SA node is the heart's natural pacemaker, the P wave should be the *first* wave form one sees in each cardiac cycle.

ATRIAL DEPOLARIZATION =

We now have a P wave, telling the monitor watcher that atrial depolarization has occurred. Not unlike other muscles, after activation there must be a rest or recovery (repolarization) period. And, just as you might suspect, during this rest period no work is done.

The period of time for atrial depolarization (activation) and atrial relaxation (repolarization) to occur presents on the monitor as a straight line —————— . This straight line is known as the P-R interval. The P-R interval further represents the time for the impulse to pass from the SA node, through the AV junction, to the ventricles. The P-R interval lies between the P wave and the R wave (which we will discuss further down the line).

P-R interval sounds like a strange name for a straight line . . . maybe a simple analogy will help.

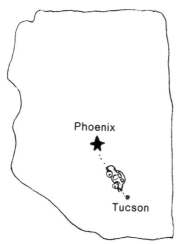

I live and work in Tucson, but I must also drive to Phoenix because I have a second job there. So I work in Tucson—my work in Tucson corresponds to atrial work, so I'll call my Tucson work P. Then, I jump in my VW and drive to Phoenix. The time it takes me to drive to Phoenix could be called my Tucson–Phoenix interval (the time it takes for me to drive from Tucson to Phoenix). This corresponds to the P-R interval which is the time it takes for the sinus impulse to travel through the atria, through the A-V junction to the ventricles.

Using this analogy further, it's easy to see that my Tucson–Phoenix interval, like the P-R interval, could vary depending on how fast I drive— or how rapidly the impulse is conducted.

If I follow the speed limit, it will take me 2½ hours to arrive in Phoenix. If the sinus impulse travels in a healthy manner, it will be 3 to 5 small squares on EKG paper. (But, we'll review this again later.)

So, when I'm looking at a monitor and see the following,

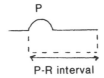

P-R interval

I know that because there is a P wave, the atria have depolarized and because there is a P-R interval, the impulse is traveling to ~~Phoenix~~ OOPS! to the ventricles.

Practice Exercise 2

    Let's review!

A. Atrial excitation (in the healthy heart) begins in the _____ .

B. As this impulse spreads across the atria, it causes atrial muscle contraction following _____

    _____ .

C. The monitor picture associated with atrial depolarization is the _____ wave.

D. Okay, now draw a P wave.

E. In the healthy heart, the _____ will note the beginning of each cardiac cycle.

F. The P-R interval looks like this: (draw one 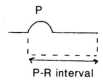)

G. The P-R interval represents the time it takes for the impulse to travel from the atria, through

    the _____ to the ventricles.

For **Feedback 2,** refer to page 35.

Input 3: The QRS Complex

    So, now what??

    So far, our EKG complex looks like this.

P

P-R interval

And, the impulse has traveled to the ventricles.

The next major event in the cardiac cycle is ventricular depolarization (the traveling impulse reaches and activates the ventricles). Ventricular depolarization is identified on the monitor as the QRS complex. The QRS will be predominantly upright in leads, I, II, III, aVL, aVF, V$_4$, V$_5$, and V$_6$. (Refer back to pages 5, 6, and 8)

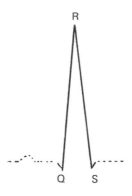

These waves (QRS) represent depolarization of the ventricular muscle. The first downward (negative) deflection is the Q wave.

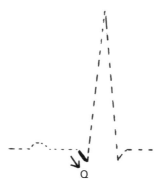

The R wave is the first upward (positive) wave or deflection . . .

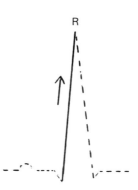

. . . and, if a negative deflection (below the baseline) follows an R wave, it is labeled an S wave.

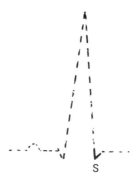

Now, our monitor picture looks like this.

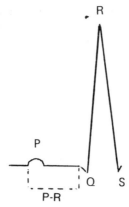

The P waves tells us the atria have depolarized. The P-R interval represents the time it takes for the SA impulse to travel from the SA node through the atria, through the AV junction, through the bundle of His, down the bundle branches to the Purkinje fibers. And voila! When the impulse reaches the Purkinje fibers, ventricular depolarization occurs—shown on the monitor as the QRS. Ventricular muscle contraction follows electrical depolarization.

Depending upon which EKG lead you are examining, you may not observe an actual Q wave. In other words, the QRS may look like this. There is no observable Q wave (negative deflection). Technically speaking, this is an Rs wave . . .

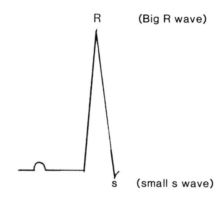

. . . but we still call it a QRS complex!

Likewise, in predominantly negatively deflected leads—V_1, V_2, and V_3—the QRS will appear different owing to the placement of the electrode, the proximity to the heart muscle and the direction of the depolarization wave. (Refer back to p. 8.)

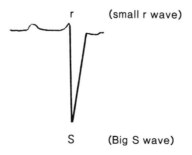

Though the above wave form is referred to as a QRS complex, technically there is only an r and an S wave! (An R wave is the first upward deflection, and an S wave is a negative-downward deflection that follows an r wave).

WHEW!

Practice Exercise 3

A. Draw and label the waves that represent ventricular activation or depolarization.

B. Ventricular depolarization begins when the SA impulse reaches _____

_____

_____

_____

For **Feedback 3,** refer to page 36.

Input 4: The ST Segment and the T Wave

Only two more *minor* details. Following ventricular activation (depolarization), there must be a period of rest or recovery (repolarization).

Simple physiology—cells work—they get tired—they rest! So the tail end of a normal EKG cycle looks like this.

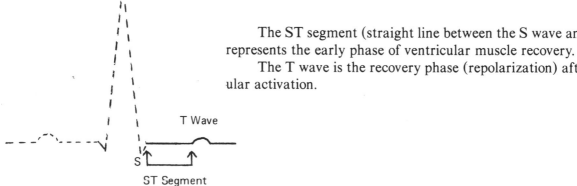

The ST segment (straight line between the S wave and T wave) represents the early phase of ventricular muscle recovery.

The T wave is the recovery phase (repolarization) after ventricular activation.

T Wave

S

ST Segment

Let's do the whole thing—an entire EKG cycle. When I see this on the monitor, I can now intellectually describe the whole physiologic process.

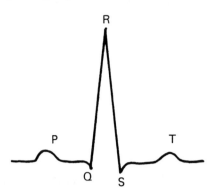

Ready? Okay. . . . "My good man/woman, EKG monitor interpretation is based on simple application of a basic physiologic principle. Ion shift at the myocardial cell membrane level allows one to record electrical potential via specially designed electrodes. Atrial excitation begins at the SA node and spreads down the conduction system. The initially recorded wave, the P wave, represents depolarization of the atria. Following the P wave is the P-R interval which represents atrial repolarization and the impulse spreading to the ventricles. The QRS complex represents ventricular depolarization. Following ventricular depolarization is the repolarization phase evidenced by the ST segment and T wave!"

Remember, the EKG is simply
a representation of the electrical events occurring within
the myocardium!

Sounds fairly intellectual, right?!

Practice Exercise 4

A. Label each wave.

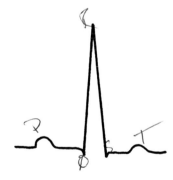

P.S. If you are unsure, look at the top of the page!

B. Atrial excitation begins in the ___Atria — SA node___

C. The P wave represents ___Depolarisation___

D. The P-R interval represents ___repolarisation time travel to AV node — Supraventricular activity.___

E. The QRS represents ___Vent. Depolarization___

    The Q wave is the first ___downward___ deflection.

    The R wave is the first ___↑___ deflection.

    The S wave is the ___↓___ deflection following the R wave.

F. The ST segment represents ___Repolarization of ventricle___
___~ Ventricular contraction occurs ~___

G. The T wave represents ___recovery phase___
_____

H. The PQRST complex 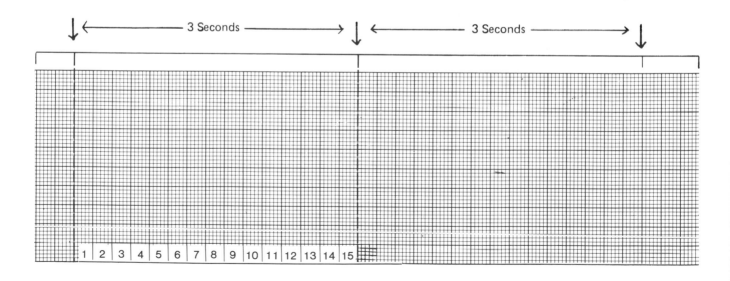 represents one ___Cardiac cycle___
_____

For **Feedback 4,** refer to page 36.

For **Feedback 4,** refer to page 36.

Input 5: Paper Time

Now that the PQRST cycle has been more or less exhausted, we need to think about EKG paper—henceforth, this will be referred to as "paper time." In order for this whole process to make good sense, some convention of measure must be applied. EKG recording paper is run at a standard speed of 25 mm per second to standardize the measurement of the various electrical events. EKG paper is subdivided both horizontally and vertically with 1 mm and 5 mm (dark lines) spaced lines. The vertical lines represent time intervals, much like a clock! ☺

So, moving horizontally across the EKG paper denotes *time*. One must understand the concept of paper time in order to calculate heart rate from the EKG paper.

In the following illustration, notice the three second marker intervals at the top of the EKG paper. Every three seconds this mark will appear. The distance between three of these markers is 6 seconds.

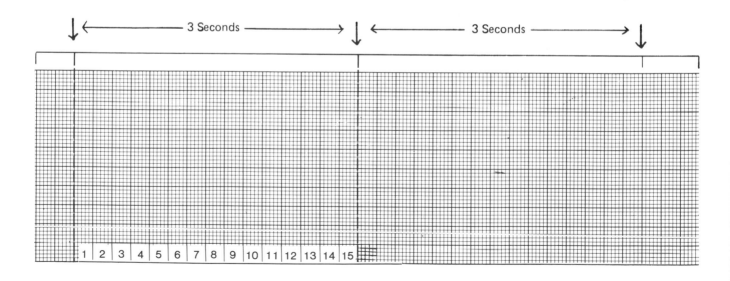

The larger squares represent *0.20 seconds* each. That makes sense if you count the number of large squares between each three second marker. (See bottom illustration page 22.)

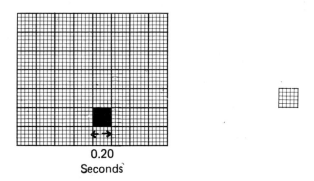

0.20
Seconds

There are 15 large squares between each three second marker.

$$15 \times 0.2 \text{ seconds each} = 3.0 \text{ seconds}$$

Now look at one of the smallest squares. Each small square represents *0.04 seconds*.

Again, that makes sense if we count the number of tiny squares across one big square.

There are five. 5×0.04 seconds $= 0.2$ seconds (one large square).

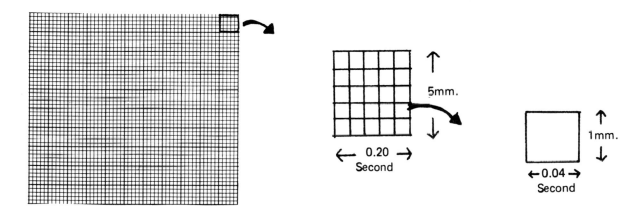

5mm.

← 0.20 →
Second

1mm.

←0.04→
Second

Practice Exercise 5

Paper time is actually quite easy . . . if you practice.

BEFORE looking back, complete the following statements.

A. Moving horizontally across EKG paper denotes __time__.

B. Every __3 second__ seconds I will see a mark on the EKG paper.

C. The amount of time between three of these marks is __6 seconds__ seconds.

D. The large squares represent __.20__ seconds.

23

E. I understand that (0.20 seconds) because there are 15 large squares between two _3_ second markers. Therefore, 15 × _20_ seconds = _3_ seconds.

F. The smallest square on the EKG paper represents _.04_ seconds.

G. There are _5_ small squares (in one row) in a large square.

H. There are _30_ large squares in a six second time interval.

I. Three tiny squares represent _.12_ seconds.

J. Four tiny squares represents _.16_ seconds.

K. Five tiny squares represent _.20_ seconds, which is the same as _____.

L. How much time is represented by five big squares? _1 second_

M. How much time is represented by 13 big squares? _2.60 second._

. . . if you can answer question N without looking back, you have a sound understanding of paper time.

N. How much time has elapsed when there are five big squares and three little squares?

1.12 seconds

For **Feedback 5,** refer to page 37.

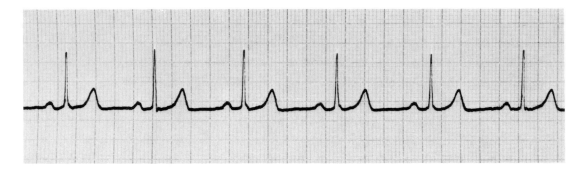

For **Feedback 5,** refer to page 37.

Input 6: Measuring P, P-R, and QRS Intervals

Although we will not go into great detail, it is important to think about *atrial activation.* You will remember that the P wave represents atrial depolarization (depolarization of both the left and right atria).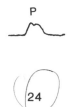

The *normal* P wave is not over 0.11 seconds in duration (less than three small squares) or over 2.5 mm. in height. Any increase in duration or amplitude suggests *atrial hypertrophy.* Though it is not always possible to distinguish right from left atrial hypertrophy on an EKG, we can make several generalizations. Basically, atrial hypertrophy represents an enlargement of one or both of the atrial chambers due to excessive strain or workload.

With left atrial hypertrophy (often seen in mitral stenosis), one may observe a wide, notched P wave called *P mitral,* best seen in leads I and II.

Right atrial hypertrophy is most commonly associated with chronic pulmonary disease. P waves associated with right atrial hypertrophy are usually tall (greater than 2.5 mm in height) and *peaked* in leads II, III and AVF.

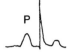

I thought this business about P waves was interesting. I don't really expect you to commit this to memory . . . however, you should be aware that abnormalities may occur in the P wave itself! *Whew!*

Remember the P-R interval? It represents the time it takes for atrial activation and impulse transmission across the atria, through the AV node, through the bundle of His, down the bundle branches, to the Purkinje fibers.

In a healthy adult heart, the impulse will travel that distance in 0.12 to 0.20 seconds.

That means that to be within normal limits, the P-R interval must be 3–5 small squares in width (or between 0.12 and 0.20 seconds).

Look at this EKG strip. The P-R interval is almost 4 small squares wide. The P-R interval is measured from the beginning of the P wave to the beginning of the Q wave . . . or if there is no Q wave, to the beginning of the upward R wave. (For assistance with measurement, see the diagrams at the top of page 26.)

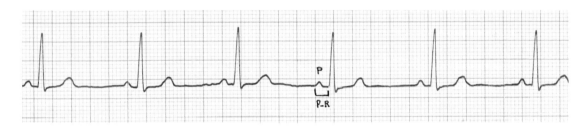

4 × .04 = 0.16 seconds. (So, the P-R interval is *almost* 0.16 seconds in duration.)

That means this is a *normal* P-R interval. In other words, the impulse is traveling through the conduction system at a healthy speed.

As a contrast, look at this strip. Here the P-R interval measures 0.24 seconds (6 × .04 = 0.24) indicating a delay in impulse conduction.

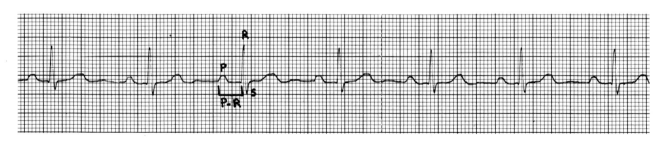

The P-R interval measures 7 little squares or 0.28 seconds (0.04 × 7 — 0.28)! Therefore, the impulse is traveling too slowly, representing pathology! A prolonged P-R interval represents a conduction defect—and a short P-R interval represents accelerated conduction . . . but we'll get to that later! Remember, *to be within normal limits the P-R interval must be 3–5 small squares in width, or 0.12 to 0.20 seconds in duration.*

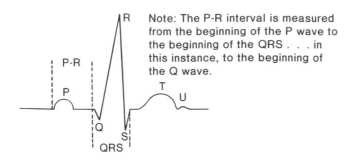

Note: The P-R interval is measured from the beginning of the P wave to the beginning of the QRS . . . in this instance, to the beginning of the Q wave.

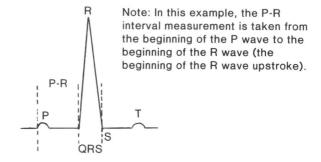

Note: In this example, the P-R interval measurement is taken from the beginning of the P wave to the beginning of the R wave (the beginning of the R wave upstroke).

We will be concerned with one other major paper time measure. The QRS, you will remember, represents ventricular depolarization. Unless a conduction defect is present (abnormal, slow conduction), the QRS should measure *less* than 3 small squares wide, or less than 0.12 seconds in duration. The QRS is measured from the beginning of the Q wave to the end of the S wave. If a Q wave is not present, measure the distance between the R and S waves. Please refer to the above diagrams.

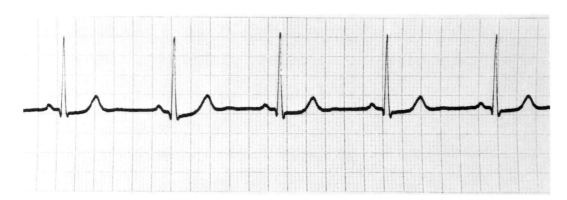

In the above rhythm strip, the QRS measures *approximately 0.10 seconds* or 2½ small boxes. Therefore, ventricular depolarization occurs within the expected period of time (*less than 0.12 seconds or less than 3 small squares*).

Practice Exercise 6

To be within normal limits, the P-R interval must be _____ to _____ small squares in width

or _____ to _____ seconds.

A P-R interval less than _____ small squares in width or greater than _____ small squares in width represents an abnormality in the impulse conduction.

Look at this EKG cycle. The P-R measures _____ small boxes or _____ seconds.

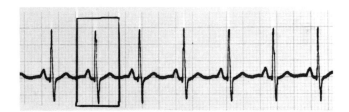

The QRS represents _____ .

To be within normal limits, the QRS must be _____ small squares or less than _____ seconds.

The QRS in the above EKG cycle measures _____ small squares which is _____ seconds.

For **Feedback 6,** refer to page 38.

Input 7: Calculating Heart Rate

Now, let's try some *fun* things with heart rate!

There are several methods for calculating heart rate. Probably the most accurate is to count the number of beats or cardiac cycles in a one minute (60 second) time interval. If you think in terms of three second time markers, that's a *long* EKG strip. Though this method is cumbersome, it should be used *when the rhythm* is *IRREGULAR* and an accurate heart rate is needed. (This is much like taking an apical pulse   if it is irregular, you must count it for one full minute . . . assuming you don't cheat!)

P.S. When in doubt about any heart rate, take the patient's pulse . . . and remember, an apical pulse is usually the most accurate.

When we are dealing with a *regular* rhythm, the process can be simplified. Every three seconds a marker appears on the EKG paper. *Count the number of EKG complexes or cardiac cycles in a six second time interval. Multiply that number by 10* to find the number of complexes in one minute. That number is the approximate heart rate.

Figure the heart rate in the following EKG strip.

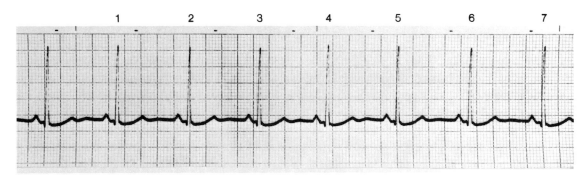

There are 7 complexes in a six second time interval.

Therefore, 7 × 10 equals 70.

This patient's heart rate is *approximately* 70 beats/minute.

The fastest method to figure a *regular* heart rate involves memorizing the following numbers: *300, 150, 100; 75, 60, 50.* Say them to yourself—300, 150, 100; 75, 60, 50. Repeat them again. Now close your eyes and repeat them.

No kidding! Close your eyes and repeat the numbers!

The next item you must know is how to recognize an R wave. The R wave is the first upward deflection in a QRS complex.

This is an R wave. *Remember* what it looks like.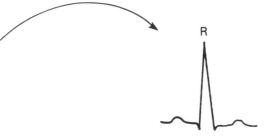

Find an R wave that falls on a *heavy vertical* line on the EKG paper.

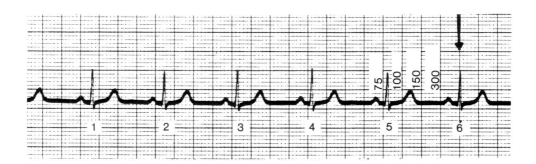

Notice that the R wave of beat 6 falls on a heavy vertical line. *Do not* count this line, but beginning with the next heavy vertical line, count 300. You may count either to the right or to the left of the complex. In this example, we will count to the left. The first heavy vertical line after the R wave is 300. Continuing on to the left, the next heavy vertical line is 150. The third heavy vertical line is 100. The fourth heavy vertical line is 75. Before the fourth heavy vertical line is another R wave. That means that this patient's heart rate is between 75 and 100, but closer to 75. Once you have become familiar with this method, it will serve to allow you a rapid estimate of the patient's heart rate. Using this method, one does not need to be concerned with the three second time markers!

Figure the heart rate in the next sample EKG strip.

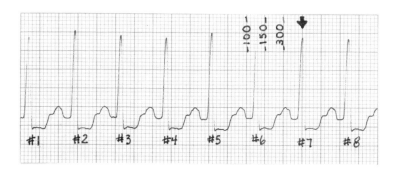

Find the R wave that falls on a heavy vertical line . . . it has to be beat 7 counting left to right. In this example, you are forced to begin counting vertical lines to the left of the R wave. *Remember,* do *not* count the vertical line that the R wave falls on. Begin counting on the next vertical line to the left.

      WHAT DID YOU GET? Me too!

This patient's heart rate falls between 100 and 150.

Now close your eyes and repeat the six numbers you have memorized.

Actually, you can use any wave (other than an R wave) that you wish when figuring heart rate in this manner. It's just that R waves are usually the easiest waves to spot.

REMEMBER: this method should *only* be used when the rhythm is **<u>REGULAR.</u>**

Note: If you are wondering why this method works, it is because there are 1500 small EKG squares per minute. If you count the number of small EKG squares between two R waves (12 in the above example), and divide 1500 by that number, you will get the precise heart rate.

$$12 \overline{)1500} = 125$$

Practice Exercise 7

Now try some practice! Figure the heart rate on each of the next EKG strips. Do not look back until you have completed the exercise.

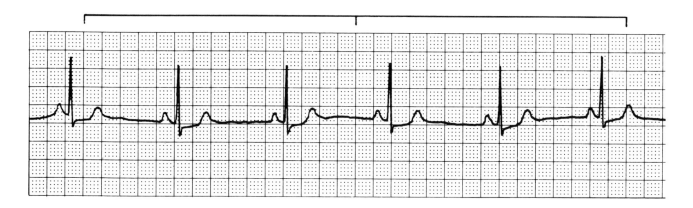

First decide if the rhythm is regular. Imagine all the tall upright waves (R waves) are sticks lying in a row. Decide if they are evenly spaced.

1. Each marker at the top of the EKG paper represents _____ seconds.

   There are _____ complexes in the six second time interval displayed. Therefore, _____

   × 10 equals _____ . The approximate heart rate is _____ beats/minute.

2. What is the heart rate on EKG strip II?

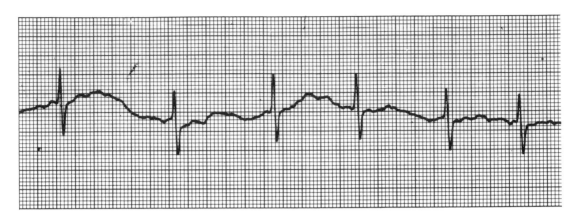

Heart rate = _____

3. Remember the six numbers you memorized? . . . 300, 150, 100; 75, 60, 50. Figure the following heart rate using that method. Step one consists of finding an R wave that falls on a heavy vertical line.

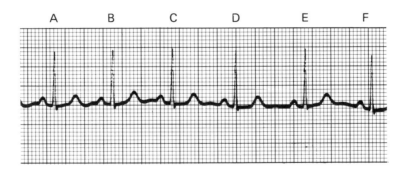

Beat _____ falls closest to a heavy vertical line. The next heavy vertical line to the left is counted as

_____ . The next heavy vertical line is counted as _____ , *etc.* The heart rate falls between

_____ and _____ beats per minute.

4. Using the same method, calculate the heart rate in the following strip.

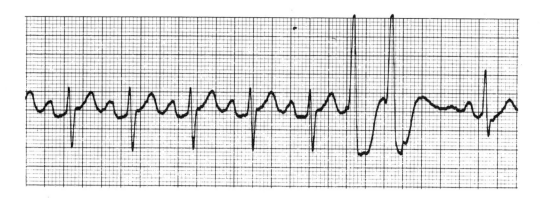

The heart rate is _____

For **Feedback 7,** refer to page 38.

Input 8: Sinus Rhythm

I forgot to tell you . . . if you get tired, you can quit. That's why the material is organized in this fashion. You can stop and go as you please. You're almost an expert now anyway!
Here is a review sheet that more or less summarizes what we have done thus far!

1. The sinus node is the pacemaker in the normal heart. Thus, the term sinus rhythm implies that the electrical impulse originates in the sinus node.
2. The P wave is the first wave formation in the normal EKG complex. The P wave represents depolarization of the atria. The P waves seen on an EKG strip should all appear identical, and should be equidistant to the following QRS complexes.
3. The P-R interval of each EKG complex represents the time that is necessary for the impulse to travel from the sinus node through the AV junction to the ventricles. In normal conduction, that time should be *0.12–0.20 seconds.* Now, how many small EKG squares is that? Remember, each small square represents 0.04 seconds . . . so, 0.12 seconds equals three small squares, and 0.20 seconds equals five small squares. Thus, the P-R interval will normally be between *3–5 small squares* in duration.
4. The QRS represents depolarization of the ventricles. Every normal rhythm should have a QRS preceded by a P wave and followed by a T wave . . . all occurring in a regular fashion. The normal QRS should be *less* than *0.12 seconds,* or less than 3 small EKG squares. (If the QRS is 3 or more small squares in width, it indicates a defect or delay in the conduction system.)
5. The T wave represents the recovery state after ventricular depolarization. The T waves should all be upright and appear identical. The ST segment will be flat, neither elevated nor depressed.
6. A normal heart rate is 60–100 beats per minute. The sinus node will fire 60–100 times per minute, and each time it fires, the impulse will be conducted down through the AV junctional tissue to the ventricles where it will cause ventricular depolarization.

Now, let's talk about a sinus rhythm or a normal rhythm. This strip illustrates a sinus rhythm.

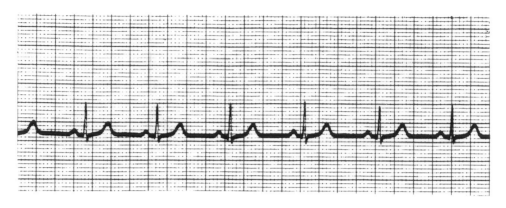

A SINUS RHYTHM WILL HAVE ALL OF THE FOLLOWING IDENTIFYING FEATURES.

> *RATE:*   60 to 100 beats per minute
> *RHYTHM:*   Regular
> *P WAVES:*   A P wave will precede each QRS complex. All P waves will be uniform in appearance.
> *QRS:*   All QRS complexes will appear uniform in configuration.
> *CONDUCTION:*   Each P wave will be followed by a normal QRS complex.

Sinus rhythm is given its name because it originates in the sinoatrial node. The SA node is the normal pacemaker of the heart because it has the highest inherent rate of discharge or automaticity (60 to 100 times per minute). Though other tissues have pacemaking capability, their inherent rates of impulse-formation are significantly less than the sinus rate. Thus, the fastest pacemaker always assumes control of the rhythm!

Here is another example of sinus rhythm.

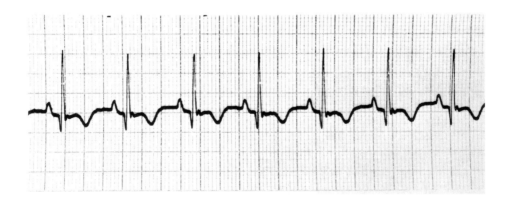

In this strip the heart rate is between 75 and 100 beats per minute, but closer to 100 beats per minute.

Practice Exercise 8

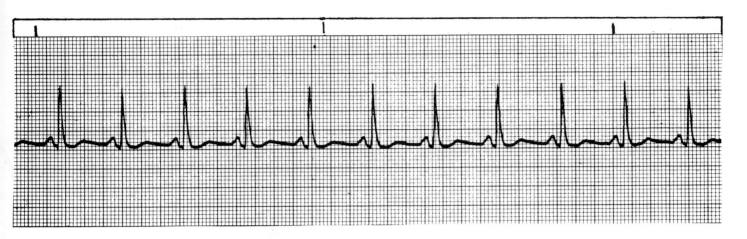

Use this rhythm strip when you answer the questions.

A. The heart rate in this strip is _____ beats per minute.

B. The rhythm is regular / irregular (Circle one.)

C. Each QRS complex is *preceded* by a _____ wave.

　　Do all the P waves look uniform or alike? _____ yes _____ no

D. Is each P wave followed by a normal QRS complex? _____ yes _____ no

E. Do all QRS complexes appear uniform? _____ yes _____ no

F. VOILA! This is a _____ rhythm!

For **Feedback 8,** refer to page 40.

Input 9: Interpreting Dysrhythmias

Following is some introductory information for Section II!

In order to accurately interpret dysrhythmias, there are *five* basic steps one must follow. As you become more proficient in EKG interpretation, you may combine, reorder . . . or even think of new steps. However, for now, it will assist you to follow these five steps when analyzing any rhythm!

FIRST, determine if the rhythm is regular. If the rhythm is irregular, try to determine what makes it irregular. Are their early (premature) beats? Are there pauses? Are there abnormal beats? The simplest method for determining rhythm regularity is to measure the distance between two consecutive R waves (R-R interval) and compare that distance with another R-R interval. In a regular rhythm, the R-R intervals will all measure the same.

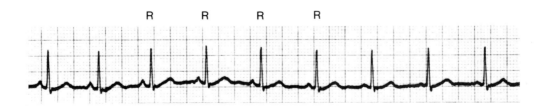

SECOND, determine the heart rate. Remember . . . if the rhythm is irregular, it is necessary to count the rate for one full minute. (In the above strip, the rate is 90.)

THIRD, we must think about the atrial activity. What are the atria doing? Are there P waves that occur uniformly across the monitor tracing? Are the P waves alike in appearance? If no distinct P waves are present, is there evidence of atrial activity, or is the baseline preceding the QRS flat? If atrial impulses are present, are they regular or irregular? Is the atrial activity occurring so rapidly that there are more atrial deflections than QRS complexes? If actual atrial wave forms are difficult to identify, does the baseline appear chaotic?

FOURTH, look at ventricular activity. What are the ventricles doing? Are the QRS's of normal duration (less than 0.12 seconds)? Do the QRS's occur uniformly across the monitor tracing?

FINALLY, it is important to *determine the relationship between atrial and ventricular activity.* Is each P wave producing a QRS, or are there P waves that are not followed by QRS complexes? Is each QRS preceded by a P wave, or is there evidence of independent ventricular activity? Is the P-R interval of all conducted beats constant, does it vary, or is there no established relationship?

REMEMBER: ONE NEED NOT APPLY A SOPHISTICATED NAME TO THE RHYTHM. A SIMPLE DESCRIPTIVE ANALYSIS (ANSWERING THE ABOVE FIVE QUESTIONS) CONVEYS THE MOST ACCURATE INFORMATION!

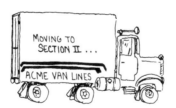

Feedback 1

Very good!

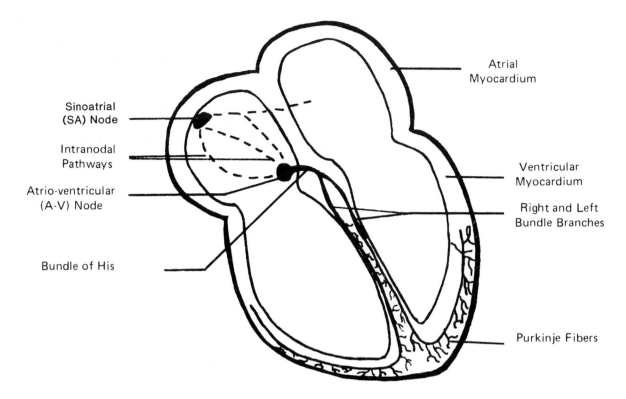

The impulse originates in the sinoatrial (SA) node and travels down the intranodal pathways, activating the atria. The impulse then travels through the AV node, slowing slightly. Impulse conduction speeds up as it leaves the AV node, passing to the bundle of His. From the bundle of His, the impulse travels rapidly down the right and left bundle branches to the Purkinje fibers.

Each cardiac cycle consists of two phases—activation or depolarization, and recovery or repolarization.

Normally, the SA node fires 60 to 100 times per minute.

Feedback 2

If your answers look like this, you're doing a super job!

1. Atrial excitation (in the healthy heart) begins in the sinoatrial or SA node.

2. As the impulse spreads across the atria, it causes atrial muscle contraction following depolarization.

3. The monitor picture associated with atrial depolarization is the P wave.

4. (a "P" wave.)

5. In the healthy heart, the P wave will note the beginning of each new cardiac cycle.

6. (a P-R interval)

7. The P-R interval represents the time it takes for the impulse to travel from the atria, through the <u>AV node</u> to the ventricles.

P.S. If your answers didn't look like this, review the material one more time!

Feedback 3

1. If you have drawn a QRS complex, good for you!

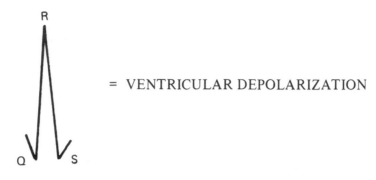

= VENTRICULAR DEPOLARIZATION

2. Ventricular depolarization begins when the SA impulse reaches the ventricles (after traveling through the atria, through the AV junction, through the bundle of His, down the bundle branches to the Purkinje fibers). Ventricular muscle contraction follows electrical depolarization.

Feedback 4

Excellent work! Your answers should be similar to mine.

1.

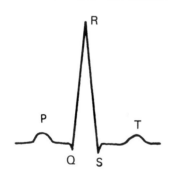

2. Atrial excitation begins in the <u>SA</u> (<u>sinoatrial</u>) <u>node</u>.

3. The P wave represents <u>atrial depolarization</u>.

4. The P-R interval represents <u>the time for the impulse to pass from the SA node, through the AV junction to the ventricles</u>.

5. The QRS represents <u>ventricular depolarization</u>.
   The Q wave is the first <u>downward</u> deflection.
   The R wave is the first <u>upward</u> deflection.
   The S wave is the negative or <u>downward</u> deflection following the R wave.

6. The ST segment represents <u>the early phase of ventricular muscle recovery</u> (<u>repolarization</u>).

7. The T wave represents <u>the recovery phase after ventricular activation</u> (<u>repolarization</u>).

8. The PQRST complex 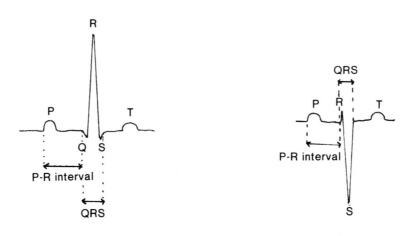 represents one <u>cardiac cycle</u>.

This is just to help tie together any loose ends.

Remember, the wave forms may be either positive or negative depending upon which lead we are viewing.

P WAVE—Atrial excitation starts at the SA node and spreads through both atria. The P wave represents depolarization of the atria. If P waves are present, and of normal size and shape, it can be assumed that the stimulus began in the SA node.

P-R INTERVAL—The period of atrial repolarization is represented by the P-R interval. It represents the time for the impulse to pass from the SA node, through the AV junction, through the bundle of His, down the bundle branches to the Purkinje fibers. The normal P-R interval is usually between 0.12–0.20 seconds.

QRS COMPLEX—These waves represent depolarization of the ventricular muscle. The initial *downward* deflection is the Q wave. The R wave is a large *upward* deflection. The S wave is the second *downward* wave. The normal QRS duration is less than 0.12 seconds.

ST SEGMENT—This segment represents the early phase of repolarization (recovery of the ventricular muscle).

T WAVE—The recovery phase following ventricular activation.

NOTE: ELECTRICAL DEPOLARIZATION OCCURS BEFORE CARDIAC MUSCLE CONTRACTION . . . AND, ELECTRICAL REPOLARIZATION FOLLOWS CARDIAC MUSCLE CONTRACTION.

Feedback 5

How did you do? Probably excellent, as usual! I hope your answers match mine.

1. <u>time</u>

2. <u>3 seconds</u>

3. <u>6 seconds</u>. That may be confusing, but |³ |³ | there are only two 3 second intervals between three markers!

4. <u>0.20 seconds</u>

5. 15 large squares between <u>two</u> 3 second markers. Therefore, 15 squares × 0.20 seconds (per square) = 3.0 seconds.

6. 0.04 seconds

7. <u>5</u> small squares

8. <u>30</u> large squares in a 6 second time interval

9. <u>0.12</u> [0.04 seconds (one tiny square) × 3 tiny squares = 0.12 seconds]

10. <u>0.16</u> [0.04 seconds (one tiny square) × 4 tiny squares = 0.16 seconds]

11. <u>0.20</u> seconds which is the same as <u>one large square</u>

12. <u>1.0</u> second [0.20 seconds (per big square) × 5 big squares = 1.0 second]

13. <u>2.6</u> seconds [0.20 seconds (per big square) × 13 big squares = 2.6 seconds]

14. <u>1.12</u> seconds. There are two ways to figure this.

    1. You could figure the 5 big squares first

       0.20 seconds per big square × 5 big squares = 1.0 second

    Then figure the tiny squares:

       0.04 seconds per tiny square × 3 tiny squares = <u>0.12</u> seconds

                            Total = 1.12 seconds

OR

    2. You could simply say there are a total of 28 tiny squares.

       So, 0.04 seconds per tiny square × 28 tiny squares = 1.12 seconds

Feedback 6

If your answers match mine, you're doing a great job! If they don't, a little more practice is in order!

1. To be within normal limits, the P-R interval must be <u>3</u> to <u>5</u> small squares in width or <u>0.12</u> to <u>0.20</u> seconds.

2. A P-R interval less than <u>3</u> small squares in width or greater than <u>5</u> small squares in width represents an abnormality in the impulse conduction.

3. The P-R interval of the EKG cycle measures <u>3</u> small squares or <u>0.12</u> seconds.

4. The QRS represents <u>ventricular depolarization</u>.
   To be within normal limits, the QRS must be <u>LESS than 3</u> small squares or less than <u>0.12</u> seconds.

5. The QRS of the EKG cycle measures <u>two</u> small squares which is <u>0.08</u> seconds.

Feedback 7

Keep up the GOOD WORK!

1. Each marker at the top of the EKG paper represents <u>three</u> seconds. There are <u>5</u> complexes in the six second time interval displayed. Therefore, 5 × 10 equal <u>50</u>. The approximate heart rate is <u>50</u> beats/minute, though it is very close to 60! This is just an estimate.

2. If you calculated a heart rate of approximately 70, you are

WRONG!!!

This method will <u>not</u> be an accurate assessment when the rhythm is <u>irregular</u>. Had you seen a full 60 second trace, you would have noticed that this was just a brief slow period in the rhythm. The patient's actual heart rate was 90 beats per minute! *Remember, when the rhythm is irregular, you must count the number of EKG complexes in a __full__ minute!*

3. Beat D falls closest to a heavy vertical line. The next heavy vertical line to the left is counted as <u>300</u>. The next vertical line is counted as <u>150</u>, etc. The heart rate falls between <u>75</u> and <u>100</u> beats per minute.

4. Did I catch you? The 300, 150, 100; 75, 60, 50 method will <u>not</u> be accurate because this rhythm is irregular. We would need to count the number of EKG complexes or cycles in one <u>full</u> minute to determine the heart rate.

*P.S. Here is a little "cheat sheet" to hang near your monitors. Count the number of small squares (small boxes) between two R waves of a regular rhythm, then read across the chart to determine heart rate.

"A TRUSTY GUIDE FOR DETERMINING HEART RATE"

No. of Boxes	Heart Rate	No. of Boxes	Heart Rate
5	300	25	60
6	250	26	57
7	214	27	55
8	187	28	53
9	166	29	52
10	150	30	50
11	136	31	48
12	125	32	47
13	115	33	45
14	107	34	44
15	100	35	42
16	94	36	41
17	88	37	40
→18	83	38	39
19	79	40	37
20	75	44	34
21	71	46	32
22	68	48	31
23	65	50	30
24	62		

Count the number of <u>small</u> EKG squares between two R waves on the following strip.

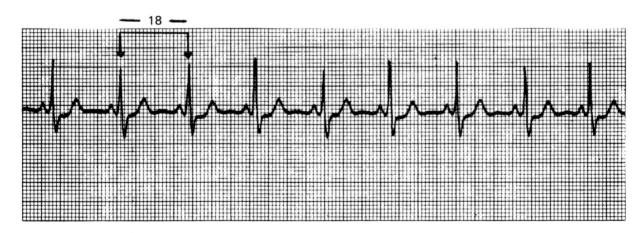

In this strip there are <u>18</u> small squares between R waves. Looking at my Trusty Guide, I can quickly see that the heart rate is <u>83</u>.

*P.S.S. This <u>ONLY</u> works with <u>REGULAR</u> rhythms.

In the event that you are wondering how this Trusty Guide came into being, the story is as follows. There are 1500 little tiny EKG squares in one minute. So, if you count the number of small squares between two R waves (i.e., 18 in the above example) and divide that number into 1500, you will arrive at the heart rate. Remember this method <u>only</u> works when the rhythm is regular.

$$18 \overline{)1500} \quad 82$$

Feedback 8

Excellent work!

1. The heart rate in this strip is <u>approximately 90</u> beats per minute.

2. The rhythm is REGULAR.

3. Each QRS complex is preceded by a <u>P</u> wave. All the P waves look uniform.

4. Each P wave is followed by a normal QRS complex.

5. All the QRS complexes appear uniform.

6. THIS IS A SINUS RHYTHM!

NOTES

Section II
Sinus and Atrial Dysrhythmias

OBJECTIVES

When you have completed Section II, you will be able to describe or identify

1. the method utilized for interpreting dysrhythmias
2. sinus arrhythmia
3. sinus bradycardia
4. sinus tachycardia
5. premature atrial contractions (P.A.C.'s)
6. atrial tachycardia
7. wandering atrial pacemaker (W.A.P.)
8. sick sinus syndrome (brady-tachy syndrome)
9. atrial flutter
10. atrial fibrillation
11. atrial flutter-fibrillation

You're back! I'm happy to see that you didn't give up after Section I! 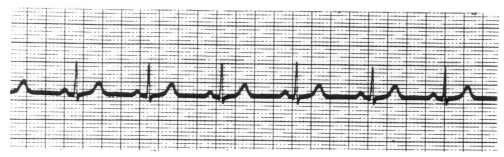 From this point forward, all that we do will involve the principles learned in the first section. All abnormal rhythm patterns that we explore will be compared to good ol' sinus rhythm.

Sinus rhythm

You'll remember, sinus rhythm is *regular* and has a rate of 60–100 beats per minute. Each QRS complex is preceded by a P wave. All P waves are uniform in appearance. All QRS complexes are uniform in appearance and each P wave is followed by a QRS.

As we begin to interpret the various abnormal rhythm patterns, *five* steps will be followed.
1. *Determine if the rhythm is regular.* If the rhythm is irregular, try to determine what makes it irregular. Are there early (premature) beats? Are there pauses? Are there abnormal beats? The simplest method for determining rhythm regularity is to measure the distance between two consecutive R waves (R-R interval) and compare that distance with other R-R intervals. In a regular rhythm, the R-R interval measurement will remain constant.
2. *Determine the heart rate.* Remember . . . if the rhythm is irregular, it is necessary to count the rate for one full minute.
3. *What are the atria doing?* Are there P waves that occur uniformly across the monitor tracing? Are the P waves alike in appearance? If no distinct P waves are present, is there evidence of atrial activity, or is the baseline preceding the QRS flat? If atrial impulses are present, are they regular or irregular? Is the atrial activity occurring so rapidly that there are more atrial deflections than QRS complexes? If actual atrial wave forms are difficult to identify, does the baseline appear chaotic?
4. *What are the ventricles doing?* Are the QRS's of normal duration (less than 0.12 seconds)? Do the QRS's occur uniformly across the monitor tracing?
5. *Determine the relationship between atrial and ventricular activity.* Is each P wave producing a QRS, or are there P waves that are not followed by QRS complexes? Is each QRS preceded by a P wave, or is there evidence of independent ventricular activity? Is the P-R interval of all conducted beats constant, does it vary, or is there no established relationship?

Practice Exercise 1

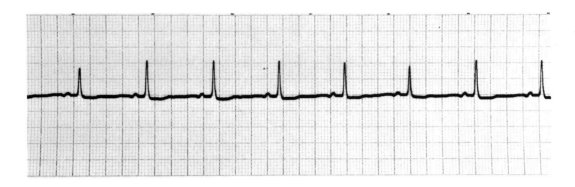

Look at this strip.

A. The heart rate is _____ beats per minute.

B. The rhythm is regular / irregular (circle one).

C. Each QRS complex is preceded by a _____ .

D. All P waves are _____ in appearance.

E. Each P wave is followed by a _____ .

F. All QRS complexes are _____ in appearance.

G. The P-R interval is _____ and measures _____ seconds.

H. Therefore, this is a _____ rhythm!

To interpret any rhythm, I use the same five principles.

1. First, I determine if the rhythm is _____ .

2. Second, I must determine the heart _____ .

3. I next ask what the _____ are doing.

4. Then I look to determine what the _____ are doing.

5. The last step involves determining if a relationship exists between _____ activity.

For **Feedback 1,** refer to page 71.

Input 2: Sinus Arrhythmia

The first dysrhythmia to be explored is *SINUS ARRHYTHMIA.*

A sinus arrhythmia is a *slightly* irregular rhythm that is initiated by the SA node. Usually the slight variation in rhythm is related to **respiration.** The heart rate will increase slightly with inspiration, and decrease slightly with expiration. A sinus arrhythmia is a normal finding in children and young adults. A *slight* sinus arrhythmia may be found throughout adulthood. Sinus arrhythmia is usually the result of increased vagal tone.

Sinus arrhythmia may be found with conditions such as rheumatic fever, atelectasis, infectious diseases, etc. Last, but not least, a sinus arrhythmia may be seen in patients receiving digitalis. Any factor which increases vagal tone will exaggerate a sinus arrhythmia.

When you look closely at this rhythm strip, you will note the following:

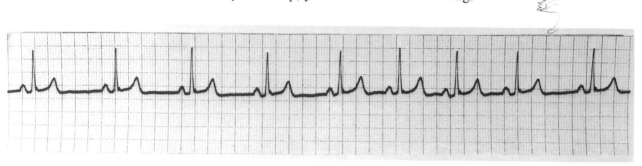

1. The heart rate falls somewhere between 60 and 100 beats per minute.
*2. The rhythm is irregular.
3. The P waves are all uniform in appearance.
4. The QRS complexes are all of normal configuration and duration.
5. Each P wave produces a QRS. The P-R interval measures approximately 0.16 seconds and is consistent across the strip (so, atrial activity is related to ventricular activity!).

*The only abnormal finding is that the rhythm is *slightly* irregular, showing irregular spacing of the normal P waves.

The easiest method for determining rhythm irregularity is to measure the distance between two P waves (P-P interval) and then compare that distance to the distance between two other P waves (another P-P interval).

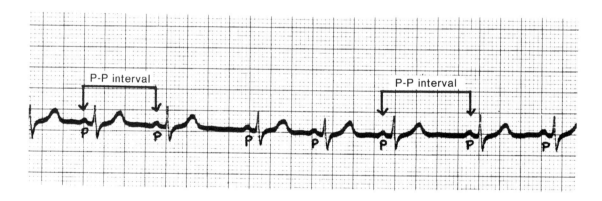

OR

Measure the distance between two R waves (R-R interval) and then compare that distance to the distance between two other R waves (another R-R interval).

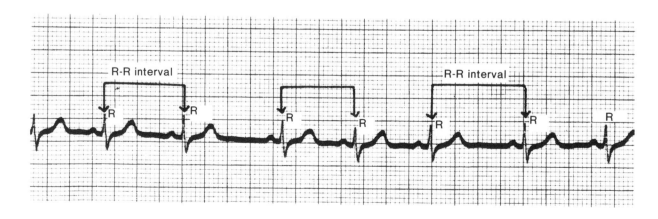

46

Easy, huh?

This strip shows the time measurement between each R-R interval. You can easily see the slight irregularity, though everything else appears normal.

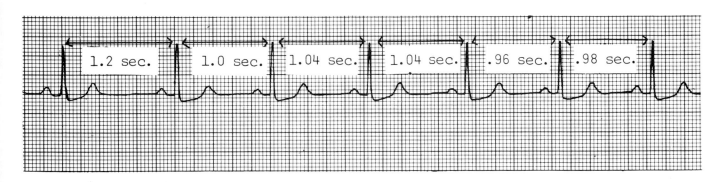

Remember, each small square on the EKG paper represents 0.04 seconds.

To review then, a sinus arrhythmia is simply a sinus rhythm that is slightly irregular! *No treatment is required.* (Just be conscious of its presence.)

Practice Exercise 2

Okay, now it's your turn! Look at these two strips, then answer the questions.

1.

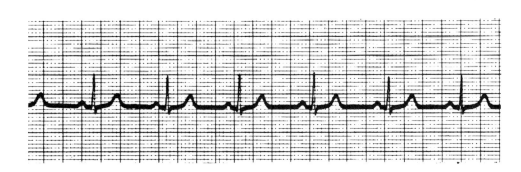

A. The heart rate in this strip is **approximately** _____ beats per minute.

B. The P waves are all _____ in appearance.

C. A _____ wave precedes each QRS complex.

D. The QRS complexes are _____ in appearance.

E. A _____ follows every P wave.

F. The rhythm is regular / irregular (circle one).

G. This is a _____ rhythm.

2.

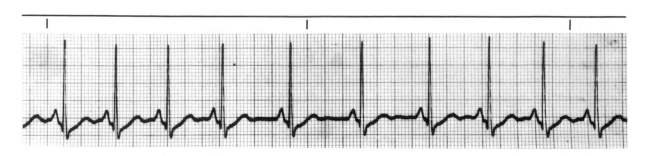

   A. The heart rate in this strip is **approximately** ＿＿＿＿＿ beats per minute.

   B. The P waves are all ＿＿＿＿＿ in appearance.

   C. A ＿＿＿＿＿ wave precedes each QRS complex.

   D. The QRS complexes are ＿＿＿＿＿ in appearance.

   E. A ＿＿＿＿＿ follows every P wave.

   F. The rhythm is regular / irregular (circle one).

   G. This is a ＿＿＿＿＿ rhythm.

3. Usually the irregularity found in sinus arrhythmia is related to ＿＿＿＿＿＿＿＿＿ .

For **Feedback 2,** refer to page 71.

Input 3: Sinus Bradycardia

Bradycardia is a term used to describe a heart rate less than 60 beats per minute. *Sinus bradycardia* is a normal rhythm with the exception that the rate falls below 60. The impulse originates in a normal fashion from the sinus (SA) node, but the impulses are fired at a slower rate due to vagal stimulation of the cardiac regulatory center.

Commonly, *sinus bradycardia* is the normal rhythm of athletes and other persons accustomed to regular physical exercise.

Sinus bradycardia may also be found when pressure is exerted on the carotid sinus or the eyeball. Likewise, a slow rate is commonly found with increased intracranial pressure, or during normal sleep.

Sinus bradycardia may be observed in conjunction with:

Obstructive disease (intestine, kidney, bladder)
Myxedema
Myocardial infarction
Drug actions (digitalis, morphine, anesthesia, or quinidine)

Here is a rhythm strip demonstrating a *sinus bradycardia.*

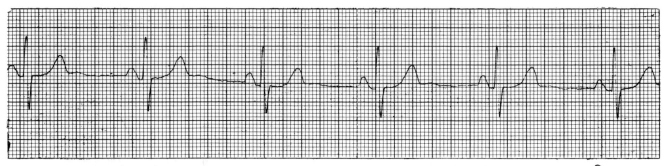

*1. The rate is approximately 48 beats per minute (I looked back at the chart on page 39 (i)).
2. The rhythm is regular.
3. The P waves are all uniform in appearance and precede each QRS complex.
4. The QRS complexes are uniform in appearance (and measure 0.10 seconds).
5. Each P wave produces a QRS. The P-R interval measures approximately 0.18 seconds and is consistent across the strip. Thus, atrial activity is assumed to be related to ventricular activity.

*The only abnormality is that the heart rate is approximately 48, which falls below the lower limits of normal, 60 beats per minute. So, we have a sinus bradycardia.

Using the five principles for dysrhythmia interpretation, one could say:

- The rate is approximately 48 per minute.
- The rhythm is slow and regular.
- The atria are activated regularly. P waves precede each QRS complex and they are uniform in appearance. (I used the Trusty Guide on page 39 to determine the heart rate.)
- There is a QRS complex following each P wave. The QRS complexes are occurring regularly at a rate of 48 per minute. All QRS complexes appear uniform and measure 0.08 seconds.
- There is a definite relationship between atrial and ventricular activity because each P-R interval is 0.18 seconds. In other words, the impulse originating in the sinus node moves down the conduction system to activate ventricular tissue in the same amount of time during each cardiac cycle.

Usually sinus bradycardia is observed and not treated. Treatment will be initiated if the patient becomes symptomatic (mental confusion or disorientation, lethargy, loss of consciousness, etc.). Should the patient become symptomatic, a physician should be notified immediately.

In most instances, atropine is the drug treatment of choice to increase the heart rate when symptoms are acute. However, make certain you monitor urinary performance following the administration of atropine! Your patient may experience urinary retention, as atropine is a smooth muscle relaxant. If the patient is receiving digitalis and his heart rate falls below 50, it is likely the digitalis will be discontinued. The physician should always be made aware of the digitalized patient with a sustained sinus bradycardia. Digitalis preparations *should be held* until the physician is notified; additional administration of digitalis may further slow heart rate or result in various forms of heart block.

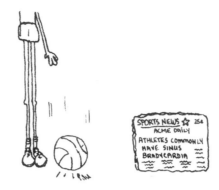

Practice Exercise 3

A. The term bradycardia implies that the heart rate is less than _____ beats per minute. Here are two strips for you to inspect.

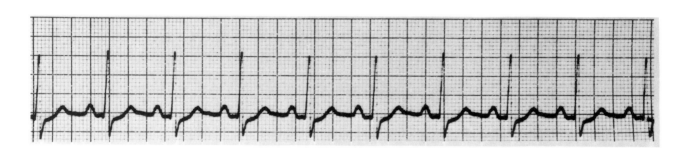

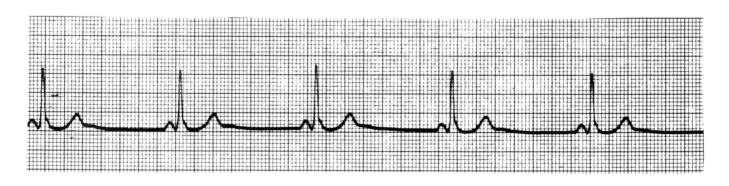

B. Strip 1 shows a sinus rhythm. Explain how strip 2 is both similar to and different from strip 1. (Use the principles that we have discussed!)

_____

_____

_____

_____

_____

_____

Strip 2 shows a _____ (rhythm).

For **Feedback 3,** refer to page 72.

Tachycardia is a term used to describe a heart rate of *greater than* 100 beats per minute. *Sinus tachycardia* is a regular sinus rhythm with a rate of greater than 100 beats per minute. *Usually a sinus tachycardia will not exceed the rate of 160 per minute.*

Sinus tachycardia is usually directly related to diminished vagal tone and may be exaggerated by increased sympathetic tone. Some of the more common causes of sinus tachycardia are exercise, excitement, anemia, fear, heart failure, pain, fever, shock, infection, and drugs—such as IV demerol, atropine or epinephrine, and foods—such as coffee or tea, and tobacco! Most authorities feel that for each Fahrenheit degree the temperature rises, the heart rate will increase approximately eight to ten beats per minute. I bet you didn't know that!

This rhythm strip demonstrates a sinus tachycardia.

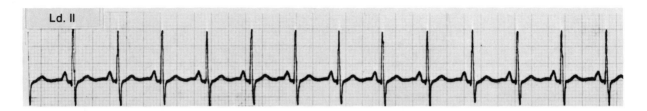

*1. The rate is rapid, approximately 115 beats per minute.
   2. ·The rhythm is regular.
   3. The P waves are all uniform in appearance.
   4. The QRS complexes are all uniform in appearance and duration.
   5. Each P wave precedes the QRS by the same interval. In other words the P-R interval is constant, measuring approximately 0.14 seconds.

*The only abnormality is that the heart rate is 115, which falls above 100 beats per minute. Thus, we have a *sinus tachycardia*. (I have used the Trusty Guide on page 39 to determine the heart rate!)

If a heart rate of exactly 100 accompanies a sinus rhythm, it is usually called a *borderline sinus tachycardia.*

Should you find your patient's heart rate greater than 100 beats per minute, you must assume the role of *detective* to discover why. The treatment for sinus tachycardia consists of *treating its cause* (i.e., lowering an elevated temperature or treating congestive heart failure.)

If the patient is extremely anxious, is cyanotic, has labored breathing or has chest pain, a physician should be notified immediately. The increased heart rate associated with a sinus tachycardia results in increased myocardial oxygen consumption, though hemodynamic imbalance usually does not occur.

Practice Exercise 4

1. Look at this rhythm strip closely, then describe *all* that you see!

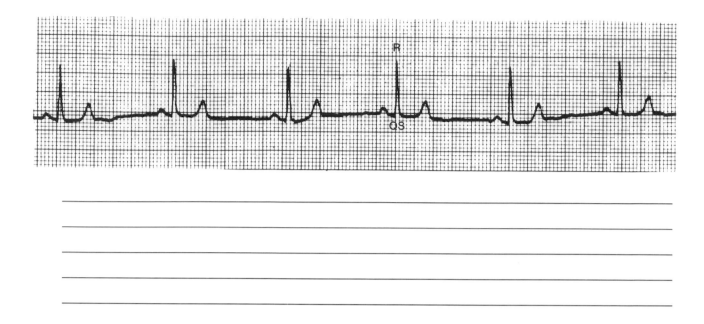

_____

_____

_____

_____

_____

_____

_____

This rhythm is a _____ .

2. Now do the same thing with this rhythm strip.

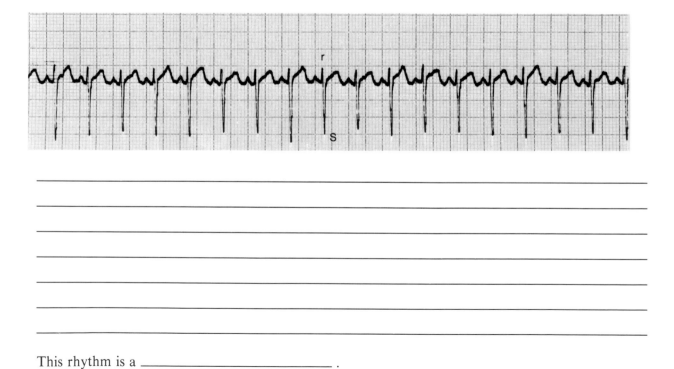

_____

_____

_____

_____

_____

_____

_____

This rhythm is a _____ .

The treatment for sinus tachycardia consists of _____

_____

_____

_____

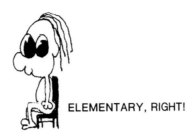

ELEMENTARY, RIGHT!

For **Feedback 4,** refer to page 72.

Input 5: Premature Atrial Contractions

Hope you enjoyed your break. I'm happy you're back for more.   We're going to begin exploring *ectopic* activity. . . . That's a fancy way to say that we're going to begin exploring stimuli for heart beats that originate in abnormal areas of the heart—outside the normal conduction system.

A *premature atrial contraction,* henceforth to be known as a P.A.C., is an impulse that arises in an ectopic or abnormal atrial focus. As the name implies, the P.A.C. is *premature* in its relationship to sinus rhythm. In addition to occurring early or prematurely, the P.A.C. has an *abnormal appearing P wave.* In other words the P wave looks distinctly different from the P wave of the sinus rhythm since the route of atrial depolarization is different for the abnormal beat.

That may sound confusing, so look at this strip.

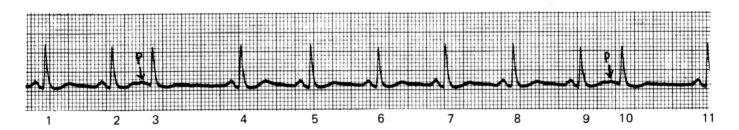

The first thing one notices is that the rhythm is *irregular.* Beat 3 and beat 10 occur early or prematurely. This is a technical interpretation based solely on quick "eyeball inspection"! You will notice the premature beats (3 and 10) have P waves . . . but they look distinctly different from the other P waves in the strip. P.A.C.'s may have P waves that are inverted, slurred, taller or wider than the normal P wave. On this strip, the P wave of the P.A.C. appears flat.

Premature atrial contraction is one of the few names used in EKG interpretation that is logical! Because the P.A.C. falls early interrupting the underlying rhythm, it is called *premature.* And because there is a P wave we know the atria have depolarized.

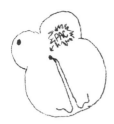

The premature atrial impulse is *usually* conducted normally through the AV junction on to the ventricles. Do you know how I know that? *Voila!* because the P-R interval of the P.A.C. is usually between 3–5 small EKG squares and because its QRS is usually narrow (*less than* 3 small squares). However, be advised that multiple rhythm abnormalities often occur together. It is not uncommon that the QRS associated with a P.A.C. will be widened, 0.12 seconds or greater. This is referred to as a P.A.C. that is *abberantly* conducted, meaning that conduction is outside the normal conduction pathway.

In this strip, every other beat is a P.A.C. (bigeminy P.A.C.'s). Notice that the P waves of the premature beats tend to be less pronounced than the P waves of the sinus beats.

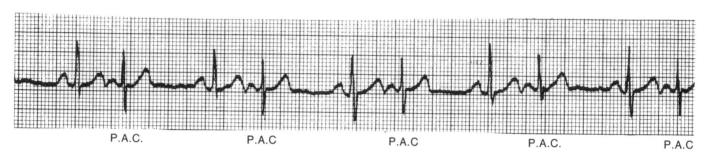

P.A.C.   P.A.C   P.A.C   P.A.C.   P.A.C

Premature atrial contractions may arise from a single or several foci within the atria. All P.A.C.'s arising from a single focus will have P waves that appear the same. Conversely, if P.A.C.'s arise from different sites, the appearance of their premature P waves will vary. When P.A.C.'s arise from a single focus, there is a *tendency for a constant coupling interval.* So what is a *coupling interval?* Well, it's simply the interval or distance between the P.A.C. and the previous sinus beat. (This business about coupling intervals is for your trivia file.)

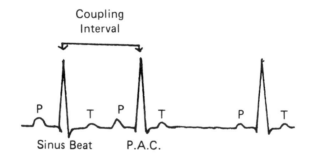

Look at this rhythm strip. Notice that the *coupling interval* is the same! (The P waves of the P.A.C.'s look the same . . . we therefore assume they are arising from the same ectopic atrial site.)

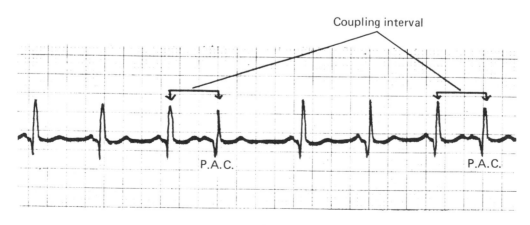

The other obvious finding with P.A.C.'s is that there is a slight pause or delay before the next sinus beat.

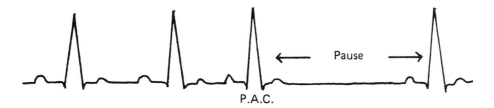

P.A.C.

This pause tends to partly compensate for the prematurity. In other words, the P.A.C. firing prematurely disrupts the regular sinus cycle; thus, the P.A.C. "resets" the sinus cycle. P.A.C.'s indicate atrial irritability and may forewarn of impending serious atrial arrhythmias.

Premature atrial contractions may be observed in healthy individuals or may be associated with heart disease. P.A.C.'s in a patient with rheumatic heart disease may be a forerunner to atrial fibrillation. P.A.C.'s may also be noted in patients with pulmonary disease, right heart disease, and myocardial infarction. Drugs such as epinephrine and digitalis, or coffee, tea, alcohol, tobacco, emotional distress, or fatigue may likewise cause P.A.C.'s. To be on the safe side, always notify a physician when a patient begins having P.A.C.'s and when they begin increasing in frequency! *The significance of P.A.C.'s is the significance of the underlying clinical condition.*

To try to pull this together, let me logically describe this strip to you.

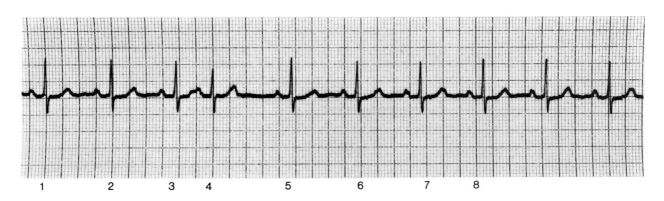

The P waves are *not* uniform in appearance. The P wave of beat 4 is premature and appears different from the other P waves. If you look closely, you will notice that the premature P wave falls on the T wave of the preceding beat. A P wave precedes every QRS complex. The QRS complexes are uniform in appearance, but do not occur regularly. There is a pause following the complex initiated by the premature P wave. The underlying rhythm is a sinus rhythm interrupted by a lone P.A.C.

Detecting P.A.C.'s is usually not difficult—but may be confusing if, for some reason, the premature atrial impulse fails to be conducted. That sounds like a mouthful, so look at this strip.

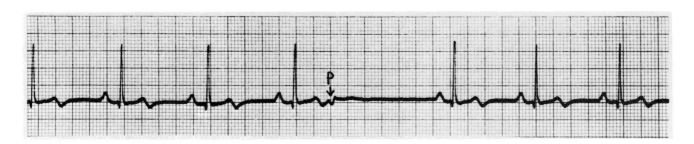

First ask yourself what the atria are doing. Refer back to the previous strip and locate all of the P waves. You will note that a premature P wave (appearing distinctly different from the other P waves) follows after beat 3. What is this? Well, it's a P wave—and P waves represent atrial depolarization. It occurs prematurely. So it's a premature atrial contraction that is not conducted to the ventricles. In other words, since a QRS does not follow the premature atrial impulse, you know that the impulse was blocked or interrupted enroute to the ventricles. So this is an example of a *blocked P.A.C.* Like conducted P.A.C.'s, there is a pause following the blocked P.A.C.

P.S.   If this is confusing to you, it may help to remember that you will never find two T waves occurring together!

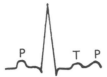

So, if a well-defined "bump" follows the T wave—most likely, it is a P wave!

Blocked P.A.C.'s are usually the result of one of two things. *First and foremost,* blocked P.A.C.'s are frequently observed in patients that are digitalis toxic. If blocked P.A.C.'s are observed, make certain to check whether or not the patient is receiving a digitalis preparation. Always be on the lookout for digitalis toxicity signs and symptoms!

Look closely at this second strip. Notice the blocked P.A.C. This strip is a tough one! By looking closely, however, you will notice that the T wave of the fourth complex is distorted . . . it has an extra "bump." This extra "bump" is assumed to be a P wave! In other words, the premature P wave is sitting on the downslope of the T wave. Thus, we have a blocked P.A.C.!

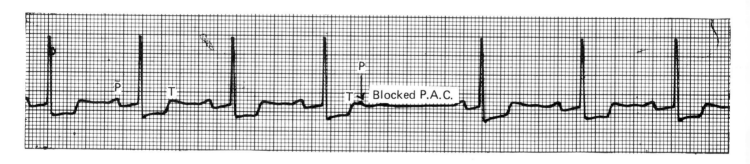

In this second example, the premature atrial impulse does not conduct to the ventricles because the cardiac tissue has not fully recovered or repolarized. In other words, if the myocardial cells do not have time to repolarize, they may be refractory to (unable to receive) the next stimulation. (The patient belonging to this rhythm strip had a digitalis level of 4.7ng/ml.!!) UGH! It is important to note that digitalis toxicity may be the culprit in either instance!

Enough on the subject of blocked P.A.C.'s Let's try some practice.

Practice Exercise 5

1. Now, you try your hand at interpretation. Describe all that you see.

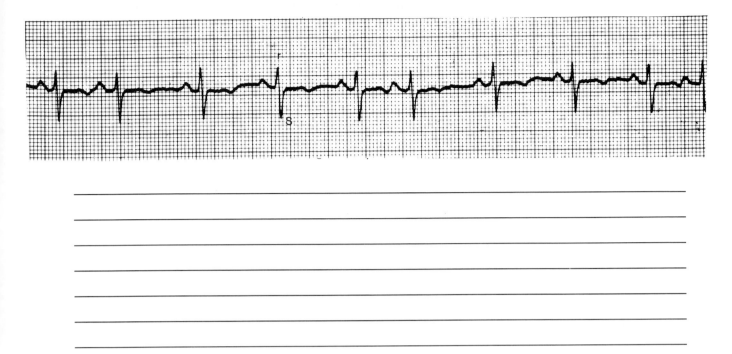

_____

_____

_____

_____

_____

_____

_____

_____

_____

_____

2. Circle the blocked P.A.C.'s and indicate any suspicions you may have.

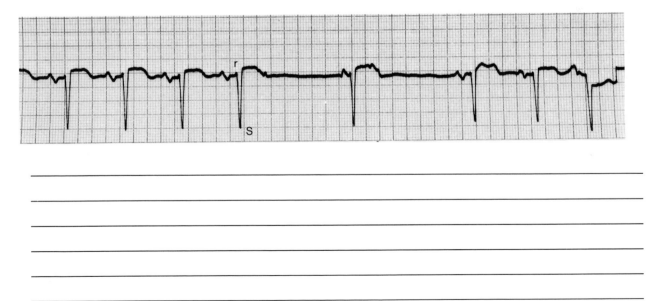

_____

_____

_____

_____

_____

It sometimes helps to sing a few bars of "KEEP ON SMILING. . . ."

For **Feedback 5,** refer to page 73.

You now have a basic understanding of ectopic activity—the P.A.C. If, for some reason, an ectopic focus in the atria fires *rapidly* and *repeatedly,* one will see an *atrial tachycardia.*

Although the SA node is the heart's natural pacemaker, it rarely fires faster than 160 times per minute. Any ectopic focus that initiates impulses faster than this rate will take control of the rhythm. *Remember, the fastest pacemaker* always *controls the rhythm!*

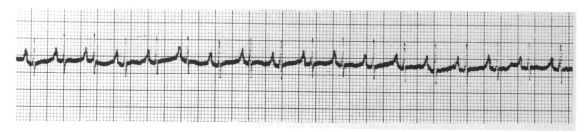

Atrial tachycardia, rate 166.

Now that I have you thinking about rapid ectopic atrial activity, we need to explore the mechanisms behind atrial tachycardia. As I indicated above, an ectopic focus within the right or left atria may discharge rapidly and repeatedly to produce atrial tachycardia. A reentry mechanism, however, is the more common cause of rapid supraventricular rhythms. When related to a reentry phenomenon, the atrial tachycardia is precipitated by a P.A.C. with a prolonged P-R interval. This P.A.C. stimulus travels down the conduction pathway normally, activating the ventricles. In addition though, the stimulus is able to reenter the bundle of His in a retrograde or backward fashion, traveling back up to the atria where it reactivates the atria and then travels down the conduction pathway again! Whew! If this reentry phenomenon persists, atrial tachycardia results. Yes, I know that is confusing . . . *it even confuses the experts!* The "bottom line" is that a rapid atrial mechanism is controlling the rhythm!

Atrial tachycardia is basically a rapid, regular *sustained* rhythm with a rate between *160 and 220* per minute. In addition to occurring in a sustained fashion, atrial tachycardia may both begin and end abruptly. When this occurs, the short runs of atrial tachycardia are said to be occurring in *paroxysms.* Hence, short bursts or runs of atrial tachycardia are referred to as P.A.T. (*paroxysmal atrial tachycardia*).

Atrial tachycardia may be associated with coronary artery disease, valvular disease (e.g., rheumatic mitral disease) . . . or may be found in otherwise healthy individuals! In fact, any of the following factors may precipitate atrial tachycardia: emotional stress, drug actions of digitalis or quinidine, coffee, tea, tobacco, alcohol, and so forth.

Most patients with a sustained atrial tachycardia experience a fluttering sensation in the chest along with light-headedness due to the rapid ventricular rate. The rapid heart rate reduces cardiac output because the volume of blood ejected with each contraction (stroke volume) is decreased as a result of the shortened ventricular filling time. That sounds a bit complicated! Actually it's a great deal like your average household toilet. If you stand there flushing your toilet 180 times per minute, you can imagine what happens . . . not much! You must allow time (between flushes) for the reservoir to refill; otherwise, there's not much action or "toilet output" at the bottom. . . . Right? . . . Just like cardiac output—there must be an appropriate ventricular filling time.

58

This decrease in cardiac output can lead to left ventricular (LV) failure. The rapid rate also increases the oxygen demand and consumption of the cardiac muscle which may cause ischemia of the myocardium and may precipitate an anginal attack (chest pain).

Let's examine a rhythm strip of atrial tachycardia.

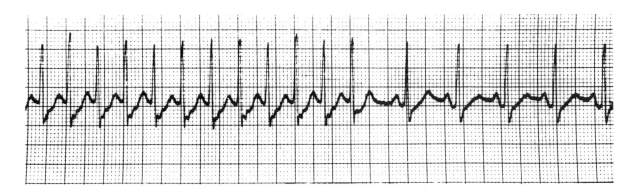

The first two-thirds of this rhythm strip demonstrates atrial tachycardia at a rate of approximately 200 per minute. The rapid rhythm breaks spontaneously into a sinus rhythm. You will recall that characteristically, atrial tachycardia has a heart rate that falls between 160 and 220 per minute. Whenever one finds a rapid rhythm with *clearly distinguishable upright P waves* occurring before the QRS's, the rhythm is assumed to be of atrial origin! You will notice that the QRS complexes in both the atrial tachycardia and the sinus rhythm are of normal duration (*narrow*), since ventricular activation occurs normally. A word of caution: because underlying pathology may complicate electrical activity, one may find an atrial tachycardia with a widened QRS.

Now, look at this strip.

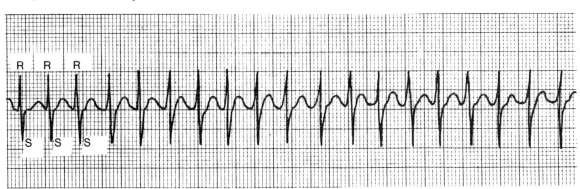

The heart rate in the above strip is approximately 187 beats per minute which makes me think of atrial tachycardia. But, where are the P waves? P waves may or may not be there! If *definite* P waves are not observable, one cannot call the rhythm *atrial* tachycardia. So what will we call it?

How about just describing what we see?

This is a rapid rhythm with a heart rate of 187 beats per minute. The QRS complexes are narrow.

Oftentimes, rapid regular rhythms with normal duration QRS's are referred to as supraventricular rhythms. The term *supraventricular* implies that the rhythm originates above the level of the ventricles.

Atrial tachycardia may terminate abruptly without treatment. If it persists, a physician should be notified immediately. If the patient is alert, he or she may be asked to perform the Valsalva maneuver. This maneuver requires that the patient hold his breath and bear down—it's basically like having a bowel movement. This maneuver increases vagal tone which may terminate the rapid rhythm. Another technique for increasing vagal tone (a vagotonic maneuver 🫕) is to place a *cold* or *ice* compress on the patient's face. By stimulating a vagal response, the AV junction may slow its rate of impulse conduction, thereby slowing the heart rate. This application of cold or ice water to the face stimulates the *diving reflex,* a primitive reflex which may result in slowed conduction! If these techniques are unsuccessful, the physician may elect to apply carotid massage or carotid sinus pressure which is an attempt to increase vagal tone. If carotid massage is unsuccessful in breaking the fast rhythm, and the patient's condition is deteriorating, the physician may perform synchronized cardioversion.

If the rapid rhythm is being tolerated, drugs such as digitalis or verapamil may be used. Both drugs serve to slow AV conduction, although their properties are very different!

Always alert the physician to even *brief* periods of atrial tachycardia.

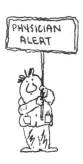

Practice Exercise 6

Just relax. Okay, now look at this strip. Describe to me everything that you see. I don't expect you to be an expert, so I'll help you.

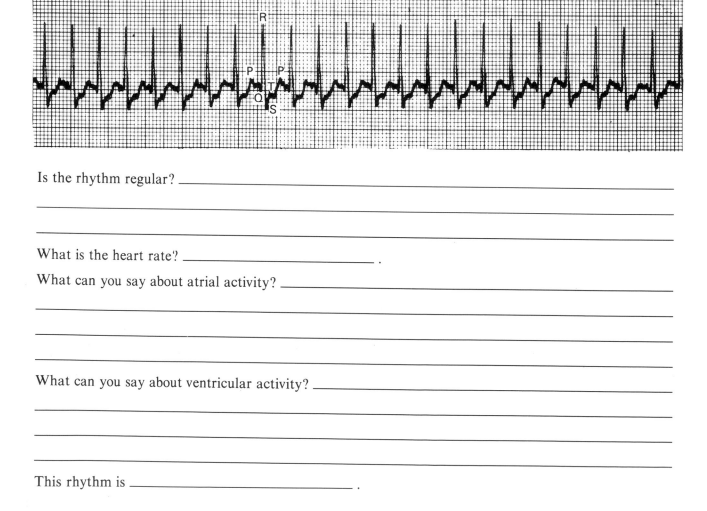

Is the rhythm regular? _____

_____

_____

What is the heart rate? _____ .

What can you say about atrial activity? _____

_____

_____

_____

What can you say about ventricular activity? _____

_____

_____

_____

This rhythm is _____ .

Treatment is aimed at slowing down the heart rate. A method that might be used is the Valsalva maneuver. Describe this maneuver. _____

_____

_____

For **Feedback 6,** refer to page 74.

Input 7: Wandering Atrial Pacemaker (W.A.P.)

not x for this. Its Rc

Before moving forward, we should look briefly at *wandering atrial pacemakers*. Basically, a *wandering atrial pacemaker* rhythm is a variation of a sinus rhythm that has no clinical significance. Rather than seeing uniform P waves across the EKG strip, the *P waves tend to vary in appearance.* This P wave variation suggests that the pacemaker is wandering within the sinus mechanism and the surrounding atrial tissue.

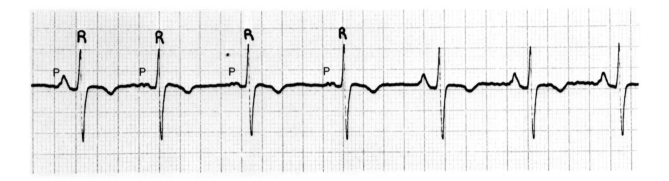

Commonly, a *wandering atrial pacemaker* is observed when the sinus rate slows. You will remember that other tissues within the atria have pacemaking capabilities. . . . <u>but</u>, it is always the pacemaker with the *fastest* rate of discharge that controls the rhythm. In a wandering atrial pacemaker rhythm, various pacemakers (located within the atrial) are discharging at similar rates. Thus, no single pacemaker site is dominant.

As you look at the above strip, you will notice that the rhythm is slightly irregular. (If you are unsure, measure the P-P or R-R intervals.) Looking further, the P waves tend to vary in shape or contour. Because of this variation, we assume that no single pacemaker within the atria is dominant. *How do I know that the various pacemakers are located within the atria? . . .* Because each cardiac complex begins with a P wave . . . and P waves represent atrial depolarization!

The other thing you should be aware of is that the P-R interval may vary throughout a wandering atrial pacemaker rhythm. Since the P-R interval represents the time for impulse conduction from the pacemaker site through the system to the Purkinje fibers, it makes sense that if the pacemaker site changes, so will the time for impulse conduction!

Since ventricular activation is unaltered, the QRS complexes are of normal duration (0.12–0.20 seconds). Owing to the fact that a wandering atrial pacemaker is a variation of normal, no treatment or intervention is required. Whew!

Practice Exercise 7

1. Without looking back, draw a rhythm strip demonstrating wandering atrial pacemaker. Sounds like fun . . . right? ☺

For **Feedback 7,** refer to page 74.

Input 8: Sick Sinus Syndrome (Brady-Tachy Syndrome)

Sick sinus syndrome is more a classification category rather than a specific diagnosis. Sick sinus syndrome is thought to be related to degeneration of the SA node cells, and is therefore usually found in patients with coronary artery disease and other degenerative processes. Because of this degeneration, the monitor picture of a patient with sick sinus syndrome displays such disorders as sinus bradycardia, sinus tachycardia, sinus pause, atrial or supraventricular tachycardia, escape beats, etc. In other words, the monitor tracing is a "*mixed bag*" of slow and rapid rhythms arising *above* the level of the ventricles (this means that the QRS duration is within normal limits indicating normal ventricular depolarization. ☺

Let's look at a sample strip.

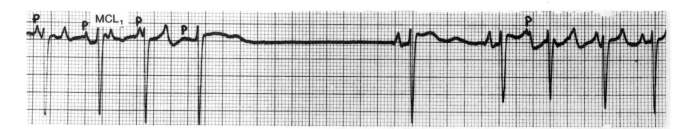

Notice the inconsistent and erratic nature of the sinus pacemaker. If you think this is a difficult rhythm strip, you are absolutely right!

Many times the patient exhibiting a sick sinus syndrome presents with a history of syncope and fluttering sensations in the chest. In many cases, diagnosis is made from the analysis of continuous Holter monitor tracings (the patient wears a portable monitor while he or she goes about normal activities). Once sick sinus syndrome is identified, the object of treatment is to maintain a stable heart rate. Drugs such as atropine have little long term success in speeding up a slow sinus pacemaker discharge rate. Suppressive drugs utilized to slow rapid rhythms would further suppress the slow phases of the rhythm. Gets complicated, right? ☺

Because of the varying nature of sick sinus syndrome, the treatment of choice involves the combination of a ventricular pacemaker (to augment heart rate during slow rhythms) and suppressant drugs (to control the rapid periods of the rhythm).

Since sick sinus syndrome is a collection of other dysrhythmias, there is no practice exercise! Such a deal!

Input 9: Atrial Flutter

Remember the normal conduction system?

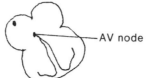

—AV node

Before we go any further, you must commit the following to memory.

The AV node *is unable* to conduct greater than approximately 220 impulses per minute. (This is a *general* rule.) If the heart rate exceeds 220 impulses per minute, some of the impulses will not be conducted through to the ventricles. This is called a normal *physiologic block*. Physiologic block is a protective mechanism that *guards* the ventricles from the effects of rapid stimulation!

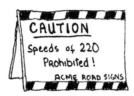

We are going to explore atrial ectopic activity even further to become familiar with *Atrial Flutter*.

Atrial flutter is a rapid *regular* atrial rhythm that arises from an excitable ectopic site (focus) in the atria. Although experts differ in their opinions, atrial flutter is commonly thought to result from a *reentry mechanism* rather than from a single ectopic focus firing rapidly and repeatedly. (You may want to reread the section on reentry . . . see page 58.)

It is important to remember that the fastest pacemaker will control heart beat. The *atrial rate* in atrial flutter is usually between *220–350* impulses per minute. Following what we said above, all of these impulses will not be conducted to the ventricles because the AV node is incapable of conducting more than 220 impulses per minute.

The rapid *atrial* impulses appear *saw-toothed* in shape and are labeled "F" waves. ("F" waves stand for flutter waves.) Flutter waves are continuous—they never stop. Consequently, they may even distort the QRS's! Flutter waves are more pronounced in leads II, III, and aVF . . . in other leads, the "saw-toothed" appearance is masked.

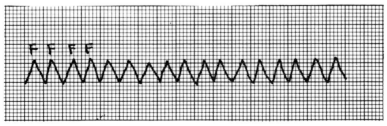

Saw-toothed atrial flutter waves

Since the AV node is unable to conduct greater than 220 impulses per minute, certain flutter impulses will not be conducted or will be blocked. *Usually,* only ½, ⅓, or ¼ of the atrial impulses will be conducted through the AV node to the ventricles.

To make this easy to understand, *let's say that the atrial flutter rate is 300.*

If ½ of those atrial impulses are conducted (2:1 conduction), the ventricular rate will be 150.

For every two flutter waves, there is one QRS. The first flutter wave is blocked; the second flutter wave conducts to the ventricles producing ventricular depolarization (a QRS).

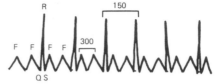

If ⅓ of those impulses are conducted (3:1 conduction), the ventricular rate will be 100.

For every three flutter waves, there will be one QRS. The first two flutter waves are blocked; the third one conducts to the ventricles producing ventricular depolarization.

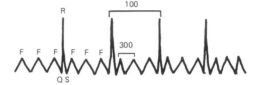

Or, if ¼ of those atrial impulses are conducted (4:1 conduction), the ventricular rate will be 75.

For every four flutter waves, there will be one QRS. The first three flutter waves are blocked; the fourth flutter wave conducts to the ventricles producing ventricular depolarization.

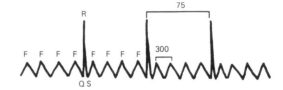

So, the atrial activity is saw-toothed in appearance in leads II, III, and aVF. There are flutter waves *rather than* P waves! The QRS complexes are normally *narrow* (less than 0.12 seconds), and the ventricular rhythm is *usually regular.* If, however, the degree of *physiologic block* in the AV node varies, the ventricular rhythm may be somewhat irregular. In other words, the AV node may arbitrarily allow flutter impulses to be conducted to the ventricles.

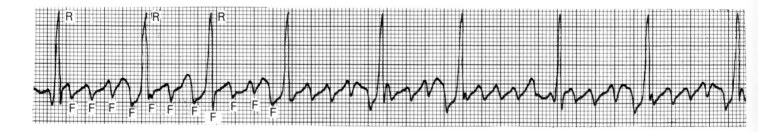

A picture like this would indicate atrial flutter with variable physiologic block in the AV node (irregular atrial flutter). As you can see, with variable block, the ventricular response is irregular. You know what this means . . . to determine an accurate heart rate you would need to count for one full minute!

Regardless whether the QRS complexes occur regularly or irregularly, the rhythm is atrial flutter. *The diagnosis of atrial flutter is based on the rapid, regular atrial impulses occurring at a rate of 220–350 per minute.*

When describing atrial flutter, it is important to specify the rate at which the atrial flutter waves are occurring and indicate both the *rate* and *regularity* of the ventricular response.

Atrial flutter is commonly associated with rheumatic heart disease, particularly with mitral stenosis, coronary artery disease, corpulmonale, hypertensive heart disease, hyperthyroidism, and pneumonia.

Here is a strip demonstrating atrial flutter with a regular ventricular response (4:1 atrial flutter—four flutter waves for every QRS).

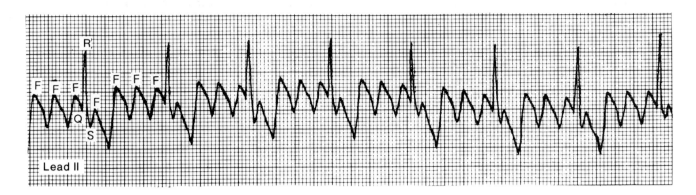

Let's describe what is happening!

Oh! I forgot to tell you something. This is going to sound *really* dumb, but . . . if I turn an atrial flutter tracing upside down, it's easier for me to see the flutter waves. When no one is watching, try it!

Okay. What are the atria doing?

Well, there are no P waves. Instead, there are saw-toothed flutter waves. Use the "300, 150, 100; 75, 60, 50" method to figure the *atrial (flutter)* rate. Find a *flutter wave* that falls on a heavy vertical line. Do not count that vertical line. The next one is 300 . . . right?

So the atrial flutter rate in this strip is 300! Because the AV node cannot conduct greater than 220 impulses per minute, some of those 300 impulses will be blocked. If you look closely, there are four flutter waves for every QRS (4:1 conduction).

What are the ventricles doing? The ventricular rate is regular at a rate of 75 per minute. The QRS complexes are narrow (less than 0.12 seconds). In atrial flutter, the *ventricular rate will usually be between 60–150 per minute.* Atrial and ventricular activity are related because the interval between the conducted flutter wave and its QRS is always constant. . . .

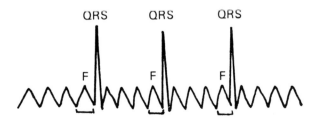

The distance between the atrial flutter wave preceding each QRS and the QRS measures the same indicating that atrial activity is related to ventricular activity. In other words, the atrial impulse (flutter wave) prior to the QRS, conducts down through the AV node to the ventricles producing ventricular depolarization (QRS).

drugs of choice Verapamil , IV cardizen

65

Vagotonic maneuvers, such as carotid massage or the Valsalva maneuver, may interrupt atrial flutter . . . or may assist in the diagnosis of atrial flutter.

Look at this next strip!

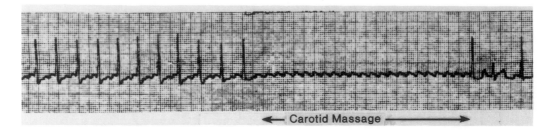

←— Carotid Massage —————→

Note the prominent flutter waves during carotid massage.

Atrial flutter may be treated in a variety of ways, but the *object* of initial treatment is to slow the rapid ventricular response. Similar to the discussion on atrial tachycardia, a rapid heart rate may predispose the patient to a diminished cardiac output, LV failure, ischemia, and angina. The best method of treatment is synchronized cardioversion using a low current setting. This interrupts the chaotic firing of the ectopic atrial focus, allowing the sinus pacemaker to resume control.

Some physicians will employ digitalis as the primary mode of treatment. Digitalis will produce further block in the AV node, thus slowing down the ventricular response. In other words, digitalis might change a 2:1 conduction to a 4:1 conduction. (If an atrial rate was 300 per minute, the ventricular rate would be 150 in a 2:1 conduction. If digitalis resulted in a 4:1 conduction, the ventricular rate would be 75. ($4\overline{)300}$ = 75)

Digitalis may also increase the atrial rate, and/or convert the rhythm to atrial fibrillation. Once the ventricular rate has been slowed, quinidine may be given in attempt to convert the atrial fibrillation to sinus rhythm.

One should remember, however, if digitalis is used as the first line of treatment, and if it is *not* effective, cardioversion is dangerous. When a patient has digitalis on board, cardioversion may produce ventricular fibrillation. Most authorities feel that digitalis should be held several days before cardioversion is attempted.

Only one other major point to make about atrial flutter. This is really a *secret* . . . a method to impress your friends!

Bonus ▶

Any time you see a regular rhythm with a heart rate between 150–190, always think about atrial flutter!

Flutter waves may be hiding . . . see for yourself!

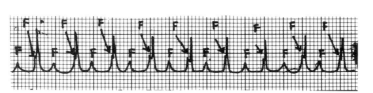

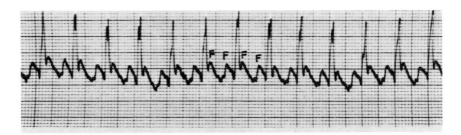

Note the atrial flutter waves occurring at a rate of 300 per minute!

Practice Exercise 9

Atrial flutter is a fun rhythm to detect.

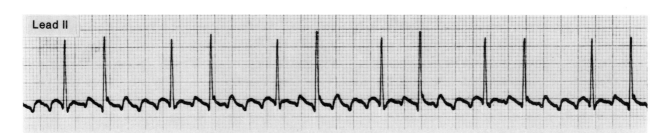

1. Use your skills to describe this strip in detail!

   P waves, Sawtooth appearance, Vent. rate irregular / Sirregular Flutter waves at 300 min. Vent rate 60-80.
   QRS .08
   Flutter waves: Rate 300

2. The atrial rate in atrial flutter varies between ___220___ and ___350___ impulses per minute. Characteristically, the ventricular rate will vary between ___60___ and ___150___ beats per minute. The AV node is unable to conduct greater than ___220___ impulses per minute. Beyond this rate, a ___Physiological AV___ block occurs.

For **Feedback 9,** refer to page 75.

Input 10: Atrial Fibrillation

By now, you may be feeling a bit overwhelmed! That, however, is a natural reaction. Knowing that this exercise is near the end of Section II may improve your outlook! We have saved the easiest dysrhythmia until last.

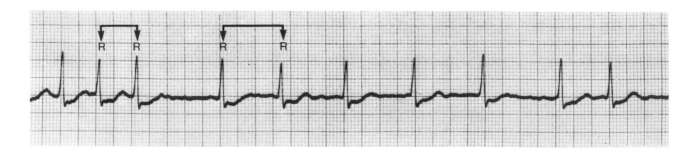

This is *ATRIAL FIBRILLATION*. There are no P waves; instead there are *bizarre* and *irregular* deflections referred to as fibrillation or "f" waves. The "f" waves have no rhythmic pattern; thus *atrial activation is chaotic*. The "f" waves in atrial fibrillation occur at a *rapid and irregular rate* which varies from *400–600* impulses per minute. In atrial fibrillation, the baseline appears to *undulate*.

We must refer back to the rule concerning physiologic block. The AV node is incapable of conducting more than *220* impulses to the ventricles per minute. Thus, we know that the 400–600 atrial impulses cannot all be conducted. Most usually, this physiologic block will permit 120–160 impulses through to the ventricles each minute. The ventricular response (QRS's) will occur irregularly due to the fact that the AV node has varying refractory periods (rest periods) following conducted impulses. Thus, the R-R interval will *always* vary. Because the "f" waves occur *continuously,* they may deform the QRS complexes, the ST segments, and the T waves!

In atrial fibrillation, there is no coordinated activation process in the atria. The tissue within the atria is electrically fragmented into various stages of excitation, refractoriness (resting state), or responsiveness. In other words, the tissues *haven't got it together*! The tissues are "out of phase" with each other. Normally, all the fibers within a heart chamber will be in essentially the same electrophysiologic state—they will all be in a state of excitation, all in a state of refractoriness, or all in a partial state of responsiveness.

Atrial fibrillation may be associated with the following conditions: hyperthyroidism, rheumatic heart disease, cardio-respiratory disease, hypertensive heart disease, arteriosclerotic heart disease, myocardial infarction, surgery, infection, etc. Patients with congestive heart failure (C.H.F.) are prone to atrial fibrillation. With C.H.F. the atria are distended and stretched which can precipitate atrial ectopic activity.

In many instances, the ventricular rate will be rapid (120–160 beats per minute). Like the previous rapid rhythms discussed, a rapid ventricular response may decrease cardiac output and precipitate LV failure, ischemia, and chest pain. Remember the toilet example . . . page 58.

With uncontrolled atrial fibrillation, cardiac output is compromised because of both the rapid ventricular rate and the loss of synchronized atrial beat (atrial kick). It is common to find a *pulse deficit* associated with atrial fibrillation. A pulse deficit exists when the apical pulse is faster than the radial pulse, when the two pulses are counted simultaneously. When the cardiac output is compromised, not all cardiac contractions will be felt radially.

Let's try describing what we see, using our rules for dysrhythmia interpretation.

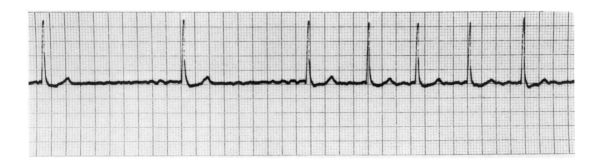

What are the atria doing? There are no P waves or P-R intervals. In the previous strip, the baseline appears to *undulate*. There are rapid, small irregular waves with no common pattern.

What are the ventricles doing? The QRS complexes are normal in shape and duration (less than 3 small squares or less than 0.12 seconds), but they occur *irregularly*. The interval between R waves (R-R interval) varies. To determine the heart rate, I would need to count the number of conducted beats occurring in *one full minute*!

What is the relationship between atrial and ventricular activity? Well, the conduction is *bizarre*! Most of the atrial impulses (fibrillation waves) that reach the AV node are blocked (because the AV node cannot conduct greater than 220 impulses per minute). Those atrial impulses that pass through the AV node are normally conducted, as demonstrated by QRS complexes of normal duration.

The aim of treatment for atrial fibrillation is reduction of the rapid ventricular response and restoration of hemodynamic equilibrium. Digitalis is the drug of choice to accomplish this. You will recall that digitalis exerts its effect on the AV node, increasing the amount of block. In other words, it further prevents atrial impulses from being conducted through to the ventricles.

Once the heart rate has been sufficiently reduced, an attempt may be made to convert the rhythm to a sinus rhythm using quinidine or synchronized cardioversion.

If atrial fibrillation is a result of an enlarged heart or C.H.F., it may be impossible to convert the rhythm to a normal sinus rhythm. Likewise, if sinus rhythm is restored, it may not persist unless the underlying problem is corrected.

Cases of long-standing atrial fibrillation, especially when associated with large atria and C.H.F., are not suitable for conversion to sinus rhythm. In general, one will not synchronize cardiovert if atrial fibrillation has persisted six months or longer. If atrial fibrillation has persisted over time, small clots may have developed within the atria. If one were to synchronize cardiovert the patient restoring a sinus rhythm, the forceful atrial contractions might shear off a clot, resulting in a cerebral accident!

This is another example of atrial fibrillation.

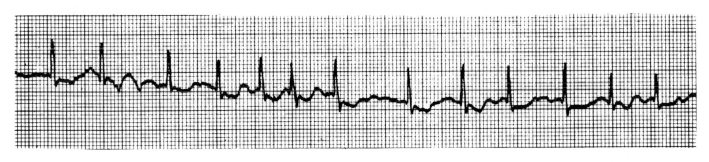

Notice how the baseline *undulates*.

Practice Exercise 10

The atrial deflections in atrial fibrillation are known as _____ waves. These atrial impulses occur _____ to _____ times per minute. Because the AV node is unable to conduct greater than _____ impulses per minute, a ____*physiologic*____ block will occur. If on a monitor tracing one sees *no clear P waves, an undulating baseline and a varying R-R interval,* one can suspect _____ .

Look at this rhythm strip. Simply, describe what you see.

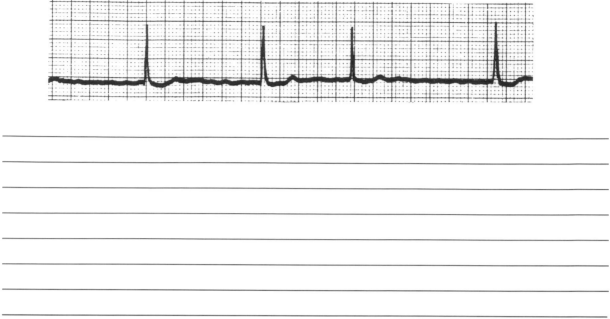

_____

_____

_____

_____

_____

_____

_____

_____

For **Feedback 10,** refer to page 75.

Input 11: Atrial Flutter-Fibrillation ("flutter-fib")

Occasionally, a rhythm strip will be encountered that looks suspiciously like atrial flutter (F waves observed across the strip). Yet, when one attempts to measure the rate and *regularity* of the F waves, they <u>do not</u> measure out! In other words, the F waves do not occur regularly. Oftentimes, this rhythm is referred to as *impure flutter,* or more commonly, *atrial flutter-fibrillation.* It is unclear whether such a phenomenon truly exists, or whether the classification has been created for convenience sake! In all probability, the underlying disorder is that of a coarse atrial fibrillation, and should be treated as such!

SEE WHAT YOU THINK! TRY MEASURING THE REGULARITY OF THE <u>FLUTTER</u> WAVES.

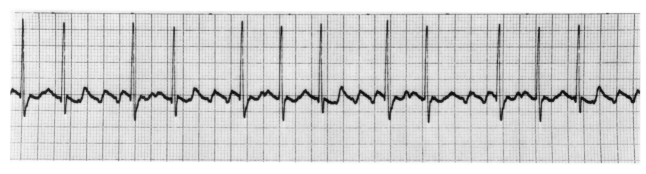

P.S. There is no practice exercise associated with input 11. Whew!

Feedback 1

    If your answers are similar to mine, you have the basics down pat! If you are "shaky" on any of the points covered, review Section I one more time. (You'll be happy you did!)

A. The heart rate in this rhythm strip is approximately <u>70</u> beats per minute.

B. The rhythm is ⟨regular.⟩

C. Each QRS complex is preceded by a <u>P wave</u>.

D. All P waves are <u>uniform</u> in appearance.

E. Each P wave is followed by a <u>QRS</u>.

F. All QRS complexes are <u>uniform</u> in appearance.

G. The P-R interval is *constant* and measures 0.16 seconds.

H. Therefore, this is a <u>SINUS</u> rhythm.

The five principles used in dysrhythmia interpretation are:
1. First, determine if the rhythm is <u>regular</u>.

2. Second, determine the heart <u>rate</u>.

3. Next determine what the <u>atria</u> are doing.

4. Then determine what the <u>ventricles</u> are doing.

5. The last step involves determining if a relationship exists between <u>atrial and ventricular</u> activity.

Feedback 2

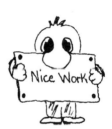

    You're doing great!

1. A. The heart rate in this strip is **approximately** <u>80</u> beats per minute.

    B. The P waves are all <u>uniform</u> in appearance.

    C. A <u>P</u> wave precedes each QRS complex.

    D. The QRS complexes are <u>uniform</u> in appearance.

    E. A <u>QRS</u> follows every P wave.

    F. The rhythm is ⟨regular.⟩

    G. This is a <u>SINUS RHYTHM</u>.

2. A. The heart rate in this strip is **approximately** <u>90</u> beats per minute.

    B. The P waves are all <u>uniform</u> in appearance.

    C. A <u>P</u> wave precedes each QRS complex.

    D. The QRS complexes are <u>uniform</u> in appearance.

    E. A <u>QRS</u> follows every P wave.

    F. The rhythm is ⟨ irregular. ⟩

    G. This is a <u>SINUS ARRHYTHMIA</u>.

3. Usually, the irregularity found in sinus arrhythmia is related to <u>respiration</u>.
   Just for review, here are the EKG criteria for a sinus arrhythmia.

normal & common in children

EKG CRITERIA FOR SINUS ARRHYTHMIA

1. Rate:	60–100 *Rate ↑inspiration / Rate ↓expiration*
2. Rhythm:	Slightly irregular. The P-P interval or R-R interval varies in duration
3. P waves:	Normal configuration
4. QRS:	Normal configuration and duration
5. Conduction:	Each P wave is followed by a QRS; the P-R interval is constant.

Feedback 3

   Nice work!

A. The term *bradycardia* implies that the heart rate is <u>less than 60 beats</u> per minute.

B. Rhythm strip 2 is similar to strip 1 in the following ways:

   1. In each strip, the P waves appear uniform.
   2. A P wave precedes each QRS.
   3. In each strip, the QRS complexes appear uniform.
   4. A QRS complex follows each P wave.
   5. The rhythm is regular in each strip.

   Rhythm strip 2 differs from rhythm strip 1 in this way:

   In rhythm strip 1 (sinus rhythm), the heart rate falls between 60 and 100 beats per minute.
   In rhythm strip 2, the heart rate is <u>41</u> beats per minute, falling below the normal range of 60–100 beats per minute. (I have used the Trusty Guide on page 39 to determine the heart rate!!)

   Strip 2 shows a <u>sinus bradycardia</u>.

   Just for review, here are the EKG criteria for a sinus bradycardia.

EKG CRITERIA FOR A SINUS BRADYCARDIA

Rate:	<u>Less than 60</u>
Rhythm:	Regular
P waves:	Normal configuration
QRS:	Normal configuration and duration
Conduction:	Each P wave is followed by a QRS; the P-R interval is constant.

MI's can cause Brady
Vasovagal Stim can
Carotid massage.

Feedback 4

   What a pro!

1. The P waves are all uniform in appearance.
   A P wave precedes each QRS complex.
   A QRS complex follows every P wave.
   QRS complexes measure approximately 0.08 seconds in duration.
   The P-R interval is constant and measures 0.16 seconds.
   The rhythm is regular.
   The heart rate is <u>50</u> beats per minute.

This is a <u>SINUS BRADYCARDIA</u>!

DID I FOOL YOU? HOPE NOT!!!

2. The P waves are all uniform in appearance.
   A P wave precedes each QRS complex.
   A QRS complex follows every P wave.
   The rhythm is regular.
   The heart rate is <u>150</u> beats per minute.
   QRS complexes (rS complexes) are approximately 0.08 seconds in duration.
   The P-R interval is constant and measures approximately 0.12 seconds.

This is a <u>SINUS TACHYCARDIA</u>.

The treatment for sinus tachycardia consists of <u>finding and treating its underlying cause</u> (i.e., fever, heart failure, anxiety, etc.).

Just for review, here are the EKG criteria for a sinus tachycardia.

EKG CRITERIA FOR SINUS TACHYCARIDA	
Rate:	100–160
Rhythm:	Regular
P Waves:	Normal configuration
QRS:	Normal configuration and duration
Conduction:	Each P wave is followed by a QRS; the P-R interval is constant.

Causes, fever, pain, anxiety, exercise, tobacco, caffeine, fear, → O₂ right away sedate them

Feedback 5

Nice work! If you are becoming frustrated, remember . . . ALL GREAT MINDS ARE FRUSTRATED!

1. Beat 2, beat 6, and beat 10 are premature. The contour of the P waves in the premature beats is slightly different from the normal P waves. The underlying rhythm is a sinus rhythm. A QRS complex follows every P wave. All the QRS complexes are uniform in appearance, measuring approximately 2½ small squares or 0.10 seconds. The P-R interval measures approximately 0.20 seconds, the upper limits of normal. A slight pause follows each P.A.C.

2. This patient may be digitalis toxic! Because the premature atrial impulses occur during the repolarization phase of the preceding beats, the ventricular tissue is unable to respond to the stimulation. Therefore, the P.A.C.'s are blocked or not conducted. The P-R interval of all conducted beats measures 0.24 seconds, indicating delayed conduction.

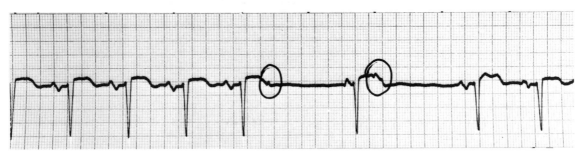

Non-conducted or blocked P.A.C.'s interrupt a sinus rhythm.

Ectopic - irritable, ectopic focus — another place other than where it should be

Just for review purposes, here are the EKG criteria for P.A.C.'s.

EKG CRITERIA FOR PREMATURE ATRIAL CONTRACTIONS

Rate:	Usually normal (60–100 beats per minute)
P Waves:	The P waves appear prematurely and differ in contour from the normal P waves.
QRS:	Usually normal configuration and duration
Conduction:	A normal QRS follows the abnormal P wave. There is a slight pause or delay before the next normal beat. This pause tends to partly compensate for the prematurity. (Of course, if the P.A.C. is blocked, it is not followed by a QRS!)

(handwritten annotations:) always early · always have a P wave in front of it · always PRS 12 ⟶ · always PR .7 · narrow QRS · Causes: Ø more than ☕ caffeine, nicotine, CHFpts.

A lot of PACs will ↑ lead pt into A Fib, tired ✓ TX: Don't drink caffeine so much, O₂, ↑ fx underlying cause

---

Feedback 6

How did you do? Sometimes this material is difficult. If you feel a bit insecure, try reading the section one more time. ☺

1. The rhythm is regular. There is a PQRST cycle in each beat.

2. The heart rate is approximately 200 beats per minute.

3. Each QRS is preceded by a P wave. All P waves look uniform.

4. Each P wave is followed by a QRS. All QRS complexes appear uniform.

5. This rhythm is atrial tachycardia.

6. The Valsalva maneuver consists of having the patient hold his breath and bear down.

Just for review, here are the EKG criteria for atrial tachycardia.

EKG CRITERIA FOR ATRIAL TACHYCARDIA *(handwritten: AKA Paroxysmal A Tach (PAT))*

Rate:	160–220 beats per minute
P waves:	May be buried in the QRS complexes or T waves and not visible; or may be similar to the contour of sinus P waves.
QRS:	Usually normal, but may be widened
Conduction:	A ventricular complex follows each P wave by the same interval
Rhythm:	Regular

(handwritten annotations:) must have electric · distinguishable p wave · uniform in appearance & have PR .12 or >

Causes: all the things that cause ST cause A Tach — ♀ in 30's, Stress, Caffeine, Tobacco, Sleeping pills

Feedback 7 ☺

How did you do? Remember, in wandering atrial pacemaker (W.A.P.), all QRS complexes will be preceded by a P wave. . . . It's just that the P waves may look different! The rhythm will be slightly irregular owing to the varying atrial pacemaker.

(handwritten:) PSVT — paroxysmal supra ventricular tach — give adenosine — P ordered

(handwritten bottom:) O₂, Vagal maneuvers, Devey reflex, Adenosine — then Verapamil, then synchronized cardiovert — then 2 Edema of choice, IV cardizem

This is what my *freestyle* W.A.P. looks like. *presence Multifocal atrial rhythm*

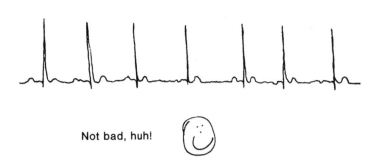

Not bad, huh! ☺

Feedback 9

Excellent work!

1. There are no P waves. Rather, there are saw-toothed atrial waves ("F" waves) occurring regularly at a rate of 300 per minute. The QRS complexes occur irregularly owing to variable physiologic block. The QRS complexes appear uniform and measure approximately 0.08 seconds. One would need to count the heart rate for one full minute!

2. The atrial rate in atrial flutter varies between <u>220</u> and <u>350</u> impulses per minute. Characteristically the ventricular rate will vary between <u>60</u> and <u>150</u> beats per minute.
The AV node cannot conduct greater than <u>220</u> impulses per minute. Beyond this rate, a <u>physiologic</u> block occurs.

Just for review, here are the EKG criteria for atrial flutter.

EKG CRITERIA FOR ATRIAL FLUTTER

Rate:	The atrial rate ("F" waves) will be between 220–350 per minute. The ventricular rate (QRS's) may vary from 60–150 depending on the number of impulses passing through the AV junction.
P Waves:	There are characteristic atrial oscillations—"saw-toothed" waves ("F" waves) that range between 220–350 per minute. <u>No isoelectric line is visible.</u>
QRS:	The QRS appears normal.
Conduction:	Usually ½, ⅓, or ¼ of the flutter (atrial) impulses will be conducted to the ventricles.

Feedback 10

What a Pro you are ☺ !

The atrial deflections in atrial fibrillation are known as "f" waves. These atrial impulses occur <u>400 to 600</u> times per minute. Because the AV node is unable to conduct greater than <u>220</u> impulses per minute, a <u>physiologic</u> block will occur.

If on a monitor tracing one sees no clear P waves, an undulating baseline and a varying R-R interval, one can suspect <u>atrial fibrillation</u>.

Interpretation

There are no clear P waves or P-R intervals. Atrial activity appears rapid and chaotic. The baseline appears to undulate. The QRS complexes are normal in shape and are less than 0.12 seconds in duration. The QRS complexes occur irregularly—the R-R interval varies. I would need a full minute strip to accurately determine heart rate. Most of the atrial impulses reaching the AV node are blocked. Those impulses passing through the AV node are conducted normally.

Just for review, here are the EKG criteria for atrial fibrillation.

EKG CRITERIA FOR ATRIAL FIBRILLATION	
Rate:	The heart rate varies according to the number of atrial impulses conducted through the AV node to the ventricles.
P Waves:	No P waves or P-R intervals; instead, there are rapid, small, irregular waves not resembling each other ("f" waves).
QRS:	The QRS's are normal in shape and duration, but occur irregularly. The R-R interval varies.
Conduction:	The conduction is bizarre. Most of the atrial impulses which reach the AV node are blocked. Those impulses that pass through the AV node are normally conducted.
Rhythm:	The ventricular rhythm is totally irregular.

apical / Radial pulse different
ie:110   ie:90

① IV Cardizem 1st drug of choice then
② Verapamil
③ Cardioversion
④ maintain on THE END...
   Verapamil po   OF SECTION II
      or Dig

76

NOTES

Section III
Junctional Escape and Ectopic Rhythms

OBJECTIVES

When you have completed Section III, you will be able to describe or identify

1. junctional escape rhythms and junctional escape beats
2. premature junctional beats
3. junctional tachycardia

Input 1: Junctional Escape Rhythm

You're back again! Persistent creature, aren't you! Though there are several other abnormal atrial rhythms, we'll save those for more advanced lessons! Whew!

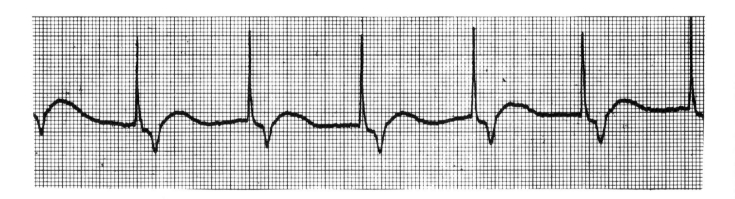

The heart has many potential pacemaker centers—the SA node, the atria, the AV junctional tissues, and the ventricles. Only the *dominant* or the *fastest pacemaker* (highest automaticity) will normally control the heart. If the sinus node fails to discharge an impulse *or* if the sinus impulse fails to be conducted *or* if the sinus rate of discharge is inadequate, a lower (more distal) pacemaker may assume the role of pacemaker. (Failure of the sinus mechanism may occur secondary to myocardial infarction, ischemia, hypoxia, vagal stimulation, etc.)

A slower pacemaker initiated rhythm is known as an *escape rhythm*—a safety mechanism of the heart. If an escape rhythm is initiated in the AV junctional tissue, it is known as an *idiojunctional rhythm* or a *junctional escape rhythm*. This junctional pacemaker *usually* discharges an impulse 40–60 times per minute (though it may discharge slower or faster . . . ugh!).

You are no doubt thinking that the term *escape* is a peculiar name for a rhythm. Basically, the term implies that a lower, more distal pacemaker has *escaped* from the control of the sinus node. In other words, although lower tissues have the ability to serve as pacemakers, their inherent rates of impulse discharge are slower than the sinus node. Therefore, the faster sinus impulse takes control of the heart. In effect, the faster sinus impulse causes depolarization before lower, more distal pacemakers have the opportunity to generate pacemaking impulses! Only when the sinus pacemaker fails (or slows) will a lower pacemaker assume control of the rhythm.

Escape rhythms *always occur* as a *secondary phenomenon,* never as a primary disorder. In other words, an escape rhythm serves as a safety mechanism when higher order pacemakers are disrupted or fail.

This rhythm strip demonstrates an idiojunctional or junctional escape rhythm. One can expect to see a junctional escape rhythm *when the sinus pacemaker fails or is depressed.* If the patient has a sinus bradycardia (less than 60 beats per minute), his heart rate may be *slower* than the AV junctional pacemaker, which has the ability to initiate a rhythm at a rate of 40–60 beats per minute. In this case, the AV junctional pacemaker might become the dominant pacemaker because it has a faster rate. It is helpful to remember that the *AV node itself has no pacemaker fibers.* Only the lower portion of intranodal pathways and the bundle of His have pacemaker properties.

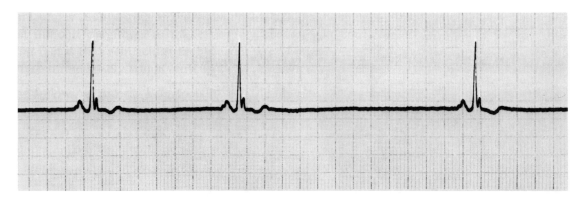

This rhythm strip demonstrates a sinus bradycardia slowing to a rate of approximately 23 beats per minute! In a *healthy* heart, one would expect a lower, more distal pacemaker to come through, taking control of the rhythm.

Before going further, let's explore a junctional escape rhythm in detail.

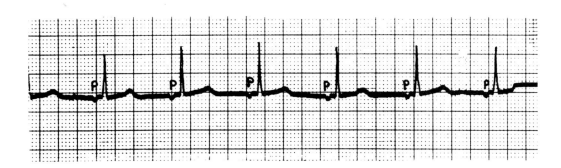

The first thing one notices is that the rhythm is *regular.* The heart rate *usually* falls between *40 and 60 beats* per minute. What are the atria doing? You will remember that P waves denote atrial depolarization. In a true junctional rhythm, the P wave (if visible) is usually inverted 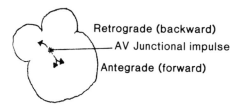 in leads II, III, and aVF. It may occur *before, during,* or *after* the QRS. Because of its location, the AV junctional impulse will be conducted both in an antegrade (forward) and a retrograde (backward) fashion.

Retrograde (backward)
— AV Junctional impulse
Antegrade (forward)

In other words, when the impulse originates in the AV junction, the impulse must travel upward across the atria to activate the atria, and downward across the ventricles to activate the ventricles. The impulse traveling down across the ventricles will be conducted in a normal fashion because the impulse travels the normal conduction pathway.

In other words, the QRS will be *"skinny"* (less than 0.12 seconds).

So, ventricular conduction occurs normally. To fully understand atrial activation, you must remember that the junctional impulse must travel in a backward or retrograde fashion.

This junctional impulse travels in the *opposite* direction of the SA impulse. Retrograde activation of the atria by the AV junctional impulse results in abnormal P waves, usually inverted 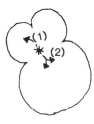 in leads II, III and aVF.

Now, we're going to do a bit of abstract thinking! The junctional impulse must travel both to the atria and to the ventricles. If the junctional impulse reaches the (1) atria before the impulse traveling downward reaches the (2) ventricles, a P wave will appear just before the QRS complex. The P wave occurring before the QRS tells the observer that atrial activation occurred before ventricular activation.

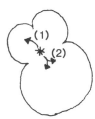
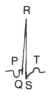

In addition, the P-R interval of the junctional beat will be of *short* duration, *less than* three small squares, or *less than 0.12 seconds*. Some authorities believe the P-R interval will be 0.10 seconds or less! No doubt you are wondering why the P-R interval is short! Since the AV junctional pacemaker is in close proximity to the atria, the impulse "travel time" is short. Therefore, the P-R interval is short!

We should point out that a P.A.C. may also have an inverted P wave occurring before the QRS if it is initiated low in the atria. However, when the ectopic impulse (P.A.C.) arises low in the atria, a sufficient time interval is required for the impulse to travel through the conduction system—in other words, it would have a normal (0.12–0.20) or prolonged P-R interval!

To review then, the above complex shows that the atria depolarize first (the P wave), followed by ventricular depolarization (the QRS). Notice that the P wave is inverted and the P-R interval is short.

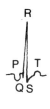

The following rhythm strip demonstrates a junctional escape rhythm with a rate of 55 per minute. Notice the inverted P wave and the short P-R before the QRS. The P wave coming before the QRS indicates that atrial depolarization precedes ventricular depolarization.

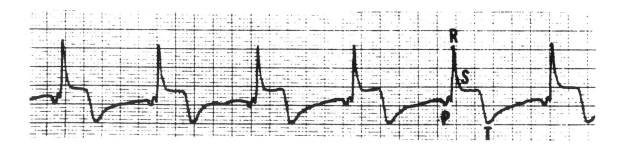

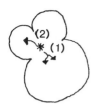

Now, let's suppose that the AV junctional pacemaker impulse reaches and activates the ventricles before it reaches and activates the atria.

The QRS represents ventricular depolarization. The P wave represents atrial depolarization. So when the ventricles depolarize before the atria, guess what we see?!

You're right. . . . the QRS coming before the P wave!

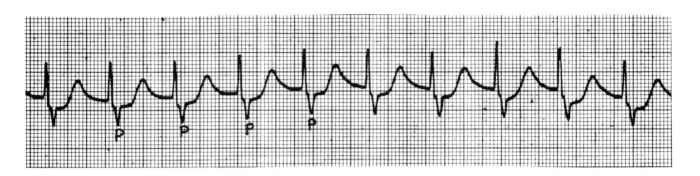

This is a junctional escape rhythm, rate 88 per minute. Since the rate of this escape rhythm is faster than the inherent AV junctional rate (40–60), one might elect to call it an accelerated junctional escape rhythm or an accelerated idiojunctional rhythm. *It is important to specify the rate of any rhythm!*

Looking at the above strip, we can now intellectually say this is a junctional escape rhythm with ventricular depolarization occurring before atrial depolarization (because the QRS comes before the P wave). If this is confusing to you, it simply means that you're in the same boat with everyone else! Usually escape rhythms occur regularly. You will notice that the rate is approximately 88 per minute, somewhat faster than a typical junctional rhythm. It is important to remember that even though a pacemaker has a common or inherent rate, the pacemaker is not limited to those rate parameters!

Now what do you think you would find if the junctional pacemaker impulse reached and activated the atria and ventricles at almost the same time?

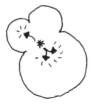

That's a tough one!

If the impulse traveling upward reaches the atria at the same time that the impulse traveling downward reaches the ventricles, the P wave will not be obvious. It is said to be "buried" or "hiding" in the QRS.

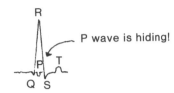

This "hiding" concept is a bit difficult to grasp, so let's get away from EKG's for a moment. Imagine that I'm in a shopping center, driving around in hopes of finding a parking space. I spy one, so I quickly drive toward it. However, I neglect to notice a big truck driving toward the empty space from the opposite direction!

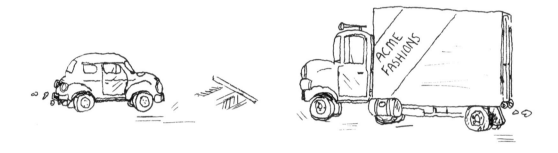

Later, when a rescue helicopter is viewing the accident scene, he only sees the truck!

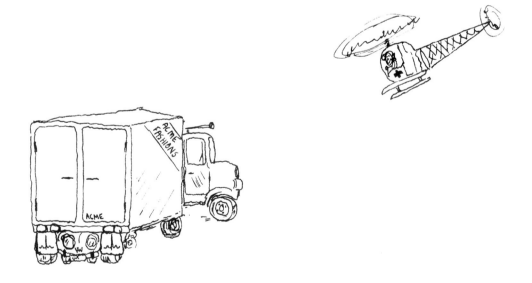

The VW is buried or hiding! But, we know it's there! It simply is not visible because the truck is so large.

The monitoring electrodes are like the helicopter! The monitoring electrodes view cardiac activity from above. When a P wave and a QRS occur close together, the monitoring electrodes only record a QRS because it's larger than the P wave.

Does that help?

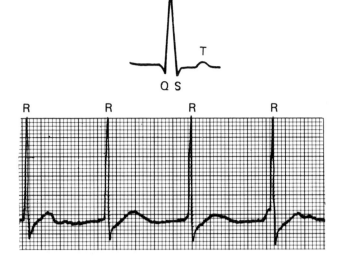

So when I see a monitor tracing like this one, I know it *cannot* be a sinus rhythm because there are no upright _⁀_ P waves occurring before the QRS complexes. But wait! There are no P waves anywhere! Yet, the QRS is of normal duration (less than 0.12 seconds), so I know the ventricles were activated in a normal fashion. Therefore, this must be a junctional rhythm with P waves "hiding" in the QRS complexes. That simply tells me that atrial and ventricular depolarization have occurred during the same period of time. ☺

Some of the more frequently encountered causes of junctional escape rhythms are digitalis toxicity, hypoxia, acute infections, vagal influence, and myocardial infarctions. A small artery nourishes the sinus node. In about 75% of the population, this small artery is supplied by the right coronary artery (RCA). It stands to reason that if the RCA is diseased or damaged, an interruption of the sinus mechanism may occur. This frequently results in a junctional escape rhythm (a lower, more distal pacemaker takes over).

If, for some reason, the SA node does not discharge (sinus arrest) or if the impulse is blocked within the sinus mechanism (sino-atrial block), an AV junctional pacemaker may take over the rhythm, as in this strip.

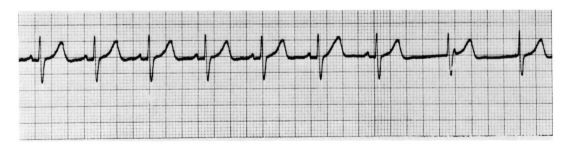

Following complex 7, the sinus mechanism is disrupted, allowing an AV junctional pacemaker to escape or take control of the rhythm.

Here is another example.

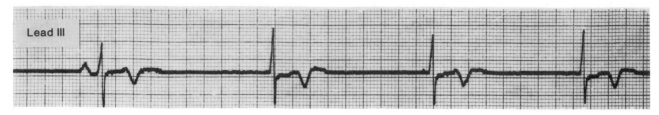

This rhythm strip demonstrates failure of the sinus pacemaker. A junctional escape pacemaker then assumes control of the rhythm. Notice that the rate of the junctional escape rhythm is approximately 33 beats per minute. There are no P waves visible either prior to or following the QRS. Thus, atrial and ventricular activation must be occurring at the same time!

To review then, any disruption or failure of the sinus pacemaker may result in an escape rhythm. To determine the origin of the escape rhythm, one must look closely at all of the wave forms. If the QRS is of normal duration (less than 0.12 seconds), we will soon learn that the rhythm cannot be initiated in the ventricles. The absence of normal, upright P waves in leads II, III, and aVF indicates that the rhythm is probably not of sinus or atrial origin. In other word, the rhythm is most likely of AV junctional origin. If a P wave is observed, it will occur prior to, or after the QRS, and will be inverted in leads II, III, and aVF. If the inverted P wave comes before the QRS, the P-R interval *must be less than* 0.12 seconds to qualify as a junctional rhythm.

Looking at this next strip, you can see that the QRS occurs before the P wave, so ventricular depolarization occurs before atrial depolarization. Easy, huh?

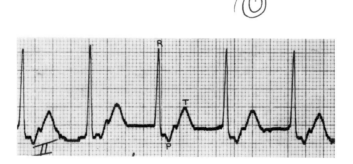

If you remember the section dealing with premature atrial contractions, you will recall that there is a pause following the P.A.C. which allows the sinus pacemaker to reset itself. With any premature beat followed by a pause, a junctional escape beat may occur before the sinus pacemaker can regain control. Do you know why that occurs?

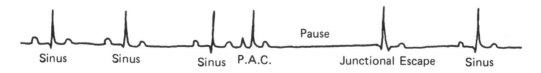

Well . . . the AV junction is behaving normally, conducting all the impulses sent down from the atria. Then all of a sudden, there is a pause—no impulse is arriving for the AV junctional tissue to conduct. The AV junction gets a little nervous wondering what's going on up there in the atria! Since the AV junction can fire from 40–60 times per minute, it slips in a junctional beat to ensure that the heart rate does not fall to an unhealthy rate. Had the sinus pacemaker failed to resume control, the AV junctional pacemaker could have maintained the heart rate at 40–60 beats per minute! Neat, huh?

The important point to remember is that escape beats or escape rhythms are *NEVER* a primary phenomenon. They always result *secondary* to another event or problem. Therefore, escape rhythms are never terminated. Rather, the aims of treatment are to support the escape pacemaker and to correct the primary disorder.

It is important to understand that a patient may experience a hemodynamic imbalance owing to both a slow rate and the loss of synchronized atrial activity (atrial kick). Therefore, it may be necessary to augment the heart rate using either atropine or a temporary transvenous pacemaker. (Atropine may promote an increase in the rate of AV junctional discharge, thereby increasing heart rate!)

Are you ready to try some practice? Hope so!

Practice Exercise 1

Look at this strip closely. I'll help!

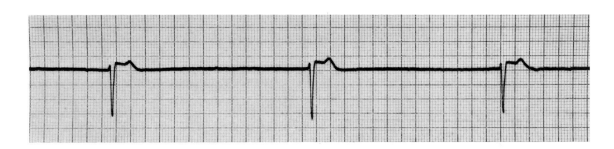

1. Is the rhythm regular? _____

The heart rate is approximately _____ beats per minute.

What are the atria doing? Are there P waves? _____

_____

_____

What are the ventricles doing? _____

_____

_____

The QRS measures _____ seconds.

Because the QRS's are of normal duration ("skinny"), I know that the impulses are conducted normally _____ .

This rhythm strip must be a _____ rhythm.

Since there are no obvious P waves, I must conclude that atrial and ventricular depolarization are

occurring _____ . Thus, the P waves are hidden in the QRS complexes.

Now, try this one on your own. Describe all that you see!

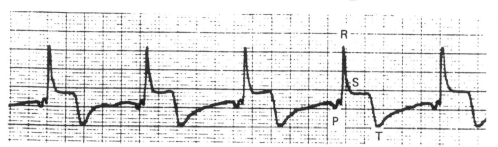

2. _____

_____

_____

_____

_____

_____

_____

For **Feedback 1,** refer to page 94.

Input 2: Premature Junctional Beats

Junctional beats can occur either early (premature) or late (escape). Escape junctional beats occur because of failure or disruption of a higher pacemaker. Premature beats, on the other hand, usually represent irritability of the involved tissue and they interrupt the normal or underlying rhythm.

A *premature junctional beat* (historically known as premature nodal beat) is an impulse that arises in an excitable or irritable site or focus in the AV junctional tissue. You will remember that the AV node itself has no pacemaking capability! The conduction of a premature junctional beat occurs in the same fashion as did a junctional escape beat—in other words, an inverted P wave may occur before, during, or after the QRS complex.

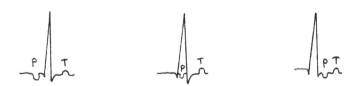

The location of the P wave has no significance other than to indicate the sequence of atrial activation.

An occasional premature junctional beat may be found in the healthy individual. However, recurrent premature junctional beats are usually associated with rheumatic heart disease or coronary artery disease. The significance of premature junctional beats is the significance of the underlying clinical problem.

Look at this rhythm strip.

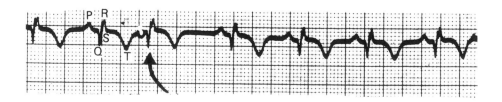

The first thing that catches the eye is an early or premature beat. Before diagnosing the premature beat, notice that the underlying rhythm is a sinus rhythm with a rate of approximately 80 beats per minute. It's always helpful to determine the basic or underlying rhythm and rate before analyzing abnormal beats.

So what about this abnormal beat? Is there a P wave? Yes, there is a P wave, but it's upsidedown or inverted. Ah-ha! Maybe this is a junctional beat! 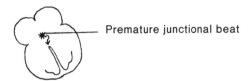 The P-R interval of the premature beat is a "hair" less than 3 small squares or 0.12 seconds. You will recall that to be qualified as a beat of junctional origin, *the P-R interval must be short*. The QRS of the premature beat appears similar to the QRS complexes in the normal underlying rhythm. This is to be expected since ventricular activation usually occurs in a normal fashion!

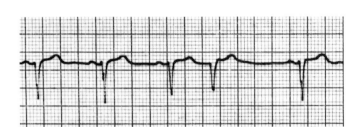

Premature junctional beat

Because the premature junctional impulse travels normally down the conduction pathway, ventricular depolarization is unaltered. Therefore, the QRS complexes are of normal duration.

Let's analyze this rhythm strip too (since we're already here 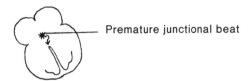).

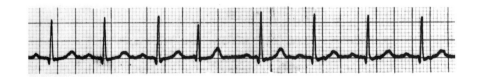

The underlying rhythm in the above strip is sinus rhythm, with a heart rate of approximately 75 beats per minute. If you have measured closely, you will notice that the QRS measures two small squares or 0.08 seconds. Beat 4 occurs prematurely. If you look closely at the premature beat, there is no obvious P wave, but the QRS is identical to the QRS complexes in the underlying rhythm. This must be a premature junctional beat! Because there is no obvious P wave in this premature junctional complex, we can assume that the atria and ventricles are depolarizing during the same period of time. In other words, the P wave is hiding in the QRS.

Our final example (see bottom of page 89) shows a premature junctional beat interrupting a borderline sinus tachycardia. You will notice that there is no evidence of a P wave either before or after the premature beat (beat #4). Thus, atrial and ventricular activation are occurring at the same time!

Usually premature junctional beats are merely observed and noted. If the patient becomes symptomatic, the premature junctional beats may be treated with digitalis or propranolol.

Practice Exercise 2

Let's try some practice.

Describe everything that you see!

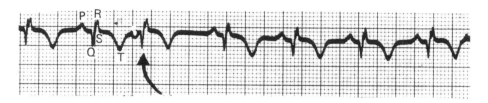

1. _____

_____

_____

_____

_____

2. _____

_____

_____

_____

_____

For **Feedback 2,** refer to page 95.

When three or more ectopic premature junctional beats occur in succession, it is termed *AV junctional tachycardia*. It may be paroxysmal in nature, or it may persist. Usually the heart rate ranges between 120–200 beats per minute. If P waves are visible, they will occur before or after the QRS complexes. The QRS is *usually* of normal duration (less than 0.12 seconds) since the impulse is conducted normally through the ventricular conduction system.

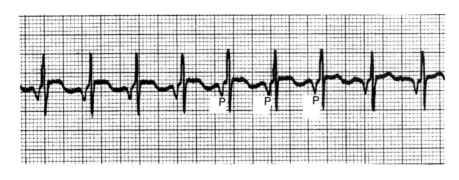

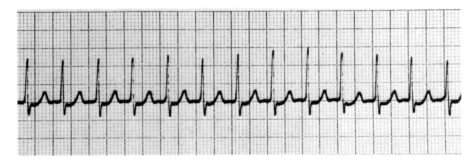

Above are two rhythm strips demonstrating AV junctional tachycardia. Notice, the rhythms are *regular* and rapid.

Strip 1 demonstrates a heart rate of approximately 125 per minute. An inverted P wave precedes each QRS complex. The P-R interval is short, measuring less than 0.12 seconds. In this example, atrial depolarization occurs prior to ventricular depolarization.

Strip 2 shows a regular rhythm with a rate of 150 per minute. There are no P waves before or after the QRS complexes, and the QRS duration is within normal limits. In this instance, the atria and the ventricles are depolarizing at the same time.

We won't dwell on the subject of AV junctional tachycardia for one *good* reason!

When the heart rate is rapid, it is usually *impossible* to determine whether a P wave is related to the preceding QRS complex or whether it is occurring before the QRS. In fact, it is often difficult to discriminate the various wave forms when the heart rate is rapid!

Look at this strip!

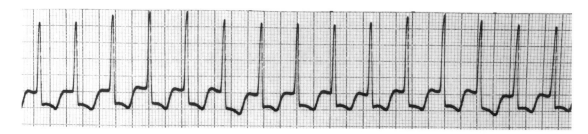

In this rhythm strip, the various wave forms are difficult to discriminate! I am uncertain if P waves are present. Because the duration of the QRS is within normal limits, I know this is either an atrial or a junctional tachycardia. Therefore, I am simply going to call this rhythm a supraventricular tachycardia with a heart rate of approximately 136 per minute. (I used the heart rate guide on page 39!)

Because it is sometimes impossible to tell atrial tachycardia from an AV junctional tachycardia, we "tag" the strip as a *supraventricular tachycardia*. That simply means that the heart rate is rapid, the QRS complexes are "skinny" (less than 0.12 seconds) and we're not going to stick our necks out by identifying *possible* P waves! Further, the term *supraventricular tachycardia* indicates that the initiating pacemaker is above the ventricles, somewhere in the atria or AV junction. Supraventricular tachycardia is one the *few* terms worth remembering!

In any event, the clinical significance of AV junctional tachycardia is similar to that of atrial tachycardia. The rapid heart rate reduces cardiac output because the volume of blood ejected with each contraction is decreased as a result of the shortened ventricular filling time . . . just like the flushing-toilet story on page 58.

However, it is important to note that the patient with junctional tachycardia will be compromised from two points of view: (1) the rapid ventricular rate, and (2) the loss of synchronized atrial activity (atrial kick).

The decrease in cardiac output can lead to left ventricular failure, and may precipitate chest pain due to the increased oxygen demand and consumption of the cardiac muscle.

The treatment for any rapid supraventricular rhythm (atrial tachycardia, junctional tachycardia) is similar. The object of treatment is to reduce the rapid ventricular rate and restore sinus rhythm. A combination of drugs . . . or synchronized cardioversion . . . is the initial treatment of choice.

Practice Exercise 3

Describe this rhythm strip in detail!

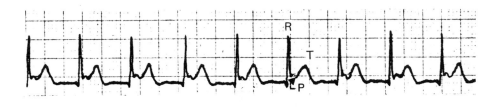

_____

_____

_____

_____

_____

_____

If you observe a rapid rhythm with narrow QRS complexes and are unable to distinguish P waves clearly, you can term the dysrhythmia a _____ .

For **Feedback 3,** refer to page 96.

Feedback 1

Pass GO and collect $200.00. You're doing a great job! 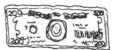 ← Color this green!

Strip 1

1. The rhythm is *slow* and regular.

The heart rate is approximately <u>21</u> beats per minute . . . 70 $\overline{)1500}$ with 21 above

I don't see any P waves anywhere!

The ventricular complexes are occurring regularly and they all appear uniform.

The QRS measures <u>0.08</u> seconds.

Because the QRS's are "skinny," I know that the impulses are conducted normally <u>across or through the ventricles</u>.

This rhythm is a <u>junctional escape</u> rhythm.

Since there are no obvious P waves, I must conclude that atrial and ventricular depolarization are occurring <u>in the same period of time</u>. Thus, the P wave is hidden in the QRS complex!

P.S. Treatment would consist of speeding up the heart rate!

Strip 2. . . . Hope your answers are <u>similar</u> to mine!

2. The rhythm is <u>regular</u>.

The heart rate is between <u>50–60</u> beats per minute.

An upside-down or <u>inverted P</u> wave preceded each QRS complex. All the inverted P waves appear uniform. The P-R interval is <u>short</u>, less than three small squares, or <u>less than 0.12 seconds</u>.

The QRS complexes are occurring <u>regularly</u>, and all are <u>uniform</u> in appearance.

The QRS measures slightly less than 3 small squares.

Because the QRS's are less than 3 small squares, I know that the impulses are conducted normally across or through the ventricles.

This is a <u>junctional escape rhythm</u>. The inverted P waves occurring <u>shortly</u> before each QRS complex indicate that the junctional pacemaker activates the atria before reaching and activating the ventricles.

Just for review, here are the EKG properties of a junctional escape rhythm.

PROPERTIES OF AN IDIOJUNCTIONAL RHYTHM

- It is a regular rhythm.
- The pacemaker impulse formation is usually slower than the sinus node (40–60 beats per minute).
- It occurs secondary to failure or disruption of the sinus pacemaker.
- P waves are usually inverted or upside down in leads II, III, and aVF.
- P waves may occur before, during, or after the QRS.
- The QRS complexes occur regularly, are uniform in appearance, and normally measure less than 0.12 seconds.

EXTRA! EXTRA! BONUS ON NEXT PAGE!

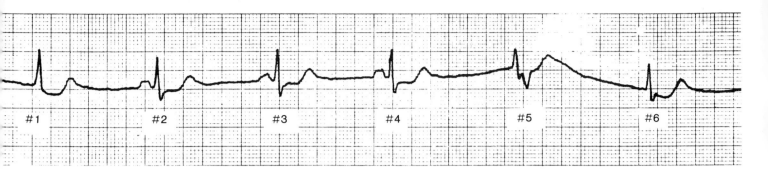

I just saw this patient today and she wasn't feeling well at all! I thought you might enjoy looking at her monitor tracing with me.

Beats 2, 3, and 4 tell me that her underlying heart rhythm is a sinus bradycardia with a heart rate of less than 50 beats per minute. Apparently, her sinus node was feeling a bit "under the weather," so it periodically failed to fire an impulse. Consequently, the good ol' AV junction came through to save the day!

Beat 1 demonstrates a junctional escape beat that has no P wave. So, in this instance, the atria and ventricles were depolarizing in the same period of time. (The P wave is hiding in the QRS.) Beats 2, 3, and 4 demonstrate the underlying sinus bradycardia. Beat 5 shows a junctional escape beat with a retrograde P wave (the P wave follows the QRS). Thus, in this instance, the ventricles have depolarized before atrial depolarization occurs. The last beat (6) is similar to beat 1.

This lady has a pacemaker wandering from the AV junction to the sinus node and back to the AV junction!

Feedback 2

Nice work!

1. The underlying rhythm is a sinus rhythm, with a rate of approximately 80 per minute. Beat 3 is premature, interrupting the underlying regular rhythm. An inverted P wave occurs before the premature beat and the P-R interval is slightly less than 0.12 seconds. The QRS of the premature beat is within normal limits. This must be a premature junctional beat interrupting a sinus rhythm! Because the premature P wave occurs before the QRS, I know that atrial depolarization preceded ventricular depolarization.

2. The underlying rhythm is a sinus rhythm with a heart rate of approximately 75 beats per minute. The QRS complexes measure 0.08 seconds. Beat 4 is premature, interrupting the underlying regular rhythm. The premature beat does not have a P wave. The QRS of the premature beat appears like the QRS complexes in the sinus rhythm. This is a premature junctional beat with atrial and ventricular depolarization occurring during the same period of time (the P wave is hiding in the QRS!).

Note: See the top of page 96 for a quick review of premature junctional beats.

Just for review, a premature junctional beat has the following properties:

PROPERTIES OF A PREMATURE JUNCTIONAL BEAT

- The premature beat interrupts the underlying rhythm.
- An inverted P wave may occur before, during, or after the QRS complex of the premature beat.
- The QRS of the premature beat is usually similar to the QRS complexes in the underlying rhythm.

Feedback 3

How are you doing? Fine, I hope!

This is a regular rhythm with a heart rate of approximately 115 beats per minute. The QRS complexes appear uniform and measure approximately 0.08 seconds. Inverted P waves follow each QRS complex, indicating that ventricular depolarization occurs prior to atrial depolarization. This is an AV junctional tachycardia!

If you observe a rapid rhythm with narrow QRS complexes (less than 0.12 seconds) and are unable to clearly distinguish P waves, you can term the dysrhythmia a <u>supraventricular tachycardia</u>.

To review then, an AV junctional tachycardia is a regular rhythm with a rapid rate. The P waves may occur prior to, during, or after the QRS complexes. The QRS complexes appear uniform and usually measure less than 0.12 seconds.

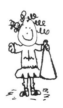

Yeah Team!
We have completed Section III

NOTES

NOTES

Section IV
Ventricular Ectopic and Escape Rhythms

OBJECTIVES

When you have completed Section V, you will be able to describe or identify

1. premature ventricular contractions (P.V.C.'s)
2. fusion beats
3. ventricular tachycardia
4. ventricular flutter
5. ventricular fibrillation
6. ventricular escape rhythm

NOW, BACK TO THE ART OF DYSRHYTHMIA INTERPRETATION!

This section addresses ventricular ectopic and ventricular escape rhythms. Sounds ominous, doesn't it? Actually, ventricular abnormalities are easy, compared to what has been dealt with previously!

Probably everyone is familiar with ventricular extrasystoles or premature ventricular contractions—good ol' P.V.C.'s! Ventricular excitation originates below the bifurcation of the bundle of His, outside the normal rhythm.

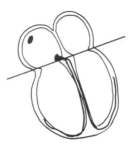

P.V.C.'s represent abnormal electrical stimulation arising from an excitable focus or site, somewhere in either ventricle. There is *no* failure of the normal rhythm, merely additional beats arising from an irritable focus.

As the name *premature ventricular contraction* implies, P.V.C.'s interrupt the normal rhythmic cycle. In addition, they may be coupled or related to the preceding sinus beats. You'll remember (from page 54) that a *coupling interval* is the distance between the premature beat and the preceding sinus beat. Remember?

Here is a rather dramatic illustration of P.V.C.'s interrupting a normal rhythm. Notice that the coupling interval is constant. One can expect the coupling interval to be constant when the P.V.C.'s are uniform in appearance, indicating that the ventricular stimulus arises from a single focus.

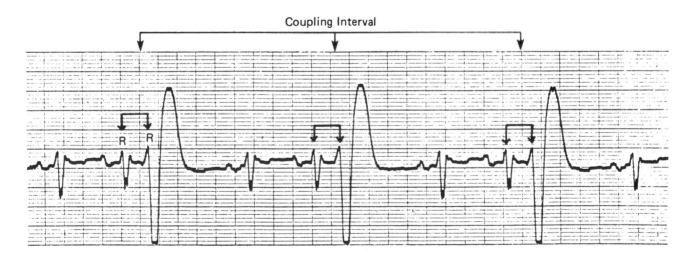

Coupling Interval

Most usually, P.V.C.'s are extremely obvious owing to their *bizarre* appearance. One needs to know very little about interpreting EKG's to recognize the abnormality!

To confirm that these abnormal beats are indeed P.V.C.'s, *they must interrupt the underlying rhythm, have a wide QRS (0.12 seconds or greater) and have no P wave prior to the wide QRS.*

Atrial depolarization is recorded on the monitor as a P wave ⌐‿⌐ ; ventricular depolarization is recorded as the QRS complex.

Since a premature ventricular impulse originates in the ventricles outside the normal conduction pathway, ventricular depolarization will occur in a backward or retrograde fashion. This abnormal activation of the ventricles causes the QRS to be wide and bizarre. Further, since the P.V.C. originates in the ventricles, there will be no P wave prior to the QRS. So where are the P waves??? . . . or when do the atria depolarize? *One of two things may happen:*

1. A sinus impulse may fire while the ventricular ectopic impulse is moving across the ventricles. If this happens, the P wave may be "buried" in the QRS complex. In this case, the atria and the ventricles are stimulated by two separate impulses—the atria by the SA impulse, and the ventricles by the ectopic impulse (the P.V.C.). On the EKG strip, no P wave is obvious in the abnormal heart cycle.

   When myocardial activation occurs in this manner, there is very little disruption of the underlying rhythm. In other words, in a regular rhythm, the P.V.C. falls almost where you would expect the next sinus impulse to occur.

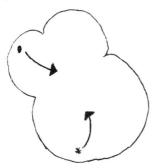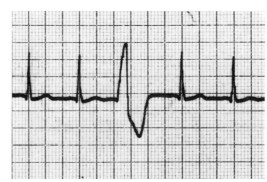

Note that there is no P wave before or after the QRS. Rather, the P wave is buried in the QRS. When the P wave is "buried," there is no pause following the P.V.C.

2. The ectopic ventricular impulse may occur early in the cycle and be conducted backward (retrograde) through the AV junctional tissue across the atria before the sinus impulse fires. In this case, ventricular depolarization occurs prior to atrial depolarization. So, one would see a wide, bizarre QRS complex followed by a P wave, like this.

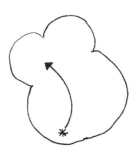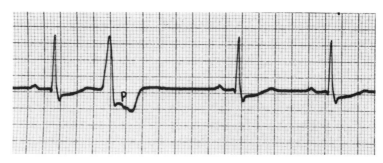

You will also notice that when this retrograde conduction occurs, a long pause follows the premature beat. This pause is called a *compensatory pause,* and measures the distance of two normal R-R intervals. This pause allows the sinus pacemaker to reset the rhythm.

If this is difficult to understand, just remember that a P wave will *never* occur before the premature ventricular beat. A P wave may occur during or after the wide, bizarre QRS complex. You're probably wondering why I did not say that to begin with . . . right? **Right!**

The important point to remember is that *all* P.V.C.'s indicate ventricular irritability. The presence or absence of a P wave indicates the sequence of atrial activation.

Now that you have an understanding of the P waves, we need to tackle the subject of the "fat" QRS. *All premature ventricular contractions will have a QRS that measures 0.12 seconds or greater.* Ventricular ectopic impulses move through the myocardial tissue from the point of origin. Since these ectopic impulses originate outside the normal rhythm, they do not travel down the specialized conducting tissue of the ventricles; rather, they travel backward. This abnormal path of conduction is *slow,* taking a longer period of time than a normally conducted beat.

You'll remember that moving horizontally across the EKG paper denotes time.

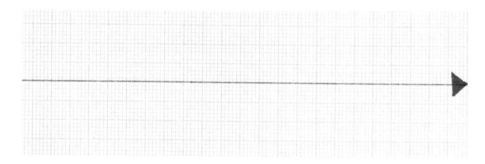

So, if the abnormal beat takes longer to depolarize the ventricles, the QRS will be wider—0.12 seconds or greater. As a matter of fact, Phibbs (*The Cardiac Arrhythmias,* C. V. Mosby, 1973, p. 25) notes that the speed of impulse movement through the myocardium varies from 0.5 to 1.0 meters per second, while the specialized conduction pathways conduct much faster, from 1.0 to 4.0 meters per second!

Easy, huh?

To review then, a premature ventricular contraction (P.V.C.) presents as a wide, bizarre QRS that interrupts the underlying rhythm. A P wave will never occur before this abnormal QRS, but may occur during or following the QRS.

P.V.C.'s can occur in normal hearts, especially during periods of fatigue or emotional distress. Likewise, persons who drink caffeine products or smoke may have P.V.C.'s. (If you have ever experienced your heart "skip a beat," you may have experienced at P.V.C.!) When listening to a heart beat or feeling the pulse, you *may* hear or feel a pause following an early beat.

Persons taking such drugs as quinidine, pronestyl, digitalis, or epinephrine, and persons with low serum potassium levels may experience P.V.C.'s. Hypoxia may also result in ectopic ventricular activity. Manipulating the heart tissue itself (open heart surgery) or catheters situated within the heart chambers (pacemaker catheters, cardiac catheterizations, Swan-Ganz catheters) may predispose to ectopic ventricular activity.

In healthy persons, P.V.C.'s are relatively harmless. However, in patients with existing heart disease and especially myocardial infarction, *P.V.C.'s may WARN OF VENTRICULAR TACHYCARDIA OR VENTRICULAR FIBRILLATION.* Ischemic tissue is thought to release a *substance* which is capable of increasing the automaticity of the Purkinje fibers. Thus, patients with ischemic disorders are prone to P.V.C.'s.

Lidocaine administered intravenously is the treatment of choice for ectopic ventricular activity. A bolus of lidocaine, usually 100 mg. I.V. push, is given initially to establish a blood level, followed by a continuous lidocaine infusion of 1–4 mg. per minute.

Usually, lidocaine therapy is instituted when any of the following scenarios are present:

[A.] P.V.C.'s occurring with increasing frequency . . . (Frequent P.V.C.'s suggest increasing ventricular irritability and serve to decrease cardiac output.)

[B.] P.V.C.'s occurring in rhythmic patterns, e.g., bigeminy P.V.C's . . . every other beat is a P.V.C.; trigeminy P.V.C.'s . . . every third beat is a P.V.C.; quadrigeminy P.V.C.'s . . . every fourth beat is a P.V.C., etc.

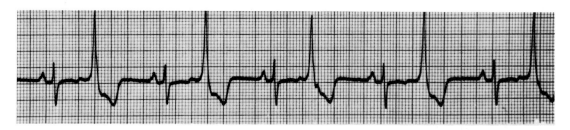

Ventricular bigeminy . . . or bigeminy P.V.C.'s. Notice that all the P.V.C.'s appear uniform or identical (unifocal).

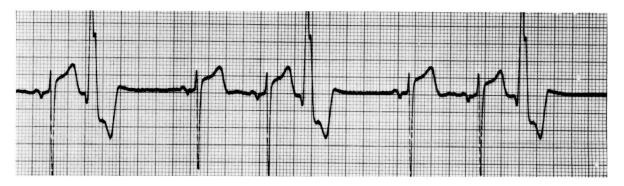

Ventricular trigeminy . . . or trigeminy P.V.C.'s.

[C.] P.V.C's falling close to the T wave of the preceding beat.

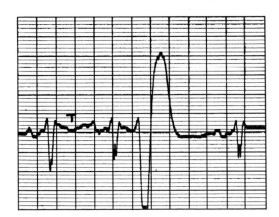

A P.V.C. falling on or near the T wave of the preceding beat is known as the *"R on T" phenomenon.* In the following strip you will notice that the T wave is inverted (upside down). That is significant too, as you will see in a later section. You will remember from Section IV, that the T wave is *vulnerable* to any electrical stimulation, particularly in the ischemic heart. A P.V.C. falling on a vulnerable T wave may precipitate ventricular tachycardia or ventricular fibrillation.

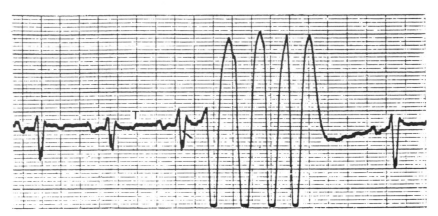

A P.V.C. falling on a vulnerable T wave produces a run of ventricular tachycardia!

(We'll discuss this later in more detail.)

D. P.V.C.'s originating from *more* than one irritable site or focus.

In other words, P.V.C.'s are different in appearance. Commonly, this is referred to as *MULTIFOCAL* or *MULTIDIRECTIONAL P.V.C.'s.*

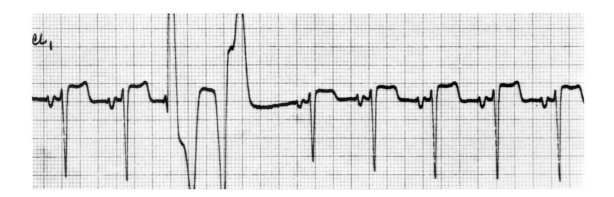

Sometimes this business of *unifocal* and *multifocal* or *multidirectional* P.V.C.'s is a bit confusing. So, to clarify the subject, I've borrowed an explanation from the Obstetrics Department!

If you can think of the ventricles as being a mama, you're all set!

Mama Ventricle has a rather unique medical history, as she has given birth to **many, many** babies, including 42 sets of twins . . . **busy lady!**

When her twins developed from separately fertilized eggs, they looked uniquely different from each other—*MULTIFOCAL.*

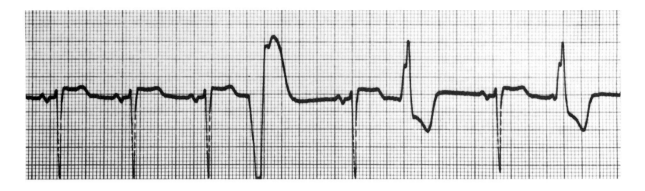

Multifocal P.V.C.'s originate from various irritable sites or foci, and appear uniquely different from each other!

When, however, her twins developed from a single fertilized egg, they appeared identical or *UNI-FOCAL.*

Unifocal P.V.C.'s originate from the same irritable site or focus and are basically identical in appearance.

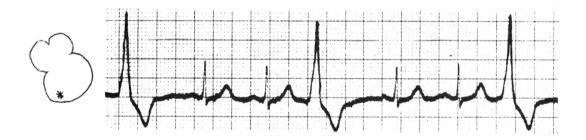

. . . Yes, I know, these analogies are a bit far-fetched . . . but, I BET YOU REMEMBER THEM!

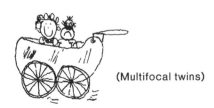

(Multifocal twins)

E. Two P.V.C.'s occurring together, referred to as *paired P.V.C.'s,* or a *couplet* of P.V.C.'s.

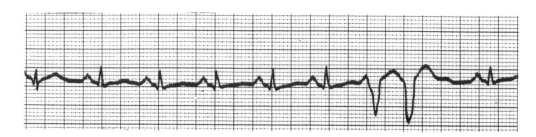

In this instance, an ectopic focus in the ventricles has discharged two impulses in rapid succession. This clues us that the ventricular ectopic site is *extremely* irritable. (If it continues to initiate rapid impulses, the ectopic pacemaker will assume control of the heart beat!!)

To review then, the following situations or patterns are indications for lidocaine therapy.
A. P.V.C.'s increasing in frequency
B. P.V.C.'s occurring in rhythmic patterns, e.g. bigeminy, trigeminy, etc.
C. P.V.C.'s falling close to the vulnerable T wave
D. multifocal P.V.C.'s
E. paired P.V.C.'s

Many physicians treat the myocardial infarct patient prophalactically with lidocaine—before any warning P.V.C.'s are noted! British research reported by Valentine, Frew, et al. (*N.E.J.M.,* Vol. 291, pp. 1324–1331) indicated that primary ventricular fibrillation did *not* occur in their experimental group of *acute myocardial infarct* (A.M.I.) patients treated with prophylactic lidocaine. Further it was their conclusion that warning dysrhythmias (P.V.C.'s) are not helpful in the decision whether or not antiarrhythmic (lidocaine) therapy should be instituted in the A.M.I. patient, since ventricular fibrillation may occur without warning. In other words, the A.M.I. patient may not have P.V.C.'s that forewarn of more lethal dysrhythmias! Thus, the patient with confirmed or suspected acute myocardial infarction is usually treated prophalactically with lidocaine.

When P.V.C.'s occur, they should be thought of as a **warning signal** until determined otherwise. They warn the observer that life threatening ventricular dysrhythmias *may* be imminent.

A physician should *always* be made aware that his or her patient is experiencing P.V.C.'s—the number per minute, their appearance (unifocal or multifocal), and their location in the cardiac cycle (i.e., falling near the vulnerable T wave). Most importantly, evaluate the patient's clinical picture!

Before leaving the subject of premature ventricular contractions, we should mention "interpolated" ventricular extrasystoles or interpolated P.V.C.'s. When a P.V.C. occurs between two normally conducted sinus beats, and the rhythm of those sinus beats is not disrupted, the P.V.C. is said to be *interpolated.* In other words, the P.V.C. is *sandwiched* between two normal beats!

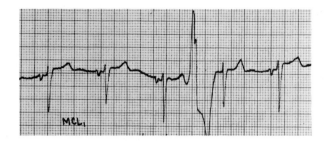

Interpolation results when the retrograde (backward) conduction of the P.V.C. is blocked from reaching and activating the atria by refractory tissue above the ventricles.

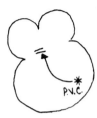

Commonly, the sinus beat following the interpolated P.V.C. will have a *prolonged* P-R interval owing to refractoriness of the AV node. The AV node has not fully recovered from the premature ventricular stimulation . . . thus, conduction takes longer! Interpolated P.V.C.'s are only observed in slow rhythms.

Interpolated P.V.C.'s have the same significance as other P.V.C.'s. I thought you might find them interesting!

IMPORTANT NOTE

Excess digitalis will frequently result in ectopic ventricular activity. In this instance, lidocaine *may* have little or no effect. Digitalis should be withheld. Dilantin therapy may be initiated to control digitalis-induced ventricular ectopic activity. Dilantin depresses ventricular automaticity and abolishes reentry arrhythmias by increasing the speed or velocity of conduction!

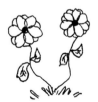

(Unifocal flowers)

Practice Exercise 1

Let's try some practice!

1. Describe this rhythm strip in detail.

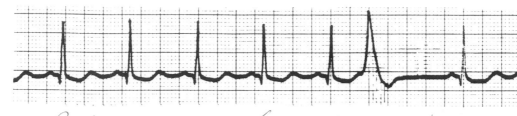

Reg, Rate approx 80 Sinus beats then a
pvc comes in early — wide QRS, Ø pwave

2. How would you describe the abnormality in this rhythm strip?

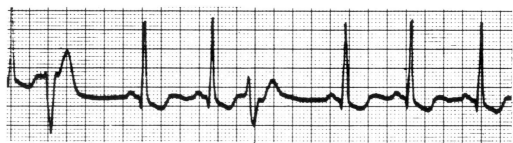

NS — multifocal pvcs

3. In this rhythm strip _____ is a premature ventricular contraction. This is known as _____ *SR c̄ unifocal pvcs bijeminal* _____

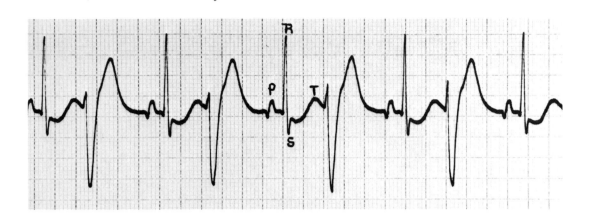

For **Feedback 1,** refer to page 125.

For **Feedback 1,** refer to page 125.

Input 2: Fusion (Dressler) Beats

To còmplicate life a bit further, we need to explore *fusion or Dressler beats*. So what's a fusion beat??

In normal conduction, the ventricles are activated by a sinus impulse traveling down the conduction system.

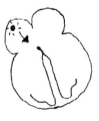
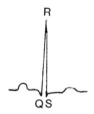

When a premature ventricular contraction (P.V.C) occurs, it initiates myocardial depolarization in a backward or retrograde fashion.

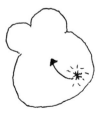
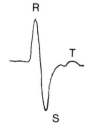

109

If a sinus impulse is initiated at the same time an ectopic focus in the ventricles initiates an impulse, ventricular depolarization (the QRS) will be produced by a double stimulation. That sounds confusing, so let's try an example. Let's say that the SA node initiates an impulse which activates the atria (producing a P wave), and that impulse travels ¼ of the way across the ventricles, beginning ventricular depolarization.

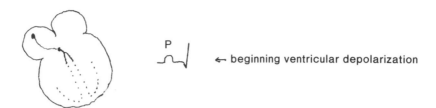

← beginning ventricular depolarization

At the same time, a ventricular ectopic focus initiates an impulse (P.V.C.) causing retrograde or backward depolarization of the lower portion of the ventricles.

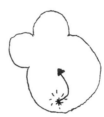

These two impulses, one traveling antegrade (forward) and one traveling retrograde (backward), collide somewhere in the ventricles.

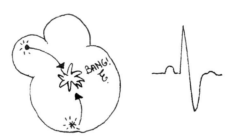

Thus, ventricular depolarization (the QRS) has been initiated by a double stimulation!

So what will the QRS look like? The QRS will resemble both the normal QRS and the wide, bizarre P.V.C. This "fused" QRS will be wider than the normal QRS, but less wide than a P.V.C.

Woops! We forgot something! What about a P wave? Will the fusion beat have a P wave? Of course! . . . because the SA impulse traveled through the atria (initiating atrial depolarization), through the AV junction into the ventricles before colliding with the premature ventricular impulse. So, the fusion beat will have a P wave, and that P wave will be equidistant from other P waves . . . in other words, the P-P interval will remain constant. Because of the double ventricular stimulation, the P-R interval, if visible, is abnormally short . . . the sinus impulse travels only part way down the conduction system!

Let's examine this strip.

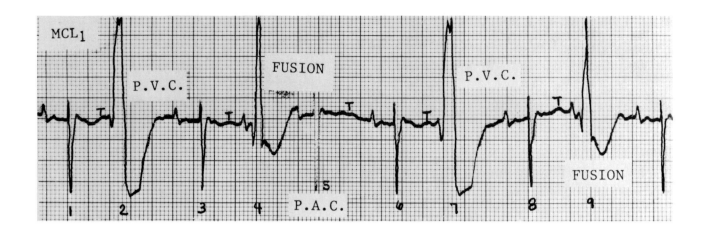

The underlying rhythm is sinus rhythm, though it is difficult to tell! The rhythm is interrupted by frequent P.V.C.'s and an occasional P.A.C. Beats 2 and 7 are P.V.C.'s—they are wide and bizarre and have no preceding P waves. *But what about* beats 4 and 9? They resemble the P.V.C.'s, except that they are not as wide. And, there are P waves preceding the QRS's! The P waves occur right on time! Beats 4 and 9 represent fusion beats *(collision beats)!*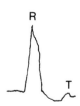

I almost forgot to tell you, fusion beats are also known as *Dressler* beats.

In review then, to identify a fusion beat:

A. There must be a supraventricular pacemaker that conducts normally, producing normal QRS complexes.

B. There must be an ectopic ventricular focus, producing wide, bizarre QRS complexes.

Then . . .

. . . if a beat with an abnormally short P-R interval and a QRS complex somewhere in between the shape of the normal and the ventricular ectopic QRS is seen, it must be a fusion beat!

Lidocaine therapy will not only abolish the P.V.C.'s, but will also abolish the fusion beats. Remember, a fusion beat is, in part, a P.V.C.!

111

Practice Exercise 2

STEP RIGHT UP AND TRY YOUR LUCK!

Look at this strip. Then label all the beats!

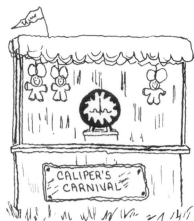

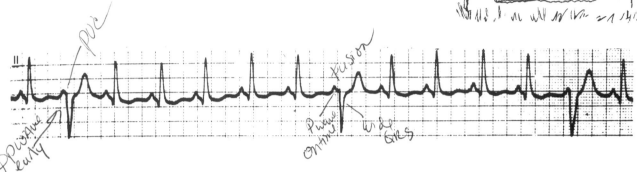

A fusion beat is _____

_____

_____

_____

_____

_____

_____

_____

_____

For **Feedback 2,** refer to page 125.

Input 3: Ventricular Tachycardia

Now, for some excitement . . . *Ventricular Tachycardia*!

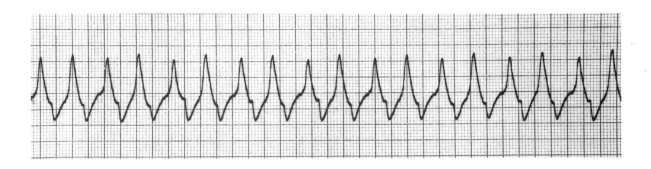

Ventricular tachycardia is *most* always associated with organic heart disease. It is probably one of the most difficult diagnoses to make, largely because one must make an instantaneous decision. The *important* fact is that ventricular tachycardia is a *LIFE-THREATENING* dysrhythmia! Treatment *must* be initiated immediately when ventricular tachycardia is suspected.

The following criteria *help* to establish the diagnosis of ventricular tachycardia.

1. The rate is usually rapid, between 140–200 beats per minute.
2. The P waves are usually buried in the QRS complexes making them obscure.
3. The QRS complexes are wide and bizarre.
4. The ventricular rhythm is *basically* regular.

IMPORTANT NOTICE

Because virtually every criteria for ventricular tachycardia can be argued, ONE MUST INITIATE TREATMENT AND *THEN* ARGUE SPECIFIC POINTS.

In ventricular tachycardia, the ventricles may be stimulated by an ectopic ventricular pacemaker firing repeatedly. Or, more likely, ventricular tachycardia is initiated by a single P.V.C. The repetitive ventricular stimulation is the result of a reentry mechanism within the ventricular myocardium.

To truly differentiate between ventricular and supraventricular activity, one must recognize atrial activity and its relationship to the QRS complexes. In ventricular tachycardia, the P waves (*if visible*) bear *no* relationship to the QRS's.

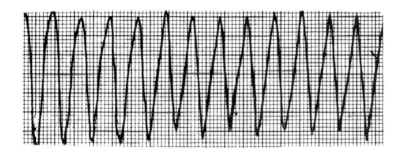

That's a difficult concept to grasp, so let's simplify it a bit! Let's say that the good ol' sinus pacemaker is firing along at a rate of 60. But, because an ectopic ventricular pacemaker is discharging an impulse at 180 times per minute, it takes control of the heart beat. (*The fastest pacemaker controls heart beat.*)

When the sinus impulses occur, they find the ventricular tissue refractory (or unable to respond) to further stimulation.

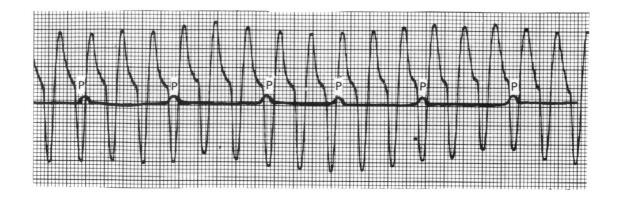

So, the P waves, *if visible,* bear no relationship to the QRS's. Usually, P waves are not visible—they're hiding within the QRS complexes!

Schamroth (*The Disorders of Cardiac Rhythm,* 1971) says the *best* evidence to support a ventricular tachycardia is the presence of a fusion beat during a tachycardia with bizarre QRS complexes. To refresh your memory, here is what a fusion beat looks like.

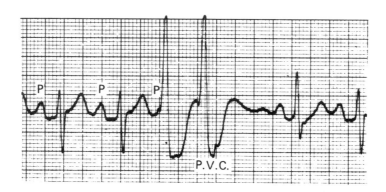

This strip demonstrates two sinus beats followed by a fusion beat and a P.V.C. The P wave of the fusion beat occurs on time . . . it does not occur early or late. The QRS of the fusion beat is wider than the normal QRS, but less wide than the P.V.C. Remember, a fusion beat is the result of a normal beat and a P.V.C. colliding!

You'll remember that a fusion beat produces the QRS by double stimulation—one impulse originating in the atria, and one from an ectopic site or focus in the ventricles. A "run" of ventricular tachycardia may begin or end with a fusion beat, or a fusion beat may be seen in the tachycardia itself.

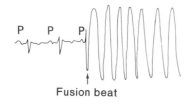

Fusion beat

Ventricular tachycardia beginning with a fusion beat.

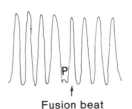

Fusion beat

Ventricular tachycardia with evidence of a fusion beat.

Why does a fusion beat occur in the middle of ventricular tachycardia? Remember the P waves that are firing along at a slower rate, bearing no relationship to the QRS's? Well, a P wave happens to find the ventricular tissue polarized, so it initiates depolarization. But *bang*! Another ectopic impulse is fired. Thus, the two impulses collide, producing a fusion beat.

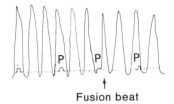

A fusion beat is produced by a dual stimulation of the ventricles (sinus beat + P.V.C.). A P wave will be obvious, and the QRS of the fusion beat will not be as wide as the QRS of the ventricular beats. The P-R interval of the fusion beat will be abnormally short.

Fusion beat

Schamroth (*The Disorders of Cardiac Rhythm*, 1971) also indicates that a capture beat is *good* evidence to support a ventricular tachycardia. So, what is a *CAPTURE BEAT*?

A capture beat is a fusion beat's Big Brother!

In essence, a capture beat is a normally conducted beat (a sinus beat) that manages to slip through during a ventricular tachycardia. One of those P waves firing along at a slower rate, bearing no relationship to the QRS's, finds the tissue polarized. So it *initiates and completes* normal conduction before the next abnormal ectopic ventricular beat occurs!

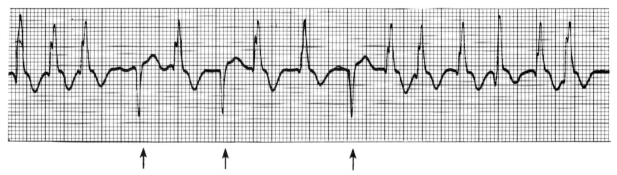

Capture Beats (three normally conducted beats occurring during ventricular tachycardia). Because the capture beats (sinus beats) are conducted normally down the conduction pathway, they are directed opposite to the P.V.C.'s (which are traveling backwards) and almost always have a visible P wave.

Because the capture beat conducts normally (in an antegrade fashion), the QRS has an entirely different contour. The capture beat depolarizes the ventricles in an orderly, antegrade fashion. *A fusion beat is an incomplete capture beat!*

One must remember that ventricular tachycardia is a *LIFE-THREATENING* dysrhythmia. It may rapidly progress to ventricular fibrillation; thus, treatment must be instituted *immediately.* Lidocaine, administered intravenously, is the drug of choice. If it is ineffective, *SYNCHRONIZED CARDIOVERSION* should be performed . . . but, we will get to that in Section VII.

The patient with ventricular tachycardia may be alert, anxious, short of breath, and have a low blood pressure—or, he may be essentially unresponsive with no attainable blood pressure. When the patient is nonresponsive, direct defibrillation is applied. There is *no* time to waste! This is a "code arrest" situation.

Ventricular tachycardia may be sustained or paroxysmal in nature. It may suddenly appear and disappear without treatment. *Three or more P.V.C.'s occurring together are considered ventricular tachycardia.*

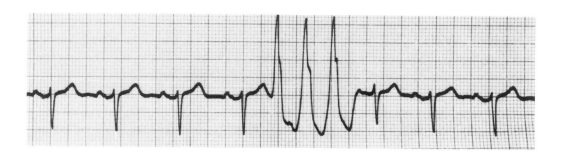

A P.V.C. falling on a vulnerable T wave may initiate a run of ventricular tachycardia. See for yourself!

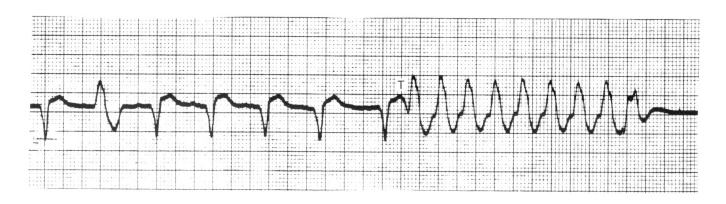

Though in the above examples, the ventricular tachycardia converted spontaneously, lidocaine treatment should have been initiated *immediately* and the physician notified!

Practice Exercise 3

Are you ready for some practice? Good!

1. Describe all that you see in this rhythm strip. What are the atria doing? What are the ventricles doing? What is the probable treatment?

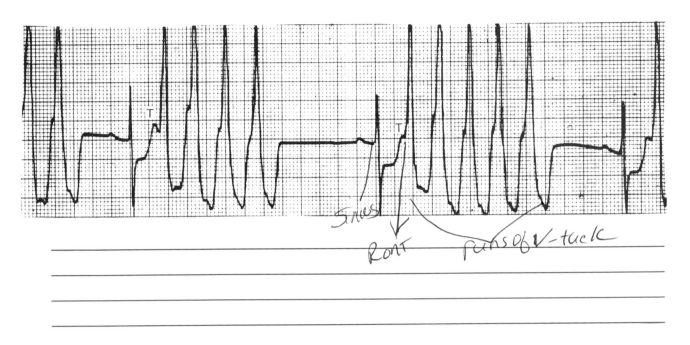

Sinus
Ront
runs of V-tach

_____

_____

_____

_____

_____

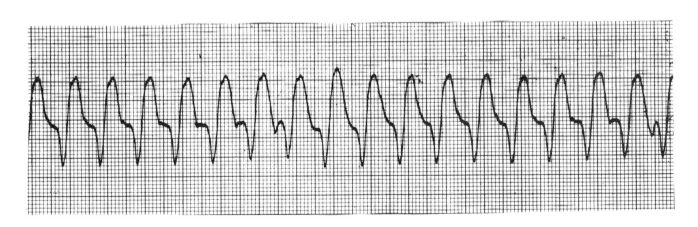

2. This strip demonstrates ___V-tach_____ with a heart rate of __150____ beats per minute.

For **Feedback 3**, refer to page 126.

Input 4: Ventricular Flutter

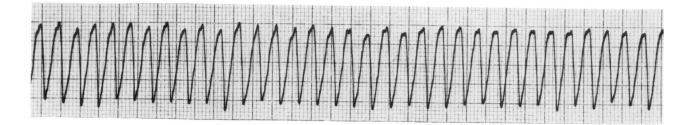

Ventricular flutter is most usually a transition rhythm from ventricular tachycardia to ventricular fibrillation. The rate of ventricular flutter is greater than 200 beats per minute. Owing to this rapid rate, cardiac output is minimal. Ventricular flutter represents a medical emergency and is an indication for defibrillation. The patient usually loses consciousness with the appearance of ventricular flutter.

Since ventricular flutter is a *transition* rhythm, we are going to make a *transition* to Input 5! There is no practice exercise associated with this dysrhythmia!

Input 5: Ventricular Fibrillation

That brings us to the lethal subject of *VENTRICULAR FIBRILLATION.*
Ventricular fibrillation is chaotic, uncoordinated ventricular depolarization.

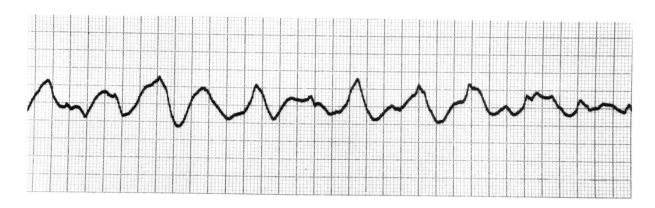

In ventricular fibrillation, there is *total irregularity* of electrical activity. There is usually constant variation in the amplitude. NO PQRST can be seen, and the baseline appears to wander.

Since there is *no* coordinated ventricular electrical activity, there is *no significant muscle contraction.* If one were to directly view the fibrillating heart, it would appear as a "bag of worms." Because the pumping action of the heart is lost, death occurs within minutes.

Usually, ventricular fibrillation does not just appear. Characteristically, myocardial irritability will first be evident—such as P.V.C.'s. However, it has been demonstrated that ventricular fibrillation may occur spontaneously when associated with acute myocardial infarction. In most instances, ventricular fibrillation is a *terminal event,* and is associated with ischemic heart disease. It may, however, be induced by quinidine or digitalis toxicity—particularly if digitalis intoxication is associated with hypokalemia. Ventricular fibrillation may also occur with *severe hypothermia*—when the body temperature approaches 28° centigrade. Further, electrical shock may induce ventricular fibrillation.

118

THE ONLY TREATMENT FOR VENTRICULAR FIBRILLATION IS ELECTRICAL DE-FIBRILLATION OR NONSYNCHRONIZED PRECORDIAL SHOCK. CPR SHOULD BE IN-STITUTED IMMEDIATELY. (Defibrillation will be discussed in Section VII, page 191.)

Commonly, one can anticipate successful defibrillation when the ventricular fibrillation occurs in a patient without heart failure or extensive myocardial damage and when the precordial shock is delivered within the first two minutes of the dysrhythmia.

* Precordial Shock

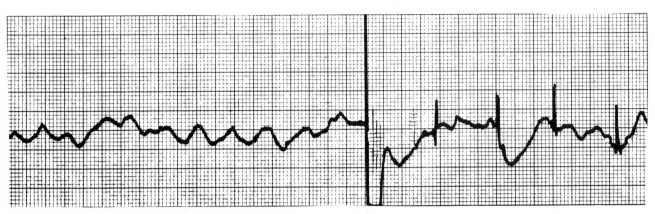

This strip demonstrates ventricular fibrillation. Non-synchronized precordial shock (defibrillation) interrupts the chaotic rhythm and a sinus rhythm resumes.

Defibrillation may be unsuccessful in the patient with long-standing respiratory or cardiac disease, or in the patient plagued with obesity!

* Precordial Shock

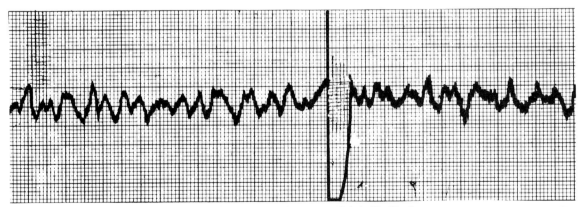

This strip demonstrates unsuccessful defibrillation.

One should bear in mind that the body *rapidly* converts to anaerobic metabolism with the cessation of circulation. There is a rapid buildup of lactic acid—resulting in metabolic acidosis. For this reason, sodium bicarbonate may be administered following the establishment of adequate ventilation. Most authorities feel that electrical intervention is more successful when the acidotic state has been altered. *ACLS Guidelines* (American Heart Association) should be consulted for the latest, up-to-date treatments for code arrest.

Practice Exercise 5

Practice time again

Describe these two rhythm strips in detail! What treatment would be appropriate?

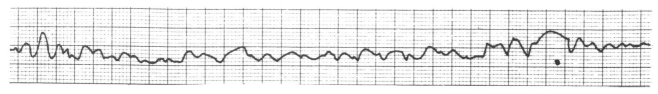

1. _____ Course V-fib _____

_____

_____

_____

_____

_____

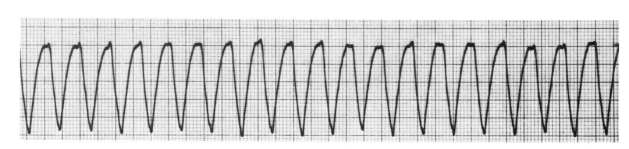

2. _____ V-tach Rate 125 _____

_____

_____

_____

_____

For **Feedback 5,** refer to page 126.

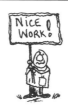

NICE!
WORK!

At this point, I'm exhausted! How 'bout you? This is the *last* exercise of this section, so we'll keep it brief. *Whew!* Since we have more or less exhausted the subject of ectopic ventricular rhythms, we need to explore *VENTRICULAR ESCAPE RHYTHMS*.

As we have discussed before, the heart has many potential pacemakers, each with its own inherent rate of impulse formation. The more distal a pacemaker is located from the sinus node, the slower its inherent ability to pace or initiate impulses.

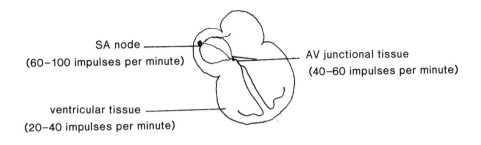

SA node
(60–100 impulses per minute)

AV junctional tissue
(40–60 impulses per minute)

ventricular tissue
(20–40 impulses per minute)

If the sinus node fails to discharge an impulse—or if the SA node discharges so slowly that the heart rate becomes inadequate—or if the sinus impulse fails to be transmitted, a lower (more distal) pacemaker may discharge spontaneously. That's a mouthful!

The SA node may be depressed by acute hypoxia, myocardial damage and/or reflex activity through the vagus nerve. In essence, an escape rhythm is a rhythm maintained by a pacemaker other than the sinus node, when the sinus node fails to activate the heart muscle or does so in an ineffective manner. Thus, an escape rhythm is never a primary phenomenon. It results *secondary* to another event or problem. Escape rhythms are *life saving mechanisms.*

Escape rhythms are generally regular and may vary in rate from 10–100 beats per minute. If the escape rhythm is initiated in the AV junction it is called an idiojunctional rhythm (narrow QRS complex). If the escape rhythm originates in the ventricles (wide QRS, 0.12 seconds or greater) it is called an *IDIOVENTRICULAR RHYTHM* or a VENTRICULAR ESCAPE RHYTHM.

Look at this example of an idioventricular rhythm.

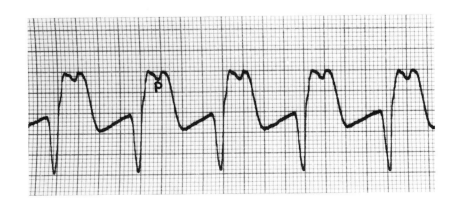

This rhythm strip demonstrates an idioventricular rhythm with a heart rate of approximately 75 beats per minute. The rate is somewhat faster than the inherent ventricular rate (20–40 beats per minute), so it would be appropriate to term this rhythm an *accelerated* idioventricular rhythm. You will notice that the rhythm is regular. Escape rhythms are *almost* always regular! There are no P waves preceding the QRS complexes because the pacemaker originates in the ventricles. You will notice however, a *retrograde* P wave is obvious following the QRS. Thus, atrial depolarization follows ventricular depolarization. (Retrograde P waves are not always obvious in an escape rhythm.)

Let's look at another example of a ventricular escape rhythm.

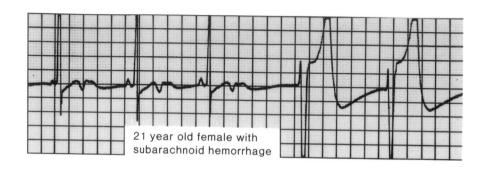

21 year old female with subarachnoid hemorrhage

The underlying rhythm here is an irregular sinus bradycardia. When the sinus pacemaker slows below 50, a ventricular escape pacemaker takes control of the rhythm. Remember, escape rhythms *never* occur as primary disorders. Thus, when observed, escape beats or escape rhythms occur *late* in the cardiac cycle (as opposed to premature), coming *after* the next anticipated beat!

As with all ventricular impulses, *ventricular escape beats are wide, the QRS measuring 0.12 seconds or greater.* It simply takes a longer period of time for the ventricular escape impulses to depolarize the ventricles because they travel backward, outside the normal conduction system. Remember, moving horizontally across the EKG paper denotes time.

The patient with an *escape ventricular rhythm* may experience hemodynamic embarrassment owing to both the slow ventricular rate and the *loss of atrial kick*. In fact, persons with diseased myocardial tissue, particularly the patient with an acute myocardial infarction, may suffer greatly as a result of the ventricular escape rhythm, even if the heart rate is within a normal range. If the atrial contraction does not precede the ventricular contraction by the normal interval, one loses the *Atrial Kick*. The atrial kick is simply the residue of blood forced into the ventricles during atrial systole (contraction), just prior to ventricular systole (contraction). In other words, the atrial kick is an extra "umph" to the distended ventricles before they contract. This essentially *supercharges* the ventricles allowing for a more forceful contraction. When heart damage is present, the absence of atrial kick may reduce cardiac output by as much as 25%. So, when a patient with heart damage presents an idioventricular rhythm, he may exhibit shock symptoms owing to the loss of atrial kick and the slow ventricular rate.

Treatment is *always* supportive in nature and is aimed at speeding up the heart rate and restoring the sinus pacemaker. If the SA node fires too slowly allowing a lower pacemaker to take control, treatment is focused on speeding up the rate of SA impulse discharge. Atropine is most usually the drug of choice.

When the escape rhythm occurs secondary to failure or blockage of a higher pacemaker, treatment is aimed at speeding up the rate of ventricular impulse formation. This may be accomplished by administering Isuprel or by inserting a transvenous ventricular pacemaker.

It is *important* to distinguish between ventricular escape beats or rhythms *and* P.V.C.'s or ventricular tachycardia. Escape beats or escape rhythms are *life saving* while P.V.C.'s or ventricular tachycardia may be *life threatening*.

Escape beats or escape rhythms are inscribed *late* in the cardiac cycle, occurring after the time of the next normal anticipated event.

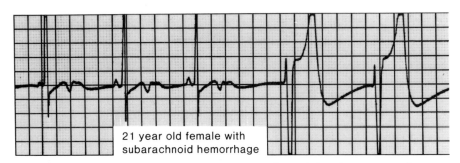

21 year old female with subarachnoid hemorrhage

As escape rhythm emerges following the failure of the sinus pacemaker.

P.V.C.'s or ventricular tachycardia interrupt the underlying rhythm and are, therefore, inscribed *early* (premature) in the cardiac cycle.

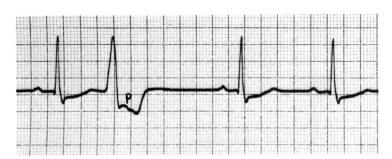

A P.V.C. interrupts the normal underlying rhythm.

The *appropriate* treatment depends upon recognizing whether the abnormal beats are "premature" or "delayed" beats!

Of course, some rhythms are *simply* complicated! See for yourself!

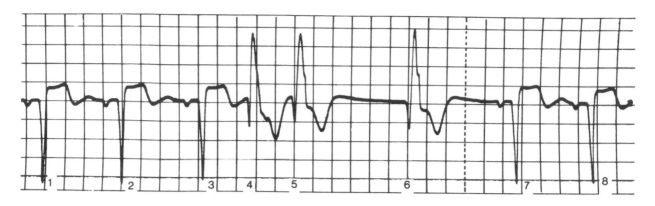

This rhythm strip belongs to a patient with an acute anteroseptal wall myocardial infarction. Notice that there is evidence of *both* "early" (*premature*) and "late" (*escape*) ventricular activity. Beats 4 and 5 are P.V.C.'s; beat 6 is a ventricular escape beat. A situation like this is truly a *treatment dilemma*! Typically, lidocaine will be administered with a transvenous pacemaker available for backup. ℰ

Practice Exercise 6

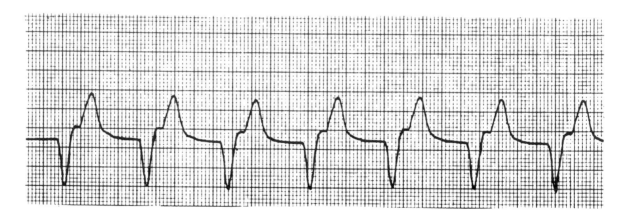

Look at this rhythm strip carefully—then describe all that you see! What treatment would be appropriate?

Ventricular Rhythm

For **Feedback 6,** refer to page 127.

Feedback 1

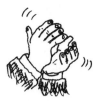

You're becoming a Pro!

1. This is a sinus rhythm with a heart rate of approximately 90 per minute. Beat 6 is premature, interrupting the normal rhythm. The P-R interval of normally conducted beats measures slightly greater than 0.12 seconds. The QRS of normally conducted beats measures approximately 0.08 seconds. There is no obvious P wave in the premature complex. The QRS of the premature beat measures greater than 0.12 seconds. This is a P.V.C. and it occurs on the T wave of the preceding beat. This could initiate ventricular fibrillation!

2. The underlying rhythm is a sinus rhythm with an approximate rate of 80 beats per minute. Beat 2 and 5 occur prematurely, interrupting the underlying rhythm. Both of the premature beats have QRS's that measure 0.12 seconds or greater. The premature beats are P.V.C.'s—but they do <u>not</u> look alike. So, we could say that there are multifocal P.V.C.'s interrupting a sinus rhythm. The QRS of normally conducted beats measures approximately 0.10 seconds. The P-R interval of these beats measures approximately 0.14 seconds.

3. In this rhythm strip, <u>every other beat</u> is a premature ventricular contraction. This is known as <u>bigeminal P.V.C.'s or ventricular bigeminy</u>!

To review then, premature ventricular contractions have the following EKG characteristics.

CHARACTERISTICS OF PREMATURE VENTRICULAR CONTRACTIONS
- They occur prematurely, interrupting the underlying rhythm.
- There may be a P wave following the QRS.
- The QRS complexes are wide and bizarre in appearance, measuring 0.12 seconds or greater.
- There may be a compensatory pause following the premature beat.

Feedback 2

We've got a winner folks!

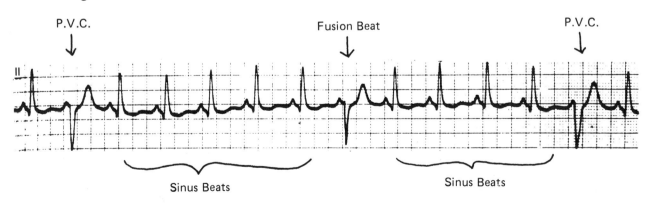

A fusion beat is an abnormal beat produced by a double stimulation. A sinus impulse is conducted normally through the atria (initiating atrial depolarization), through the AV junction, and into the ventricles initiating ventricular depolarization. At the same time, an ectopic ventricular focus fires (P.V.C.) initiating depolarization of the lower part of the ventricles. The sinus impulse and the ectopic ventricular impulses somewhere in the ventricles. Consequently, the QRS of the fusion beat looks somewhere

in between the normal sinus QRS and the P.V.C.! The underlying rhythm is a sinus rhythm with an approximate rate of 90 beats per minute.

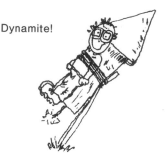 Whew!

Remember, to truly identify a fusion beat, there *must* be a sinus beat and a P.V.C. to compare it to! Fusion can only take place if the atrial impulse has started to penetrate the ventricles from above—so, *a P wave will always precede the abnormal appearing QRS*!

Feedback 3   Dynamite!

1. The underlying rhythm is probably sinus rhythm. The underlying rhythm is interrupted by frequent bursts of ventricular tachycardia! P.V.C.'s land on the vulnerable T waves initiating short "runs" of ventricular tachycardia. The QRS's of the ventricular tachycardia are wide and bizarre. Lidocaine would be the probable treatment.

2. This strip demonstrates <u>ventricular tachycardia</u> with a heart rate of <u>150</u> beats per minute.

CRITERIA THAT <u>HELP</u> TO IDENTIFY VENTRICULAR TACHYCARDIA
- The rate is usually rapid, between 140–200 beats per minute.
- The P waves are usually buried in the QRS complexes, making them obscure.
- The QRS complexes are wide and bizarre.
- The ventricles are directly stimulated by an ectopic ventricular focus firing repeatedly or through a reentry process. This action is independent of atrial activity.
- The ventricular rhythm is <u>basically</u> regular.
- Fusion or capture beats may be evident.

Feedback 5

Nice work!!

1. There is no coordinated activity in this strip. The activity is totally irregular. No PQRST can be seen. The baseline appears to wander or undulate. This is ventricular fibrillation. Treatment would consist of electrical defibrillation or nonsynchronized precordial shock. Until the electrical defibrillation is administered, full cardiopulmonary resuscitation must be done!

2. The rhythm is regular at a rate of approximately 187 beats per minute. No P waves can be identified. The atrial activity is hidden in the QRS complexes. The QRS complexes are wide (0.12 seconds or greater) and bizarre in appearance. This is ventricular tachycardia. Treatment would consist of administration of lidocaine and synchronized precordial shock. If the patient is unconscious, defibrillation may be used.

To review then, ventricular fibrillation is totally uncoordinated electrical activity. No PQRST can be observed. The baseline appears to wander.

Feedback 6

How are you doing? Sometimes it's difficult to grasp ESCAPE rhythms . . . so, you may want to reread Input 6 one more time.

The rhythm is regular with a heart rate of approximately 70 per minute. There are no P waves preceding the QRS complexes. The QRS complexes are wide, measuring greater than 0.12 seconds. This must be a ventricular escape rhythm! (One only sees an escape rhythm when higher pacemakers fail!) Typically, a ventricular escape rhythm will be slow, 20–40 beats per minute. One might call this rhythm an accelerated ventricular escape rhythm since the rate is 70 beats per minute.

The treatment for this rhythm would depend on the cause. Any suppressant drugs (i.e., digitalis) would be discontinued. Treatment would be aimed at restoring a normal rhythm. One might attempt to speed up the SA node with atropine—or speed up a slow ventricular response rate with Isuprel or a transvenous ventricular pacemaker.

Remember, there are no pacemakers distal to the ventricles! If the ventricular escape pacemaker fails, the patient's monitor picture may look like this. . . .

NOTES

Section V
Conduction Disturbances and Heart Block

OBJECTIVES

When you have completed Section V, you will be able to describe or identify

1. sinus arrest (pause) and sinus block
2. atrial tachycardia with block
3. His bundle electrocardiography
4. first degree AV block
5. second degree AV block
   a. Mobitz type I—Wenckebach
   b. Mobitz type II
6. complete heart block
7. bundle branch block

You've come a long way! I hope EKG interpretation has not become the focal point of your existence. However . . . as we said in the very beginning, once you have a good grasp of the fundamentals, it is *repeated* practice that adds finesse!

We are now going to leave behind the world of dysrhythmias and consider *conduction disturbances* and *heart block*. Before doing that, however, let's review the conduction system one more time.

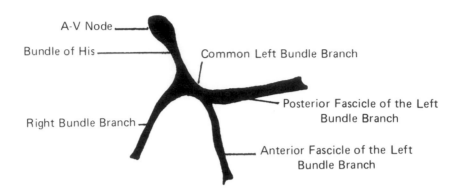

You will notice that the bundle branch system looks somewhat different than in earlier pictures. That is because *in reality* the left bundle branch has both an anterior and posterior division. Thus, the bundle branch system is composed of three fascicles . . . the right bundle branch, the anterior fascicle of the left bundle branch, and the left posterior fascicle of the left bundle branch.

The important point to be made here is that *disease* or *toxic drug manifestations* may delay normal sinus impulse transmission or result in failure of impulse transmission from the atria to the ventricles (thus, the term *AV block*). This delay or interruption may occur anywhere within the conduction system!

Conduction disturbances and heart blocks are sometimes a bit confusing, so read carefully and proceed ahead!

PROCEED AHEAD ...

Input 1: Sinus Arrest (Sinus Pause) and Sinus Block

Occasionally excessive vagal discharge, ischemic damage of the AV node, degenerative disease of the sinus mechanism or digitalis toxicity may interrupt the firing or conduction of the normal sinus impulse. Whew! That's a mouthful. When this phenomenon occurs, a normal sinus rhythm may be interrupted by a pause or pauses.

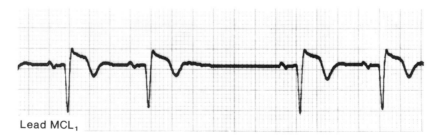

Lead MCL₁

Though there are many abnormalities in the above strip, notice the pause following two normally conducted sinus beats. The pause is thought to result from failure (arrest) of the sinus mechanism.

130

As you inspect the previous tracing, you will note the abnormal pauses. (These pauses would serve to give the patient an irregular pulse . . . therefore, you would need to count the heart rate for one full minute.) If you look closely, you will notice that the next *anticipated* event during the pause is a P wave followed by a QRS. Because that anticipated P wave did not occur in a timely fashion, we assume that the sinus pacemaker did not initiate an impulse, or, if it did, it did not cause atrial depolarization. (Remember . . . the presence of a P wave tells us the atria have depolarized . . . therefore, the *absence* of a P wave tells us the atria did *not* depolarize.)

For purposes of definition, *sinus arrest* (or sinus pause) occurs when the sinus pacemaker fails to discharge an impulse at the expected time. The resulting pause is of *undetermined length,* as is demonstrated in the previous rhythm strip. Sinus arrest may be associated with degenerative disease of the sinus mechanism or drug toxicity (quinidine, digitalis). If the pauses are of significant duration, pacemaker therapy may be required.

Sinus block, on the other hand, exists when the sinus pacemaker initiates an impulse at the expected time, but that impulse is blocked within the sinus mechanism itself. In other words, the sinus impulse does not penetrate into the atria to initiate atrial depolarization. In this case, the resulting pause is usually predictable.

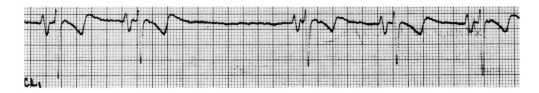

Commonly, the pause will be the same duration as the distance between two normally conducted beats. SA block may be associated with vagotonia (athletes), digitalis administration, and rarely with hypokalemia. Usually, no specific treatment is required.

Interestingly enough, a true differential diagnosis between sinus arrest and sinus block cannot be established on the basis of an EKG alone . . . because all one observes is a pause (the absence of a P wave)!

Probably the best way to describe a strip like the one above is to call it a *sinus pause,* reporting the duration of that pause. (Remember, each small square represents 0.04 seconds!) In the above strip, 2.2 seconds elapse between the R wave prior to, and the R wave following, the pause.

131

Practice Exercise 1

Look at this strip closely . . . then describe all that you see!

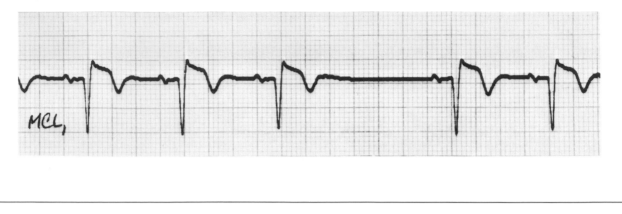

MCL,

_____

_____

_____

_____

_____

_____

_____

_____

For **Feedback 1,** refer to page 163.

Input 2: Atrial Tachycardia with Block

Remember atrial tachycardia? . . . We discussed this dysrhythmia on page 58. You will recall that atrial tachycardia is a rapid ectopic atrial dysrhythmia with an atrial rate of 160–220 per minute. Well, atrial tachycardia with rapid rates may be complicated by second degree AV block, the *physiologic* variety. This is the same *physiologic block* that we discussed earlier (page 63) . . . a protective mechanism that guards the ventricles from the effects of rapid stimulation.

Here is an artist's rendering of atrial tachycardia with block.

Atrial tachycardia with 2:1 AV block.
Ventricular rate = 100 (regular)
Atrial rate = 200 (regular)

Frequently, *atrial tachycardia with block* occurs as a manifestation of digitalis toxicity, and is therefore a contraindication for the continued administration of digitalis preparations.

Much like atrial flutter, the atrial rate in atrial tachycardia with block is described as a ratio to ventricular conduction, e.g., 2:1, 3:1, etc. In other words, there are two P waves for every QRS, three P waves for every QRS, and so forth.

In the event that you are wondering how atrial tachycardia with block differs from atrial flutter . . . remember, it's *ALL* in the atrial rate! By definition, if the atrial rate is regular at a rate of 160–220, the rhythm is atrial tachycardia. If, however, the atrial rate is regular at a rate of 220–350, the rhythm is atrial flutter! Additionally, P waves become "saw toothed" in appearance at more rapid rates. Simple enough, right? 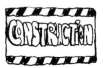 I know, it is difficult to remember all of these rates! And sometimes, even the *experts* disagree, as you can see in the above rhythm strip. (Atrial rate, 260 per minute!)

Practice Exercise 2

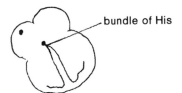

Draw an example of 2:1 atrial tachycardia or atrial tachycardia with 2:1 block.

For **Feedback 2,** refer to page 163.

Input 3: His Bundle Electrogram Studies and Related Facts

In the early days of electrocardiography, most conduction disorders were thought to occur primarily in the AV node. You will remember though that impulse transmission from the atria to the Purkinje system is electrically silent on the EKG. In other words, the P-R interval is electrically silent, representing impulse "travel time" from the atria to the Purkinje system.

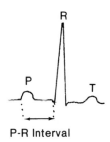

P-R Interval

Looking only at the P-R interval, it is impossible to detect where in the conduction system a delay or block is occurring. In 1969, a technique to study impulse conduction was introduced—the His bundle electrogram (HBE).

Anatomically, the bundle of His lies under the membranous portion of the intraventricular septum. By positioning a catheter electrode in this area, actual depolarization of the bundle of His could be recorded—giving a bi- or triphasic deflection during the P-R interval on the EKG.

That sounds a bit complicated, right? Essentially, by placing a catheter electrode in the area of the bundle of His, the catheter can monitor the atrial impulse and its passage through the bundle of His to the ventricles.

Let's try an analogy at the race track!

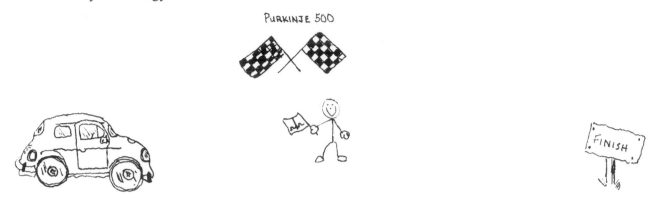

A timekeeper is positioned somewhere on the raceway to clock how long it takes the traveling racer to reach the midpoint. The timekeeper can also observe and record the start and finish of the race.

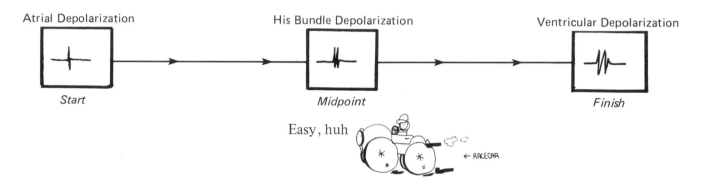

Atrial Depolarization	His Bundle Depolarization	Ventricular Depolarization
Start	Midpoint	Finish

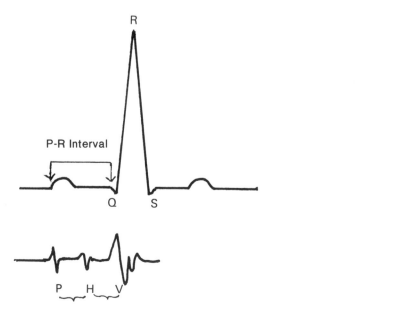

Easy, huh

The His bundle monitoring electrode allows the P-R interval to be divided into segments or intervals. One interval extends from the P wave to the His bundle deflection (representing depolarization of the bundle of His). This is known as the *P-H interval* and represents the *conduction* time from the atria through the AV node to the bundle of His.

The second interval extends from the His deflection to the onset of the QRS complex. This is known as the *H-V interval,* and measures the conduction time from the bundle of His to ventricular activation.

The His Bundle Electrogram (HBE) has been an important diagnostic tool for determining where in the conduction system defects occur. A defect may lie either above or below the bundle of His. So, the old theory that conduction disorders occurred primarily in the AV node was disproven.

Studies have shown that conduction defects or blocks occurring above the bundle of His are usually *benign,* seldom progressing to complete heart block. Conduction defects or blocks that originate below the bundle of His usually have a *grave* prognosis!

Thus, the HBE procedure has refined the classification of heart blocks, and has assisted the practitioner with both treatment and prognosis. For the most part, heart blocks can be classified in the following manner.

HEART BLOCKS ABOVE THE BUNDLE OF HIS	HEART BLOCKS BELOW THE BUNDLE OF HIS
• First degree AV block • Mobitz Type I (Wenckebach) second degree AV block • Complete AV block with a QRS of normal duration (less than 0.12 seconds)	• Mobitz Type II second degree AV block • Complete AV block with a widened QRS (0.12 seconds or greater)

Usually, AV conduction delays or blocks occurring *above* the bundle of His are *benign* in nature and are frequently associated with ischemia or toxic drug effects. Conduction delays or blocks occurring *below* the bundle of His are *commonly* associated with extensive myocardial damage and therefore have poorer prognoses.

The above chart will be a useful reference as we continue on. In the event that you are confused, be assured you are progressing in a normal fashion!

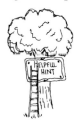

After completing Section V, reread these first few pages. It will all begin to make perfectly GOOD SENSE! HONEST!

Practice Exercise 3

How about some practice?

1. Label the parts of the conduction system.

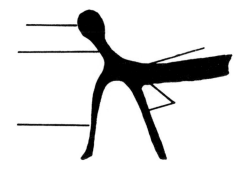

2. Atrial depolarization is represented on the EKG as a _____ wave.

The P-R interval represents _____

_____

_____

The QRS represents _____

_____

3. The P-R interval is electrically silent.

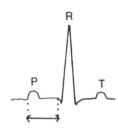

By placing a catheter electrode in the _____ , depolarization of the bundle of His can be recorded. The His bundle deflection occurs between the _____ wave and the _____ complex of an EKG cycle.

4. The His bundle monitoring electrode allows the P-R interval to be divided into segments. The interval from the P wave to the bundle of His deflection is known as the _____ interval. (Label the diagram below.)

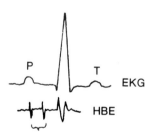

The interval from the bundle of His deflection to the onset of ventricular depolarization is known as the _____ interval. (Label the diagram below.)

IF YOU ARE CONFUSED, PLEASE [✓] THE BOX ON THE TOP OF THE NEXT PAGE! . . .

. . . it sometimes helps to decrease FRUSTRATION! ☺

For **Feedback 3,** refer to page 163.

Input 4: First Degree AV Block

On to bigger and better things. . . .

FIRST DEGREE HEART BLOCK is a technical way of saying that the *P-R interval is greater than* the upper limits of normal.

Your long term memory should now be registering that the duration of a normal P-R interval is between 0.12–0.20 seconds, or 3–5 tiny EKG squares. The P-R interval represents the time it takes for the pacemaker impulse to travel across the atria, through the AV junction, down the bundle branches to the Purkinje system. Remember?

Well, because the P-R interval is electrically silent, it's impossible to determine where in the AV conduction system the delay is occurring. We know there is a delay because the P-R interval is abnormally long, greater than 0.20 seconds. Somethin' is HOLDING UP THE SHOW!!!

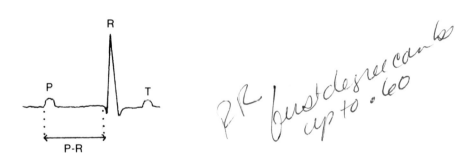

PR 1 first degree can be up to .60

This is where it's helpful to understand the His bundle electrogram. Past HBE studies demonstrated that first degree heart block (an abnormally long P-R interval) is *usually* due to a block somewhere *above* the bundle of His.

This means that it takes the pacemaker impulse an abnormally long period of time to travel through the AV node to the bundle of His—but the conduction time from the bundle of His to the Purkinje fibers is normal!

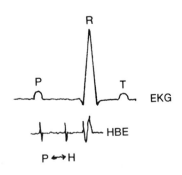

That may not excite you . . . but it excites me! . . . ! I know that when blocks or delays occur above the bundle of His, they are *usually BENIGN*!

Let's look at a rhythm strip.

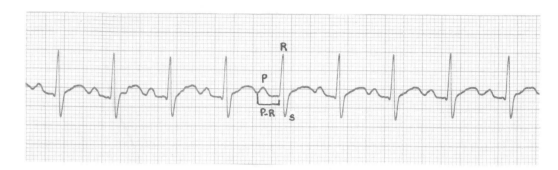

You'll notice that the P-R interval is greater than 0.20 seconds (greater than five small squares). The P waves are of normal shape. The QRS is of normal configuration and duration (less than 0.12 seconds). *All* sinus impulses reach and activate the ventricles. The sinus impulses are merely taking longer time than normal. So, this is a sinus rhythm with a first degree heart block.

That's all it takes to have a FIRST DEGREE HEART BLOCK!

Because first degree heart block is usually benign, it serves only to be watched. However, *an increasing P-R interval should always be reported.* First degree heart block is most frequently associated with coronary artery disease, digitalis administration, and all types of acute myocardial infarction.

On this strip, notice that the P-R interval measures 0.28 seconds or 7 little squares.

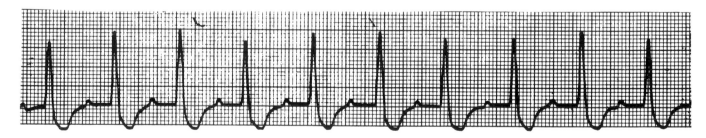

The above rhythm strip demonstrates a sinus rhythm with a first degree heart block. Most authorities note that a P-R interval may be as long as one second and still conduct! Let's look at another example of first degree AV block.

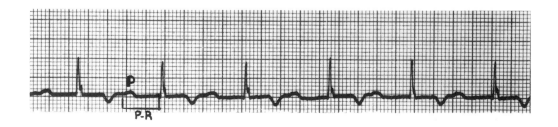

The previous strip demonstrates a sinus rhythm, rate approximately 70 per minute, with a prolonged P-R interval. The P-R interval measures *almost* two big squares, or 0.4 seconds. Thus, we have a sinus rhythm with a first degree AV block. It is always important to measure the duration of the P-R interval!

To review then, first degree heart block manifests as a *prolonged P-R interval*. Most usually, the conduction defect or block occurs intranodally, above the bundle of His. However, if we only have a standard EKG as a tool for interpretation, we cannot know where the block is—all we see is the isoelectric P-R interval. We can only assume the block is above the His bundle!

Practice Exercise 4

See what you can do with this!

1. Describe all that you see in this rhythm strip!

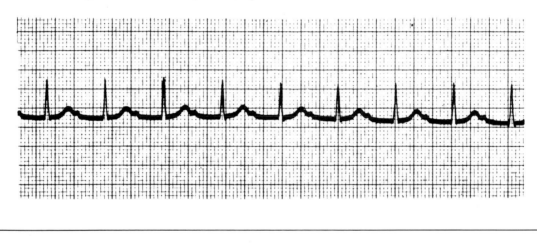

_____

_____

_____

_____

_____

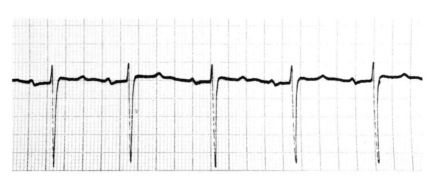

2. The P-R interval in this rhythm strip measures approximately _____ little squares or _____ seconds.

139

3. His bundle electrogram (HBE) studies have shown that the conduction defect or delay in first degree heart block usually lies _____ the bundle of His. First degree heart block is usually benign and serves only_____.

For **Feedback 4,** refer to page 164.

Input 5: Second Degree AV Block

That brings us to the subject of *Second Degree Heart Block.*

The very *best* description that I've ever heard of second degree AV block went something like this . . .

. . . "Some P's make it and some don't; those that don't, should!"

Very simple and to the point!

To complicate the understanding of second degree heart block, God created two types, Mobitz type I (Wenckebach) and Mobitz type II.

Mobitz Type I—Wenckebach

Mobitz type I, affectionately called *Wenckebach,* is a fun rhythm . . . **HONEST!**

In Wenckebach, one finds a *progressive prolongation of the P-R interval until a P wave is finally blocked . . .* or not conducted . . .

. . . like this.

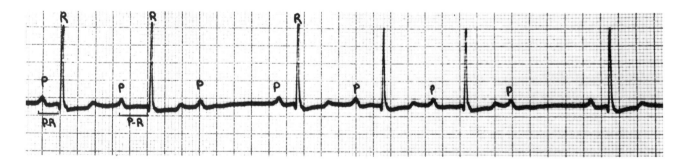

Notice that the P-R interval gets progressively longer until *finally,* a P wave does not conduct.

Because the P-R interval progressively becomes longer, the ventricular response is irregular—or, we could say that there is a *varying R-R interval . . .* (the distance between any two R waves varies). In Wenckebach, or Mobitz type I, the P-R interval lengthens, while the R-R interval shortens.

The Wenckebach rhythm is usually described as a ratio, the number of P waves to QRS complexes per cycle. The following tracing would be described as a "5:4 Wenckebach" (five P waves for four QRS complexes).

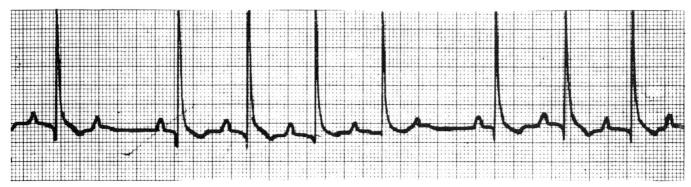

A 5:4 Wenckebach pattern

A Wenckebach type of second degree heart block is most frequently associated with acute inferior wall myocardial infarction, and is probably due to ischemic damage of the AV node. The AV junctional artery fills from the right coronary artery—and it is usually the right coronary artery involved in the inferior wall infarction. Wenckebach may also be a manifestation of digitalis toxicity.

HBE studies have shown that this conduction disturbance is usually located above the bundle of His. *If associated with acute inferior wall myocardial infarction, Wenckebach will usually develop within the first 24-hours after the infarction, and usually will not persist beyond the third day.* Since we expect it to disappear within 72 hours, we merely observe it. If Wenckebach occurs secondary to digitalis toxicity, the administration of digitalis should be discontinued.

Mobitz type I, or Wenckebach, is thought to occur because of progressive fatigue in the AV junctional tissues. In other words, a sinus beat is conducted normally through the AV junction. The next impulse conducts more slowly because the AV junction is tired. Each additional impulse tends to be conducted progressively slower—until *finally* the AV junction says, "I'm going to sit this one out boys!" The AV junctional tissues become so fatigued that they are incapable of transmitting the impulse. Thus, the atrial impulse finds the AV junctional tissues *refractory* (unable to receive the next impulse), and the impulse is blocked. This gives the AV junctional conducting tissues a rest! Then, the whole process begins again!

With Wenckebach, the cycle of dropped beats may vary, giving the patient a varying radial pulse—similar to that of atrial fibrillation.

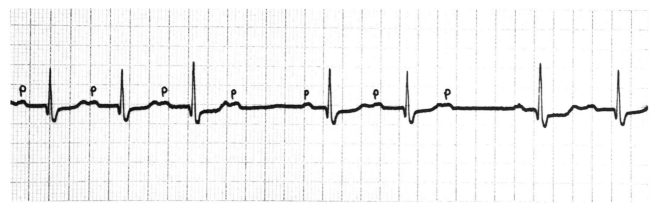

Variable cycle Wenckebach

Another significant feature of the Wenckebach cycle is that it may begin with a junctional escape beat. . . .

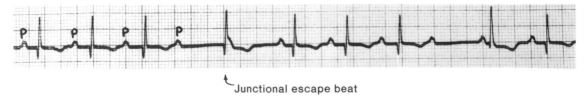

Junctional escape beat

Why does that occur? Well, if the pause following the blocked P wave is prolonged, a lower, more distal pacemaker (with a potential rate of 40–60 per minute) will fire an impulse. Remember, **IF THE SINUS NODE FAILS TO DISCHARGE AN IMPULSE—*OR* IF THE SA NODE DISCHARGES SO SLOWLY THAT THE HEART RATE IS INADEQUATE—*OR* IF THE SINUS IMPULSE FAILS TO BE TRANSMITTED, A LOWER (MORE DISTAL) PACEMAKER WILL DISCHARGE SPONTANEOUSLY!**

WARRANTY
July 4, 1944

. . . THIS ESCAPE FEATURE ACCOMPANIES EACH HEART. IT IS GUARANTEED FOR THE LIFETIME OF THE UNIT, WITH CERTAIN EXCEPTIONS . . .

ACME ENTERPRISES

P.S. If you need review of junctional escape beats, refer to page **80**.

That about wraps up the subject of Mobitz type I (Wenckebach). So let's explore Mobitz type II.

Mobitz Type II

Most always, Mobitz type II blocks originate below the level of the bundle of His (in the bundle branches or the Purkinje system) and are of organic origin. Frequently, Mobitz type II is associated with acute anterior wall myocardial infarction (extensive myocardial damage).

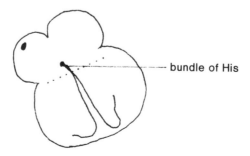
bundle of His

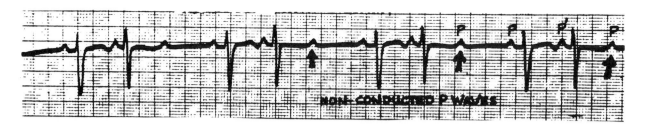

On EKG, one sees a *sudden* blocked P wave without warning! The P-R interval of all conducted beats is constant. The P wave that fails to conduct is neither premature nor late . . . *it occurs in rhythmic sequence with the other P waves.* The ventricular response is irregular owing to the nonconducted P waves. The duration of the QRS complexes are usually within normal limits, though the QRS may be widened depending upon the underlying pathology. In other words, the QRS's are generally skinny, but may also be fat!

To definitely identify Mobitz II, there must be *two or more consecutively conducted* sinus impulses with a constant P-R interval before the blocked P wave.

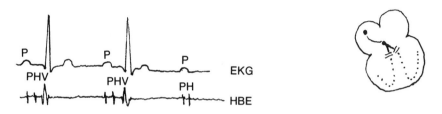

Notice the constant P-R interval of the two consecutively conducted sinus beats!

HBE studies have shown that impulse transmission failure occurs distal or below the bundle of His. Since the impulse never reaches the ventricles, the problem is due to bilateral blockage of the bundle branches!

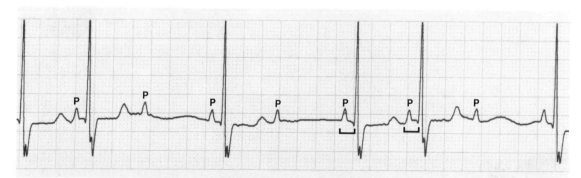

This strip demonstrates a Mobitz type II block. Notice that the P-R interval of all conducted beats is constant and measures approximately 0.14 seconds. The nonconducted P waves occur in rhythmic sequence with the other P waves. The QRS complexes are of normal duration.

The patient with Mobitz type II must be watched closely and constantly. At any point he or she could develop complete heart block or ventricular standstill!

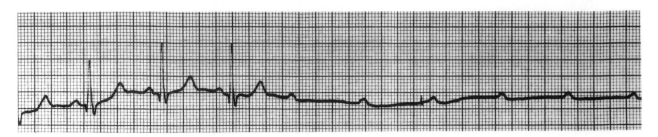

This strip demonstrates ventricular standstill. There is no cardiac output. CPR must be instituted immediately.

Some physicians will prophylactically insert a ventricular pacemaker wire—on a standby basis . . . *just in case*! If this is not done, Isuprel should be kept close at hand. Isuprel is a cardiac stimulant and may produce P.V.C.'s. (When there is no, or limited, ventricular activity, P.V.C.'s will generate cardiac output.)

A ventricular pacemaker is the treatment of choice, because administering Isuprel may increase the area of myocardial infarct! Isuprel increases the myocardial oxygen consumption, which further compromises the ischemic myocardial tissue.

You'll remember from the first part of this section that the prognosis for a patient with Mobitz type II second degree AV block is usually grave. Mobitz type II is *most usually* associated with extensive myocardial damage. It is the *extent of myocardial damage* that determines the prognosis!

To review then, to *definitely* identify Mobitz type II, there must be two or more consecutive sinus impulses with the same P-R interval conducted to the ventricles before a blocked impulse occurs. The blocked sinus impulse is neither premature nor delayed.

Owing to the fact that Mobitz type II is commonly associated with extensive myocardial damage, there is usually evidence of intraventricular conduction defects. In other words, even when the sinus impulses are conducted normally, there may be some delay in ventricular activation. Therefore, the QRS's seen in Mobitz type II are *commonly* widened.

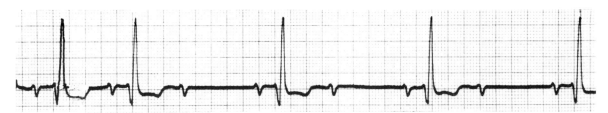

Mobitz type II second degree AV block with widened QRS's.

This "cookbook method" of looking at EKG's is not always a sure method. A patient's heart rhythm may appear like this.

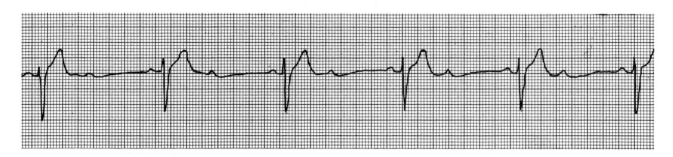

This rhythm strip demonstrates a 2:1 conduction pattern, two P waves for every QRS. One cannot say whether the P-R interval increases or stays constant, because there is *only* one conducted beat occurring before each blocked beat. In this case, we would simply describe what we see . . . there are *two* P waves for every QRS (2:1 conduction). The QRS complexes measure 0.12 seconds and the ventricular rate is 38 per minute! Because the P-R interval of the conducted beats is constant, we know that the atrial and ventricular activity are related.

REMEMBER two conducted P waves must occur *consecutively* in order to identify either Wenckebach or Mobitz type II. Although the above rhythm is a form of second degree heart block, it is *unclear* which type, since there are *never* two consecutive impulses conducted through to the ventricles.

This rhythm strip also demonstrates a 2:1 conduction, but in this instance, the QRS complexes are widened (0.12 seconds or greater).

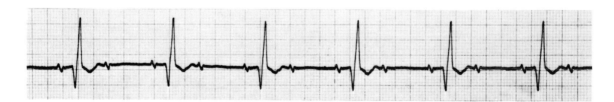

A 2:1 AV conduction pattern associated with *narrow* QRS complexes *usually* represents a form of Wenckebach. A 2:1 AV conduction pattern associated with *wide* QRS complexes (0.12 seconds or greater) is *usually* associated with a delay in conduction below the bundle of His—thus, it is *usually* a Mobitz type II block. If only the 2:1 conduction pattern is observed, further study would be warranted to identify the origin of the block (above or below the bundle of His). Oftentimes, if one continues to observe a 2:1 conduction pattern, there may be a point where two sinus impulses are *consecutively conducted* to the ventricles. When this occurs, the P-R of the two consecutively conducted beats can be measured. If the P-R interval *increases,* you are *no doubt* looking at a Wenckebach rhythm! On the other hand, if the P-R interval of the two consecutively conducted beats *remains the same,* the rhythm is *probably* Mobitz type II.

In either instance, the slow ventricular rate may require augmentation. Since the sinus mechanism is healthy, atropine may serve to increase the sinus rate. Although atropine will not reduce the block, it may serve to increase overall rate of those beats which are conducted. Whew!

Practice Exercise 5

It's funny how it **always** seems to be practice time! Time passes fast when you're having a good time. . . . right?

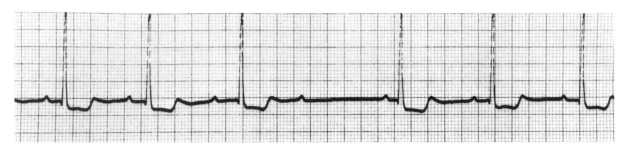

1. Look at this rhythm strip . . . describe what you see!

_____
_____
_____
_____
_____
_____
_____
_____
_____
_____
_____

2. Describe this rhythm strip in detail!

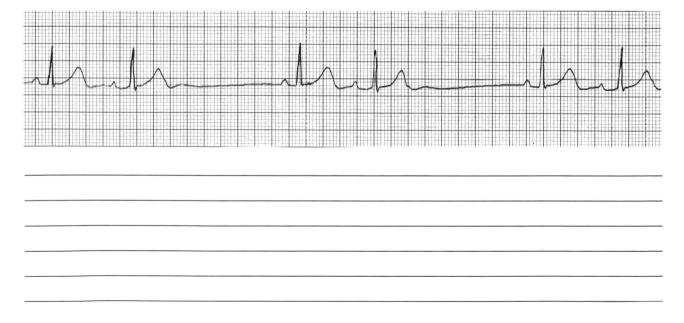

_____
_____
_____
_____
_____
_____
_____

3. What would you say about this rhythm?

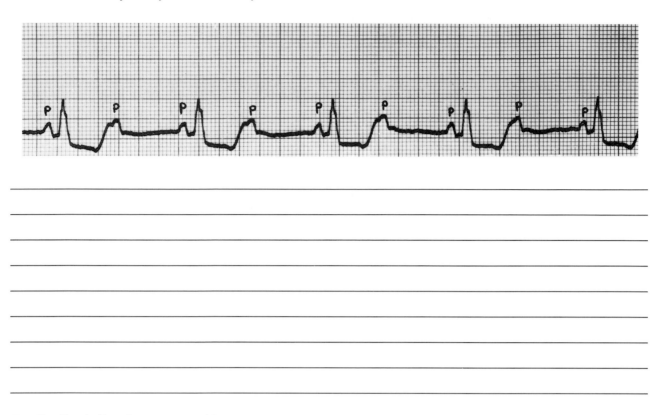

_____

_____

_____

_____

_____

_____

_____

_____

_____

For **Feedback 5,** refer to page 165.

Input 6: Complete Heart Block (CHB)

Now that you have an appreciation for first and second degree heart blocks, let's explore third degree, or complete, heart block.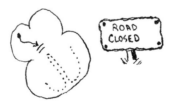

Complete heart block (CHB) is a good descriptive term. It simply means that *all* atrial impulses are blocked—none of the atrial impulses conduct through to ventricles to initiate ventricular depolarization.

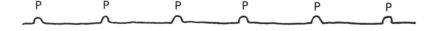

In other words, the sinus pacemaker is usually discharging at a normal rate (60–100 per minute) causing atrial depolarization, but none of these impulses are conducted through to the ventricles.

Thus, the patient's EKG *could* look like this!

However, you'll remember . . . if a sinus impulse fails to discharge or *fails to be transmitted,* a lower (more distal) pacemaker will take control of heart beat! Hurray for escape pacemakers!

That's just what happens in complete heart block! Because none of the sinus impulses are conducted, a more distal pacemaker takes over.

If the AV junction is healthy, it will initiate the escape rhythm. Remember what idiojunctional or junctional escape rhythms look like?

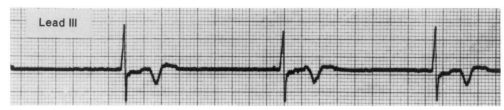

Junctional escape rhythm.

The heart rate is usually 40 to 60 beats per minute. A P wave may occur before, during, or after the QRS complex. The QRS complexes are narrow, measuring less than 0.12 seconds!

If the AV junction is diseased or damaged, it may be unable to take over as the escape or safety pacemaker. When this occurs, the next lower (more distal) pacemaker takes control. This would be a ventricular escape pacemaker!

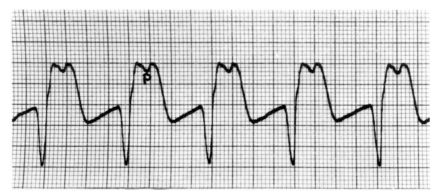

Accelerated ventricular escape rhythm.

You'll remember that idioventricular or ventricular escape rhythms are usually slow, though they may occur at a rate of 10–100 beats per minute. Ventricular escape rhythms have no P waves preceding the QRS complexes—P waves may be hidden in the QRS complexes, or follow the QRS complexes. Ventricular impulses are *wide,* measuring 0.12 seconds or greater . . . that's because it takes a longer period of time for the ventricular escape impulses to depolarize the ventricles.

(If you need some review of idioventricular rhythms, turn back to page 121.)

In complete heart block, none of the sinus impulses are conducted through to the ventricles . . . so, a lower (more distal) pacemaker assumes control of ventricular activation.

THERE IS ONE THING YOU NEED TO REMEMBER . . . both the sinus P waves and the escape rhythm will be obvious on the EKG recording. There is no failure of the sinus pacemaker or atrial activation, only a failure of impulse transmission to the ventricles. Thus, P waves will be present!

Let's look at an EKG strip.

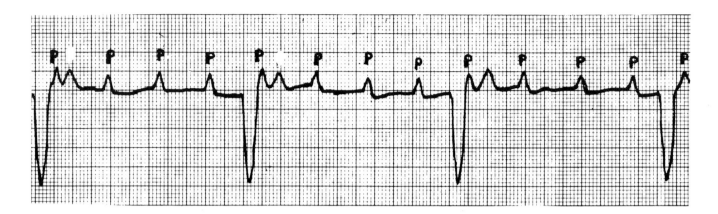

First, let's locate all the P waves and ask the question, "What are the atria doing?" Well, atrial activation is occurring at a rate of approximately 107 per minute (count the number of tiny squares between P waves . . . there are 14 tiny squares between P waves. So, I looked back to the chart on page 39 and found that 14 tiny squares is a rate of 107 per minute).

Now, "What are the ventricles doing?" The QRS's are occurring regularly and slowly at a rate of less than 30 per minute. If I wanted to know the exact rate, I could count the number of small squares between the QRS complexes . . . that comes to 55 small squares. The chart on page 39 does not give the rate for 55 small squares, so I could do the calculation myself! Divide 55 into 1500 . . . there are 1500 small squares in a one minute time interval.

$$55\overline{)1500}^{27}$$

So, the ventricular rate in this strip is about 27 beats per minute. *Ugh!*

The QRS complexes measure 0.16 seconds in duration. Thus, we know the escape rhythm is most likely of ventricular origin.

Now comes the big question, "Are atrial and ventricular activity related?" *No!* because the P-R interval is *never* constant in complete heart block.

There are two *independent,* or asynchronous, pacemakers bearing no relationship to one another! Thus, the two pacemakers are dissociated. Hence, we have a new term . . . *AV dissociation.*

CRITERIA FOR COMPLETE HEART BLOCK

- The atrial and ventricular rates are different—the atrial activity is independent of, or dissociated from, ventricular activity (*AV dissociation*).
- The atrial rate (P waves) is faster. No sinus impulses are conducted through to the ventricles.
- The ventricular rate (QRS complexes) is slow and regular.
- The QRS complexes may be narrow (less than 0.12 seconds) or wide (0.12 seconds or greater).

JUNCTIONAL ESCAPE RHYTHMS HAVE NARROW QRS COMPLEXES;
VENTRICULAR ESCAPE RHYTHMS HAVE WIDE QRS COMPLEXES.

- The P-R interval is never constant.

IMPORTANT NOTE: The term *AV dissociation* is a nonspecific generic term that may be applied to any rhythm when the atria and ventricles are activated independently. AV dissociation is never a primary disorder; rather, it is a descriptive term.

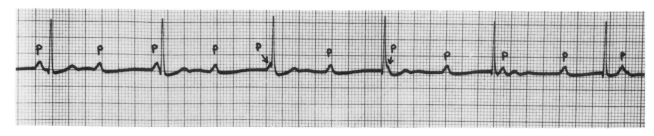

Complete heart block with QRS complexes of normal duration (less than 0.12 seconds).

Sometimes, in a complete heart block, the P waves are hidden in other wave forms. We assume they are really there! *P WAVES ARE SAID TO BE "MARCHING" THROUGH THE RHYTHM.* (Personally, I didn't know that P waves marched . . . but I bet John Phillip Sousa would have been happy to know that.)

His bundle studies have demonstrated that when QRS complexes are within normal limits, the defect in complete heart block is *usually* in the AV node. In this case, complete heart block usually develops *gradually* as a *progression* from *Wenckebach, Mobitz type I*. Commonly, ischemia resulting from an inferior wall myocardial infarction or digitalis toxicity are the *culprits* responsible for this rhythm! When complete heart block is intranodal in origin, the QRS complexes are narrow and the ventricular rate generally averages 40–60 per minute. Past studies have indicated that complete heart block of intranodal origin has a lower mortality rate than any other form of complete heart block, averaging 25%.

Complete heart block associated with wide QRS complexes (0.12 or greater) is usually a manifestation of bilateral bundle branch block (Mobitz type II) and is almost always associated with *extensive* myocardial damage. The ventricular rate in this instance is usually less than 40 per minute. This type of complete heart block can lead to ventricular standstill with dramatic suddenness. The mortality rate has been estimated to be 80%.

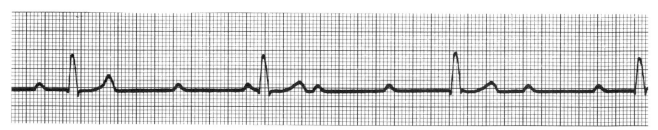

Complete heart block with QRS duration of 0.12 seconds. The ventricular rate is 29 beats per minute!

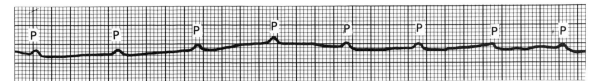

Ventricular Standstill (no evidence of ventricular activity).

In ventricular standstill, none of the atrial impulses reach and activate the ventricles, and a lower more distal pacemaker fails to emerge. This is an extreme emergency warranting immediate C.P.R.

When looking at rhythm strips, a nice *general rule* to remember is . . .

. . . if the P-R interval is *never* constant, the rhythm can only be *Wenckebach* or *complete heart block* (CHB). Wenckebach has a *varying* R-R interval or irregularly occurring QRS complexes. CHB usually has a *regular* R-R interval—the QRS's occur in a regular pattern.

BONUS: Remember atrial fibrillation, the irregularly irregular rhythm with an undulating baseline? (If you don't, turn to page 68.)

There is *one* instance where you will find an atrial fibrillation with a *REGULAR* ventricular response. When a complete heart block exists, all chaotic atrial impulses will be blocked. A lower more distal pacemaker will then assume the role of pacemaker. Thus, the monitor tracing will show undulating atrial activity and a slow, regular ventricular response!

Let's try some practice!

Practice Exercise 6

1. Complete heart block means that _____

   _____

   _____

   _____

2. Because none of the atrial impulses are conducted to the ventricles, a lower more distal pacemaker will usually initiate ventricular activation. This is an _____ .

3. If the escape rhythm has narrow QRS complexes and a rate of 40–60 beats per minute, it is probably a/an _____ rhythm. If the escape rhythm has a slow rate (20–40 beats per minute) and wide QRS complexes, it is a/an _____ rhythm.

4. Describe this next rhythm strip in detail. What are the atria doing? What are the ventricles doing? Are the two activities related?

BEWARE OF OBSCURE P WAVES!

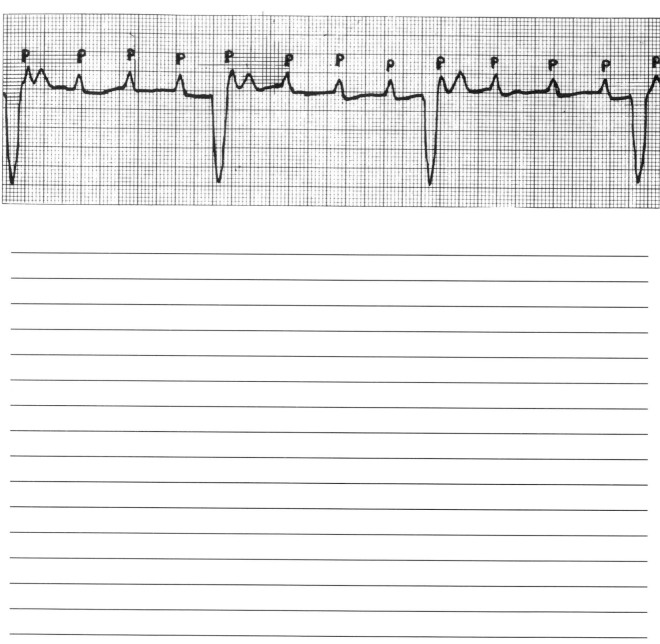

_____
_____
_____
_____
_____
_____
_____
_____
_____
_____
_____
_____
_____
_____
_____
_____
_____

NICE WORK!

For **Feedback 6,** refer to page 165.

Blocks, blocks and more blocks!

You'll probably be happy to know that this is the last exercise in this section.

We now need to think about BUNDLE BRANCH BLOCKS (BBB).

When one speaks of bundle branch blocks, he or she is actually referring to a trifascicular system. You'll remember that the left bundle branch has two branches or fascicles. So, the two bundle branches (right and left) have three conducting segments or fascicles. That's where we get the term *trifascicular*!

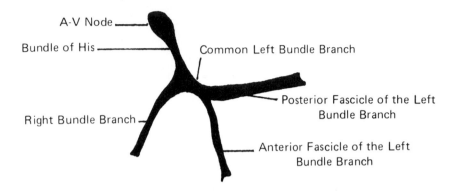

The left bundle branch divides into two separate fascicles early in its course through the ventricles. The anterior fascicle is longer, thinner, and has a single blood supply. In contrast, the posterior fascicle is shorter, thicker, and has a double blood supply.

Using these three fascicles, there are *11* types of block which could exist: bundle branch blocks, hemiblocks, bifascicular blocks, and trifascicular block! To *simplify* this matter, we will concentrate on right bundle branch block (RBBB) and complete left bundle branch block (LBBB)!

Complete bundle branch block means that for some reason, conduction through either of the bundle branches has been delayed or interrupted. This delay causes ventricular activation and depolarization to occur more slowly, causing the QRS to widen to at least 0.12 seconds.

Bundle branch blocks have a *multitude* of causes. Probably the more *frequent* causative factors are: coronary artery disease, myocardial infarction, hypertensive heart disease, excessive potassium intake, rapid tachycardia, and quinidine, pronestyl, or digitalis toxicities. Treatment of either right or left bundle branch block consists of managing the *underlying* disorder.

We will consider right bundle branch block (RBBB) first, since it occurs twice as commonly as left bundle branch block.

Right Bundle Branch Block (RBBB)

Right bundle branch block (RBBB) occurs when conduction through the right bundle branch is delayed or interrupted. This delay or interruption may be associated with almost any type of heart disease, hypertensive cardiovascular disease, right ventricular hypertrophy, or congenital lesions involving the septum. Occasionally, RBBB may be found in an otherwise healthy individual!

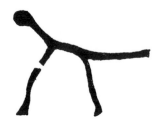

In RBBB, an atrial impulse is conducted normally through the atria and through the AV junction. A blockage in the right bundle branch, however, causes right ventricular activation to occur more slowly.

Slow ventricular depolarization is recorded as a "FAT" QRS . . . . . . 0.12 seconds or greater.

So, on the monitor, we would see a P wave and a normal P-R interval because the defect is confined only to the right bundle branch. The left ventricle is activated in a normal fashion. The right ventricle is stimulated by an impulse from the left bundle branch which passes to the right side of the septum below the block. This *abnormal* activation of the right ventricle requires a greater duration of time . . . thus, the QRS is widened.

Let's see if we can put that into perspective.

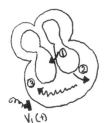

(1) Septal activation occurs normally, from right to left. If we are monitoring from a right chest lead V_1, the force of septal depolarization moves toward the positive electrode. Thus, the initial part of the QRS is directed upward. (2) Secondly, the free wall of the left ventricle depolarizes. This time, the direction of depolarization is away from the positive electrode, so the next part of the QRS is directed negatively. (3) Last, the right ventricle is stimulated abnormally, with the direction of depolarization moving toward the positive electrode.

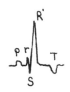

Lead V_1

So, what does the QRS look like . . . you guessed it! In lead V_1, there are two R waves! And, because of the abnormal right ventricular activation, the QRS is widened! Neat, huh! Remember, when the force of depolarization moves *toward* a positive electrode, the resulting deflection is *upright,* or positive. Likewise, when the force of depolarization moves *away from* a positive electrode (toward a negative electrode) the resulting deflection is *downward,* or negative. If you need a quick review of leads, turn back to page 4!

One can identify a bundle branch block on a tracing by the widened QRS. Everything else about the rhythm is usually normal (at least in "textbook" cases)!

In order to *distinguish* right from left bundle branch block, however, it is necessary to look at the V leads. V leads (V_1-V_6) are the chest leads that look directly at the heart (for a refresher, see page 7).

EKG CRITERIA FOR RBBB

- QRS measures 0.12 seconds or greater.
- Wide and slurred S waves in lead I, V_5 and V_6.
- rsR' (M pattern) in V_1 and V_2.
- PQRST relationship is normal.
- Secondary ST and T wave changes.

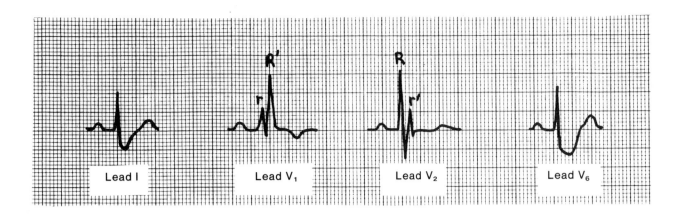

Lead I   Lead V₁   Lead V₂   Lead V₆

Remember, to distinguish right from left bundle branch block, one must look at the V leads! I have difficulty remembering all of that, so I just remember . . .

In RBBB, the QRS in lead V_1 will appear wide and positive.

No matter which lead you look at, the QRS will be fat! . . . at least 0.12 seconds!
Here is a lead V_1 monitor trace showing RBBB.

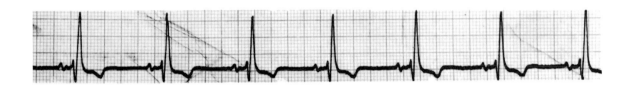

The rhythm is regular at a rate of approximately 80 beats per minute. P waves precede each QRS complex. All P waves are uniform. The P-R interval is of normal duration. The QRS complexes are uniform, occur regularly, and measure approximately 0.16 seconds.

The QRS is wide and positive. In lead V_1 a positive, wide QRS characterizes right bundle branch block.

So, this is a sinus rhythm with RBBB!

Right bundle branch block is twice as common as left bundle branch block and frequently develops with changes in heart rate—especially tachycardias. RBBB is *generally* a consequence of occlusion of the anterior descending coronary artery, and is generally associated with extensive myocardial damage. Most authorities agree it is probably the extent of myocardial damage that determines the patient's prognosis.

Now, a look at rate dependent bundle branch blocks. Conducting tissues that are diseased may only be capable of conducting normally when the heart rate is slow. If that rate is speeded up, there may be delayed conduction or no conduction at all. The involved conducting tissue must have time to recover from its refractory period if it is to conduct normally. If recovery time is not sufficient, conduction will be delayed. When conduction through a bundle branch is delayed, the monitor shows a widened QRS complex (a bundle branch block pattern). This delay in a bundle branch is due to unequal refractoriness of the bundle branches.

Anyway . . . what happens is . . . a patient will have a normal rhythm. If his heart rate increases over a certain point, he will exhibit a bundle branch block pattern. His diseased conducting tissues are unable to recover as quickly at faster rates, so conduction occurs abnormally (wide QRS complexes). When his heart rate slows, conduction will again be normal. This is known as *Rate Related or Rate Dependent Bundle Branch Block*. Most commonly, the defect in rate related bundle branch blocks is in the right bundle branch. That's a mouthful.

Look at this patient!

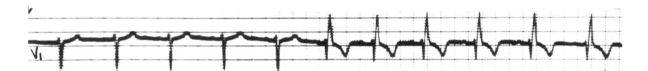

The first five beats show a sinus rhythm with a rate of 75. When the heart rate speeds up to 80 beats per minute, conduction is *abnormal*. When this patient's heart rate approaches 80 beats per minute, his diseased conducting system requires *more* time for recovery. Notice that at the faster rate, the QRS is widened and positive. Since this is V_1, we are looking at a rate related right bundle branch block. Neat huh?

Left Bundle Branch Block (LBBB)

Left bundle branch block (LBBB) occurs when conduction through both segments or both fascicles of the common left bundle is *delayed* or *interrupted*. This delay or interruption is often associated with coronary artery disease, diseases that produce left ventricular hypertrophy, and congenital lesions involving the septum.

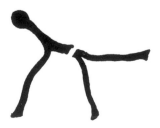

In LBBB, the atrial impulse conducts normally through the atria and through the AV junction. A blockage in the left bundle branch causes depolarization of the septum and left ventricle to occur *more slowly*. In left bundle branch block, the right ventricle is activated in a normal fashion. The left ventricle is then activated by an impulse from the right bundle branch which passes to the left side of the septum below the block. Thus, activation of the left ventricle is delayed causing a widening of the QRS!

Again, let's put this into perspective!

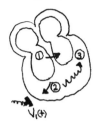

(1) Septal activation is abnormal, moving left to right. The force of septal depolarization moves away from the positive V_1 electrode. Thus, the initial part of the QRS is directed negatively. (2) The right ventricle depolarizes normally, with the direction of depolarization moving toward the positive electrode. So, the second part of the QRS will be upwardly directed. (3) Left ventricular activation occurs abnormally, moving away from the positive electrode!

The "textbook" picture of LBBB in a V_1 lead is that of a distorted W. Usually, however, the W is not well defined. Rather, the picture presents as follows.

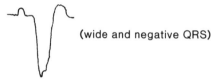

(wide and negative QRS)

To distinguish left from right bundle branch block, one must look at the V leads.

EKG CRITERIA FOR LBBB

- QRS measures 0.12 seconds or greater.

- QRS is wide and may be notched—the T wave is usually inscribed in the opposite direction to the R wave in most leads.

- W or V pattern seen in leads V_1 and V_2.

- M pattern (rsR') seen in leads V_5 and V_6.

- Secondary ST and T wave changes.

If this is complicated, just remember . . .

In LBBB, the QRS in lead V_1 will appear wide and negative.

No matter what lead you observe, the QRS will be widened . . . measuring 0.12 seconds or greater! Here is a V_1 monitor tracing showing LBBB. Notice that the QRS measures 0.14 seconds.

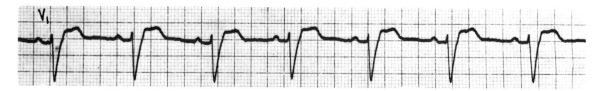

In the previous strip, the rhythm is regular at a rate of 62 beats per minute. P waves precede each QRS complex. All P waves appear uniform. The P-R interval is of normal duration. The QRS complexes are uniform, occur regularly, and measure 0.14 seconds. The QRS is wide and negative. In lead V_1, a widened and negative QRS characterizes left bundle branch block.

So, this is a sinus rhythm with **LBBB**!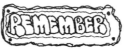

Though *rate dependent* bundle branch block is usually the result of delayed right bundle branch conduction, it occasionally occurs because of delayed left bundle branch conduction! See for yourself! Here is a rate dependent left bundle branch block.

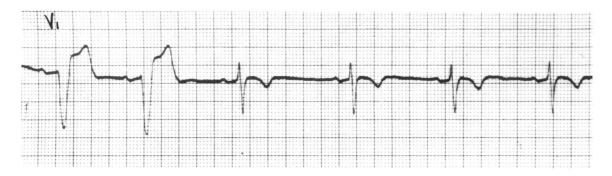

Rate dependent left bundle branch block. It is easy to be fooled by wide QRS's . . . always look for P waves! If a P wave comes before the widened QRS, a bundle branch block exists. (If no P wave is observed before the QRS, the beat is of ventricular origin.) Notice that as the heart rate slows, conduction becomes normal.

To clarify any confusion . . . **REMEMBER** . . .

if a rhythm is normal except for a QRS that measures 0.12 seconds or greater, the patient has a bundle branch block.

To distinguish between a right and left bundle branch block, look at lead V_1!

> LBBB = QRS is wide and negative in lead V_1
>
> RBBB = QRS is wide and positive in lead V_1

It is the extent of myocardial damage causing a bundle branch block that determines patient prognosis.

Practice Exercise 7

Are you ready for more practice? PRACTICE, PRACTICE, PRACTICE . . . This is worse than piano lessons!

1. This is a patient's monitor strip (lead 2):

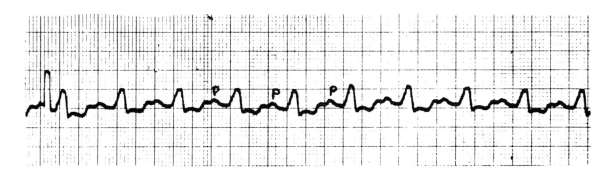

The rhythm is regular with a heart rate of approximately 100 beats per minute. Each QRS complex is preceded by a P wave, and all P waves appear uniform. The QRS complexes, however, are FAT!

BONUS

Generally speaking . . .

there are only two types of rhythm patterns with FAT QRS's . . . ventricular beats and bundle branch block beats. Ventricular beats DO NOT HAVE P WAVES PRECEDING THEM!

Neat, huh?

So, since there are P waves in the above strip, this must be bundle branch block.

BUT WHICH TYPE . . . RIGHT OR LEFT????

To distinguish right from left bundle branch block, one must look at the V leads—particularly V_1 and V_6.

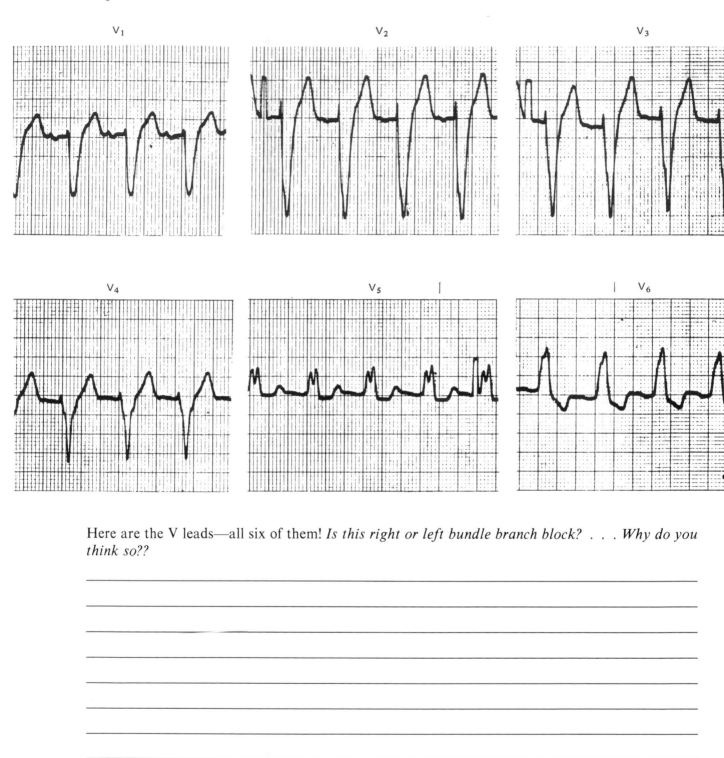

Here are the V leads—all six of them! *Is this right or left bundle branch block? . . . Why do you think so??*

_____

_____

_____

_____

_____

_____

_____

_____

2. Another patient has a monitor picture that looks like this (lead 2):

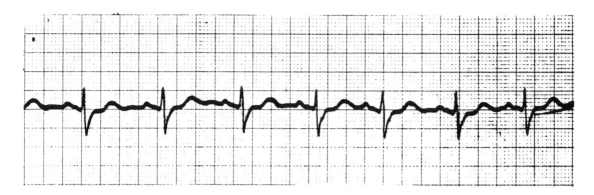

Everything looks normal—**except** that the QRS's measure 0.12 seconds. To be normal, the QRS duration must be less than 0.12 seconds!

Because you are a *suspicious* creature, you look at the patient's chart—at his 12-lead EKG. Here are the V leads! What do you think???

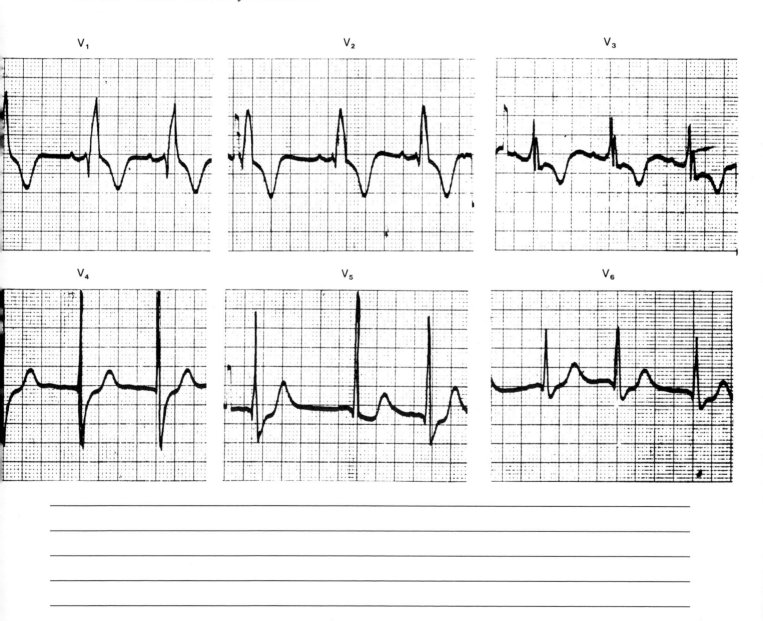

_____

_____

_____

_____

3. This is a little lady with a rate related ___Bundle___ bundle branch block.

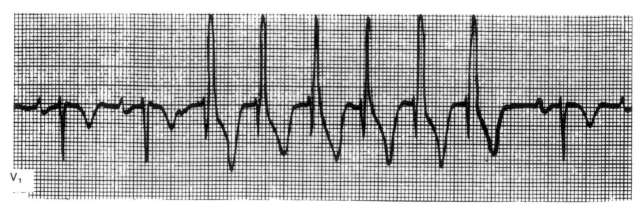

V₁

What do you think she is doing?

_____

_____

_____

_____

_____

For **Feedback 7,** refer to page 166.

Feedback 1

How did you do? Hope your interpretation resembles mine!

The rhythm is irregular, but the heart rate is probably within normal limits. There are P waves preceding each QRS and the P-R interval is constant, measuring slightly greater than 0.16 seconds. The QRS duration is within normal limits measuring 0.06 seconds. There is a pause in the sinus mechanism. A P wave fails to occur at the expected time. The pause measures greater than 1.4 seconds.

Feedback 2

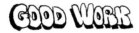

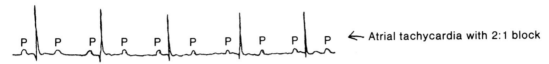

← Atrial tachycardia with 2:1 block

Atrial rate regular between 160-200 per minute.
(Don't forget, the P-R is always constant!)

Feedback 3

How did you do? Like I said before . . . if Input 1 is confusing, try rereading it **again** when you have completed this section!

1.

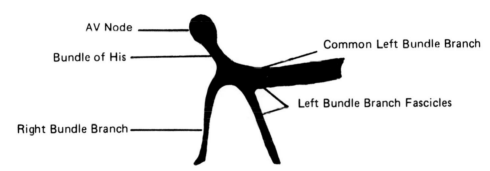

AV Node

Bundle of His

Common Left Bundle Branch

Left Bundle Branch Fascicles

Right Bundle Branch

2. Atrial depolarization is represented on the EKG as a <u>P</u> wave. The P-R interval represents <u>the transmission of the pacemaker impulse from the atria to the Purkinje system.</u>
   The QRS represents <u>ventricular depolarization</u>.

3. By placing a catheter electrode in the <u>bundle of His</u>, depolarization of the bundle of His can be recorded. The His bundle deflection occurs between the <u>P</u> wave and the <u>QRS</u> complex of an EKG cycle.

4. The interval from the P wave to the bundle of His deflection is known as the <u>P-H</u> interval.

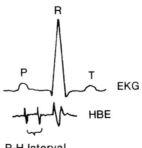

R

P   T

EKG

HBE

P-H Interval

The interval from the bundle of His deflection to the onset of ventricular depolarization is known as the <u>H-V</u> interval.

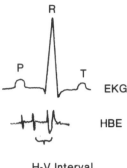

H-V Interval

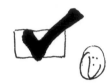

Feedback 4

Excellent work!

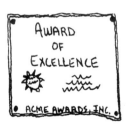

1. The rhythm is regular with a heart rate of approximately 100 beats per minute. P waves precede each QRS. The P waves are uniform in appearance, sitting on the down slope of the T waves. The QRS complexes are narrow, less than 0.12 seconds. But, voila! The P-R interval is prolonged. The P-R interval measures approximately 7½ small squares or approximately 0.30 seconds. The QRS measures 0.08 seconds. So, this is a borderline sinus tachycardia with a first degree heart block!

$$\begin{array}{r} 0.04 \\ \times 7.5 \\ \hline 0.30 \end{array}$$

2. The P-R interval in this rhythm strip measures approximately <u>6</u> little squares or <u>0.24</u> seconds. The QRS measures approximately 0.08 seconds.

$$\begin{array}{r} 0.04 \\ \times 6 \\ \hline 0.24 \end{array}$$

3. HBE studies have shown that the conduction defect or delay in first degree heart block usually lies <u>above</u> the bundle of His. First degree heart block is usually benign and serves only <u>to be watched</u>.

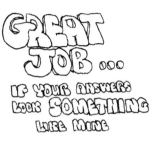

Feedback 5

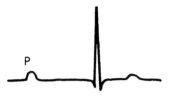

1. The rhythm is irregular. Some of the P waves are not followed by QRS complexes. The P-R interval gradually lengthens until finally a P wave is not conducted. The R-R interval shortens. The cycle then repeats. This is "OUR FRIEND" WENCKEBACH! usually a <u>benign</u> arrhythmia.

2. This rhythm is irregular and one must become a detective to discover why. There are three cycles that appear identical. The P-R interval of the first beat measures 0.20 seconds. The P-R interval of the second beat measures almost 0.24 seconds. This same pattern is evident in complexes 3 and 4, and 5 and 6. This is a Wenckebach (Mobitz type I) rhythm. The P wave that fails to conduct (after beats 2, 4 and 6) is somewhat obscured, though it follows the T wave and is flat in appearance.

3. The rhythm is regular with a heart rate of approximately 45. There are two P waves for every QRS. Atrial activity is regular. The QRS complexes are widened, measuring approximately 0.11 seconds. This is a 2:1 AV conduction with widened QRS complexes. This may be a Mobitz type II AV block, so it should be observed *closely*! In order to distinguish between a Mobitz type I and type II, two beats *must* be conducted consecutively so one can determine the constancy or progression of the P–R interval.

Feedback 6

Nice work.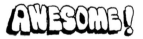

1. Complete heart block means that <u>none of the sinus impulses are being conducted to the ventricles to initiate ventricular contraction</u>.

2. Because none of the atrial impulses are conducted to the ventricles, a lower more distal pacemaker will usually initiate ventricular activation. This is an <u>ESCAPE RHYTHM</u>.

3. If the escape rhythm has narrow QRS complexes and a rate of 40–60 beats per minute, it is probably an <u>idiojunctional or junctional escape rhythm</u>. If the escape rhythm has a slow rate (20–40 beats per minute) and wide QRS complexes, it is an <u>idioventricular or ventricular escape rhythm</u>.

4. P waves are occurring in a regular pattern at a rate of 105 per minute. The P waves appear to be "marching" through the rhythm strip. The QRS complexes are occurring regularly at a rate of approximately 28 per minute. The QRS complexes are wide, measuring 0.16 seconds. There is no relationship between the P waves and the QRS complexes. The P-R interval is <u>never</u> constant. This is complete heart block with an idioventricular escape rhythm.

To review, complete heart block has the following features:

A. Atrial and ventricular rates are different.
B. The atrial rate is faster.
C. The ventricular rate is slow and regular.
D. The QRS complexes may be narrow or wide.
E. The P-R interval is <u>never</u> constant—the P waves appear to be "marching" through the rhythm strip.

Feedback 7

Outstanding achievement! You win the key to the city!

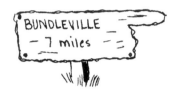

1. This is left bundle branch block because the QRS in V₁ is wide and negative.

2. I think this is a sinus rhythm with right bundle branch block! The QRS measures greater than 0.12 seconds and V₁ shows a wide, positively directed QRS.

3. <u>Right</u> bundle branch block (wide, positive QRS in lead V₁).

   The little lady is sitting in a rocking chair. When she rests, her heart rate is approximately 70 beats per minute and conduction is normal. When she rocks, her heart rate speeds up . . . and voila! A rate related RBBB!

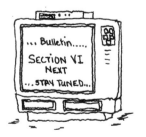

NOTES

NOTES

Section VI
Artifact . . . To Be, or Not To Be . . .

OBJECTIVES

When you have completed Section VI, you will be able to describe or identify

1. electrical artifact encountered in monitoring
2. appearances and sources of artifact
   a) 60-cycle interference
   b) motion artifact
   c) signals from other electrical equipment
   d) "off the monitor"
3. problems caused by artifact
4. principles of artifact recognition
5. steps to reduce or eliminate artifact

Text by:

DELORES D. SCHULTZ

Input 1: Introduction to Artifact

Now that you have been through all of the basic dysrhythmias (yes, all of them), you may need a change of pace.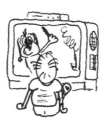

Sometimes you will encounter "things" on a monitor tracing that have nothing whatsoever to do with the heart. These are commonly known as *artifact* or *electrical interference*. Other popular words are "glitches" or "noise." Artifact, then, is an electrical signal which appears on the tracing and which originates from sources other than the heart!

Let's try a simple analogy.

This is a kid watching cartoons on Saturday morning:

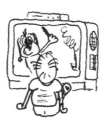

Here is the mother in the next room cleaning . . . and . . . she turns on the vacuum.

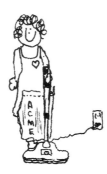

Instantly, above the noise of the vacuum, the mother hears, "OKAY, WHAT'S WRONG WITH THIS PICTURE?"

The picture looks like this:

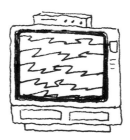

What is a mother to do???
  a. Kick the television.
  b. Send it off for repair.
  c. Turn off the vacuum.

Fortunately, this mother chose alternative c. The picture now looks like this:

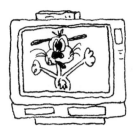

And the kid looks like this:

In this case there was nothing wrong with the television *and* there was nothing wrong with the vacuum. Simply stated, *the impulses generated by one electrical device in operation interfered with the correct operation of a second electrical device.* The precise electrical theory behind all of this is very complicated . . . at least, *I* think so.

If the mother plugs the vacuum into a different outlet, she may discover that the T.V. is working fine and the kid still looks like this:

. . . or, she may elect to finish vacuuming at some later time!

A monitoring system attached to a patient acts a lot like the television. The monitoring system picks up electrical signals form the heart and transmits them to an oscilloscope. If another electrical device is in operation nearby, electrical signals generated from that device may be picked up by the monitoring system, thus interfering with the monitor picture. What you see on your tracing may look like this.

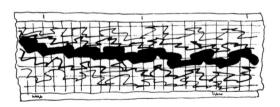

Like the T.V. and the vacuum, the patient's heart <u>and</u> the electrical device are probably operating cor-

rectly . . . it's just that the electrical device is altering the monitor picture. 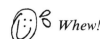 *Whew!*

To monitor your patient effectively, you will need to be able to recognize artifact when it appears, distinguish it from a patient's rhythm, and take appropriate steps to minimize the artifact.

Practice Exercise 1

Now for a short practice session:

FILL IN THE BLANK

1. "Glitches" or "noise" on the monitor tracing is known as _____ , or electrical interference.

True or False

2. ___ The presence of artifact is a signal that there is a disturbance in the heart's electrical activity.

3. ___ The presence of artifact is an indication that an electrical device in proximity to the patient is malfunctioning.

FILL IN THE BLANK

4. To monitor a patient's rhythm effectively, you will need to be able to _____ artifact when it appears, _____ it from the patient's rhythm, and take appropriate steps to _____ it.

Not too difficult so far, huh?

For **Feedback 1,** refer to page 188.

Input 2: Sixty-cycle Interference

There are several different kinds of artifact commonly encountered in monitoring. This tracing shows 60-cycle interference.

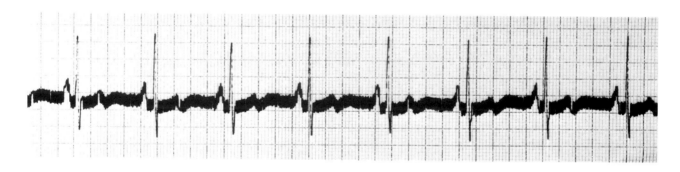

Sixty-cycle interference is characterized by a *wide, fuzzy baseline* which makes atrial activity difficult to recognize. A "good" tracing should have a narrow, distinct baseline. Monitors may normally show a few seconds of 60-cycle interference when they are first turned on. If the interference persists, it is usually related to *faulty electrode contact*. Poor electrode contact is usually the result of inadequate skin preparation techniques, dried electrode gel, or defective wires or patient cable.

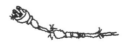

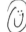 The source of 60-cycle interference is the current which supplies power to the electrical wall outlets.

The 60-cycle energy is given off by the electrical wiring in the patient's room and is picked up by both the lead wires and the patient. This is *normal,* and this radiant energy *cannot be eliminated.* Although monitors are designed to reduce 60-cycle interference, there must still be good contact along the path from the patient skin to the monitor, *and* the electrical path must be well shielded.

Specific interventions (*anti-artifact techniques*) include checking to see that the EKG cable is not draped across, or parallel to, other cables (such as call-light, electric bed, or transducer cables). Also, the EKG cable must not touch the metal parts of other electrical equipment such as side rails of electric beds or metal portions of ventilators.

To determine the origin of, and to correct, electrical interference (artifact), try momentarily *pulling the plug* of any other electrical equipment in contact with the patient. Also, make certain there are no loose connections in the monitoring system. It may be helpful to apply new electrode patches using correct skin prep (more about that later). If these techniques are unsuccessful, check for defective wires using a leadwire continuity tester, and replace any which do not produce a steady glow . . .

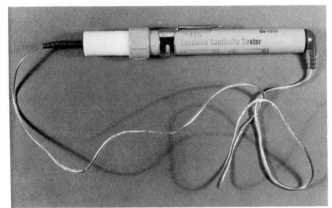

A leadwire continuity tester

or check for a defective monitor cable by trying a different cable. Whew!

Now, it's your turn. You are officially commissioned as a "troubleshooter" or a detective. This is your patient's monitor tracing:

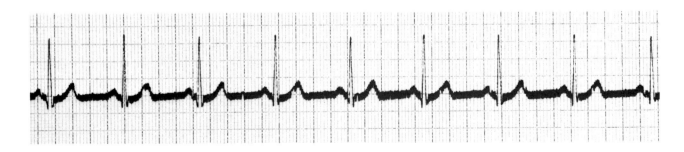

Here is your patient: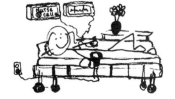

What should you do?

    a. Yell, "What's wrong with this picture?"
    b. Notify the doctor, "Your patient's gone into atrial fibrillation."
    c. Try moving the cable away from the call light cable.

If you chose c, your patient's tracing now looks like this:

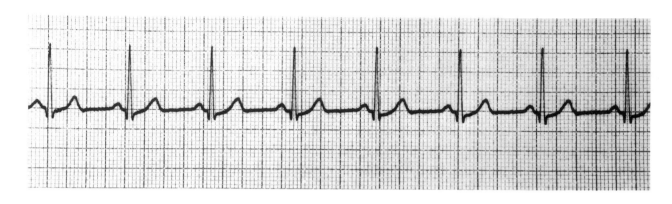

Nice work! ☺

Practice Exercise 2

1. Sixty-cycle interference is characterized by a _____ baseline.
2. Identify at least five ways to reduce 60-cycle interference:

    a. _____

    b. _____

    c. _____

    d. _____

    e. _____

For **Feedback 2,** refer to page 188.

Input 3: Motion Artifact

This is an example of motion artifact:

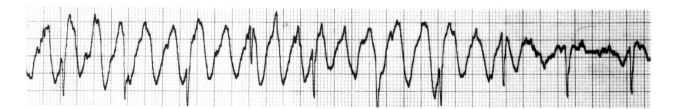

A Fairy Tale:

Long, long ago in a CCU far away, a nurse saw this tracing on the monitor. Mr. Jones, the patient, had not been looking too well prior to this "picture." The nurse raced to the room and administered a resounding thump on the patient's chest. Mr. Jones stopped brushing his teeth, leaped from the bed, and was out of the door in a flash, never to be seen again. 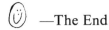 —The End

The moral of the story . . . *look (before) the patient leaps!*

Motion artifact can be the *most troublesome* and *confusing* type of artifact, even for the "so-called" experts! Many patients have undeservedly been thumped on the chest or given lidocaine for this kind of tracing. If the nurse had looked at the patient before thumping, she would have had the first clue that this was artifact and *not* ventricular tachycardia. If she had checked his pulse, she would have noted that his pulse was regular at a rate of approximately 80.

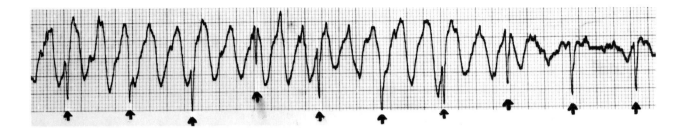

In this strip, you will notice (see arrows) that there are sharp deflections throughout the entire tracing (which just happen to coincide with the patient's pulse). These deflections are QRS complexes. Since ventricular contraction follows ventricular depolarization (QRS), and ventricular contraction results in a pulse, you can usually verify the presence or absence of QRS complexes by checking the patient's pulse. (Neat trick, huh?)

Believe it or not, the *skin* is the source of the small electrical signals which produce motion artifact. A voltage of several millivolts can be generated by stretching the outer layer of skin, the epidermis. It is the stretching which results in the artifact. *Large baseline shifts* occur when the patient turns over in bed, brushes his teeth, taps an electrode, etc.

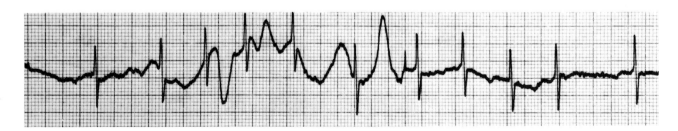

This strip demonstrates an example of a shifting baseline. If an electrode is placed close to the diaphragm, even the skin movement produced by breathing will cause artifact!

Here are some examples of motion artifact:
The notorious toothbrush artifact . . .

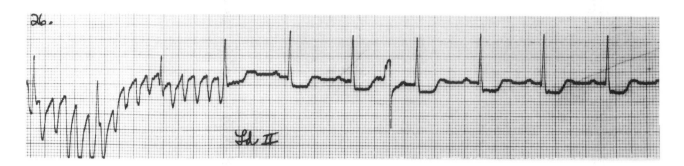

Here the artifact might be mistaken for atrial flutter. Did you notice, though, that the R-R interval (the distance between any two R waves) remains precisely the same when the "supposed flutter" converts to sinus rhythm? In other words, measure the R-R interval at the beginning of the strip and compare that to an R-R interval at the end of the strip. Voila! It's the same! This would *seldom* occur if an actual atrial flutter were converting to a sinus rhythm! There is usually a pause when atrial flutter stops, and then, a different ventricular rate when the sinus node takes over. Makes sense, right?

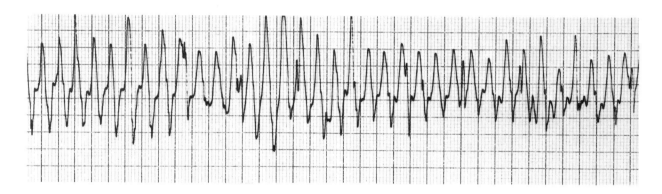

This is another patient (like the one in the fairy tale), brushing his teeth. This strip sent a "rescue squad" rushing to the patient's room in belief that the patient was in ventricular flutter. Can you find the narrow spikes appearing in the tracing at a rate of approximately 95? Those are the patient's normal QRS complexes . . . and correspond to the patient's pulse. When in doubt, check the patient's pulse. If the patient is alert and in no distress, it is highly unlikely that he or she has a heart rate of 300!

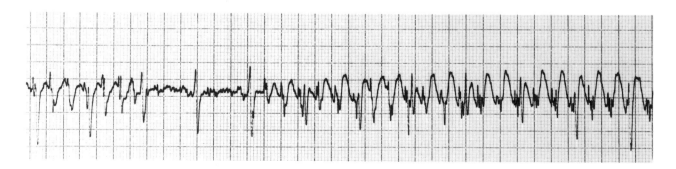

This is the same patient a few seconds later still brushing his teeth, but now his underlying rhythm is more visible! Notice that there is no change in the QRS rate from the previous strip. This constant rate strongly suggests that the underlying rhythm is the same as in the previous strip. If there is any doubt in your mind about a rhythm, always assess the patient. *It is especially important to compare the patient's pulse with the monitor picture.*

Here are two other tracings which contain artifact that mimics ventricular dysrhythmias. In strip A, the patient is swinging his monitor cable. In strip B, an electrode is being tapped. (*Some smart patients learn that if they tap their electrode, someone will appear immediately.*) By now, you can easily discern artifact! The narrow electrical spikes "walk through" the artifact and correspond to the normal QRS complexes.

A.

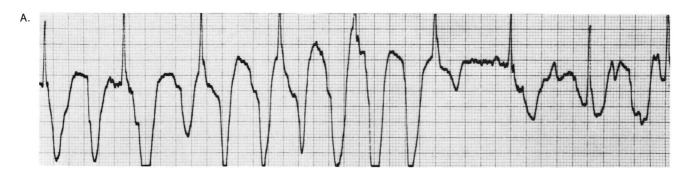

B.

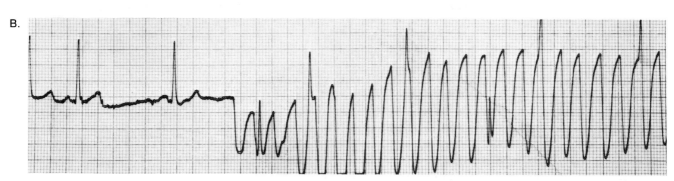

The next strip is more difficult!

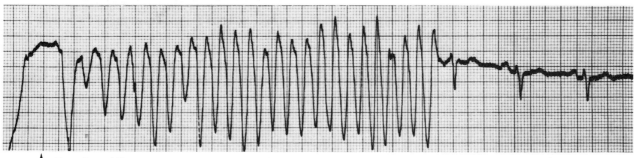

↑ Baseline shift

177

This tracing would send almost anyone running for lidocaine, *including* me. There are two clues that indicate this might possibly be artifact. The first clue is the shift in the baseline that occurs before the onset of what appears to be "ventricular tachycardia." This shifting baseline strongly suggests that the patient is moving. The second clue relates to the termination of the "ventricular tachycardia." When a patient converts from a ventricular tachycardia to a sinus rhythm, there is *almost always a pause* after the ventricular tachycardia. It is important to note that in this tracing, the ventricles would not have sufficient time to repolarize before we see the first normal QRS. If this were a true ventricular tachycardia (rather than artifact), the sinus beat following the termination of the "ventricular tachycardia" would *usually* be widened since the ventricular recovery period is not complete!

What should you do if you cannot decide between artifact and what might be a run of ventricular tachycardia? Here are four *possible* actions, although step 3 is most important.

1. Get someone else's opinion. Two or three, or more, heads are often better than one when it comes to deciphering a puzzling strip.
2. If the patient's physician happens to be present, let him or her diagnose the rhythm and determine the treatment.
3. Check with the patient. He may admit to the fact that he was idly *tapping* his electrode . . . or you might catch him brushing his teeth!
4. If you are still unable to decide, lidocaine would be the treatment of choice. It is better to treat the rhythm than to risk the consequences of further serious ventricular dysrhythmias.

Following are other examples of motion artifact:

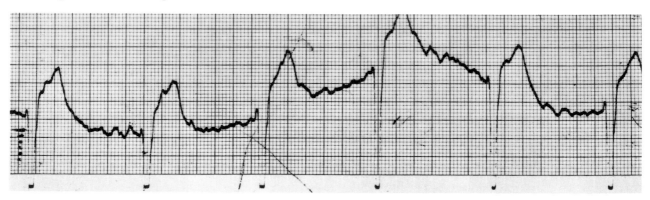

This is called *wandering baseline*. It is the result of pronounced, slow, patient movements, such as stretching, turning over in bed, and so forth.

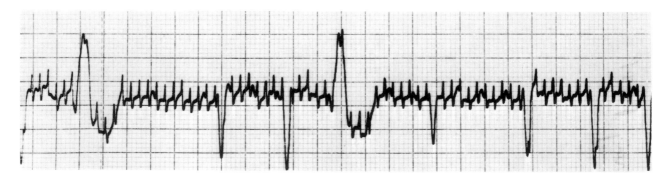

This patient is receiving *chest percussion* and drainage (for respiratory disorders). *Motion* from seizure

178

activity or muscle tremor could also produce this pattern. It is usually impossible to diagnose atrial dysrhythmias with this type of artifact. (Brilliant, right?!)

This tracing demonstrates one type of respiratory artifact:

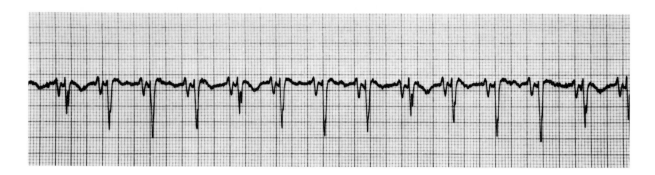

Notice that there is a *cyclic* variation in the QRS amplitude and configuration, as well as in the T waves. Chest wall movement during normal respiration can produce cyclic changes in the baseline, the QRS amplitude, and the T wave appearance! When assessing the patient, one can usually correlate his respiratory cycle with the changes that appear on the monitor.

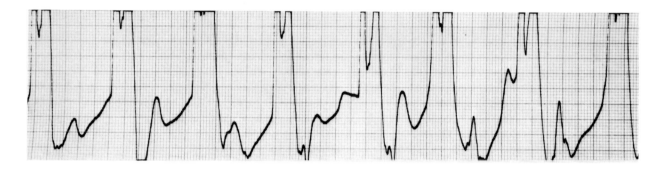

The above tracing is an example of what may be seen when a patient is coding. The artifact is produced by chest compression, or CPR. In order to visualize the underlying rhythm, compression must be stopped momentarily. See for yourself!

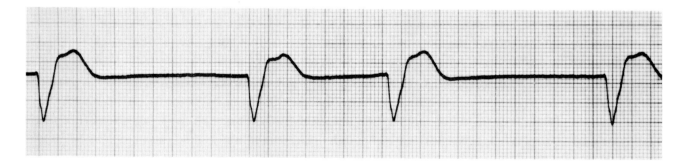

The underlying rhythm is obvious when chest compression is momentarily interrupted.

The foremost responsibility in dealing with motion artifact is to *recognize it* as artifact! Accurate analysis will prevent unnecessary patient treatment and will prompt you to take steps to eliminate the artifact. *It is important to eliminate the artifact so that any underlying dysrhythmias will not be masked.*

Some of the same *principles* for eliminating 60-cycle interference also apply to motion artifact. Correct skin preparation and an ample quantity of gel on the electrode patches can effectively reduce motion artifact. To prevent cable and wire movement, clip the cable to the patient's clothing. Perhaps there is an underlying clinical problem which may need medical treatment. Check to see if the patient is having tremors, seizure activity, or an increase in movement because of discomfort or confusion. Ask the patient to lie quietly or assist him in doing so if you need to analyze an underlying rhythm. You may reduce respiratory artifact by monitoring on a lead where the positive electrode is *not* over the diaphragm, for example, lead I. (Remember the bedside version of lead I? . . . If you need a quick review, turn back to page 10.) You may reduce motion artifact in general, by *attaching the electrodes over bony areas* rather than over skin folds, large muscle masses, joints, or large amounts of fatty tissue!

Always check the patient before treating any dysrhythmia. Remember, one should . . .

TREAT THE PATIENT, NOT THE MONITOR

Practice Exercise 3 . . . Your Turn

1. Motion artifact usually results from electrical signals produced by the _____ .

2. Describe how you can tell this tracing shows motion artifact rather than ventricular tachycardia.

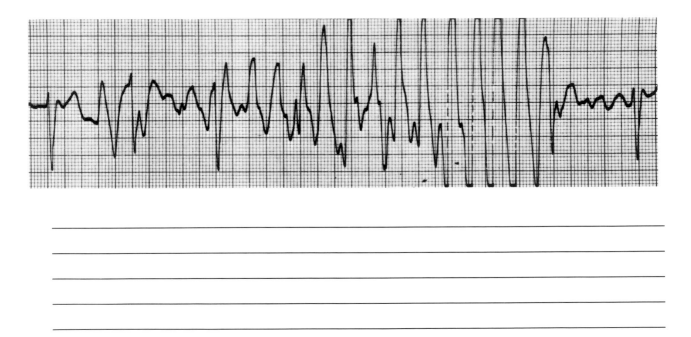

_____

_____

_____

_____

_____

3. List at least three steps you could take to reduce the motion artifact in this tracing to create a better "picture."

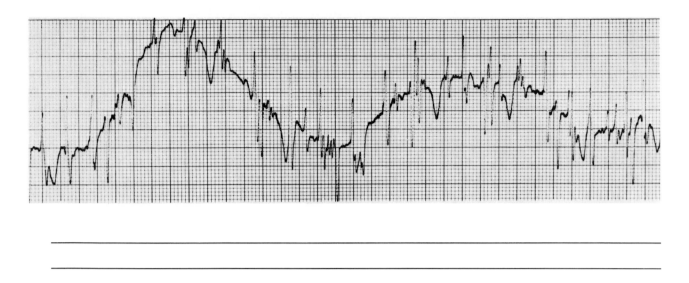

_____

_____

_____

For **Feedback 3,** refer to page 188.

Input 4: Artifact Produced by Electrical Equipment

More artifact . . . ugh!

The next type of artifact that we will discuss originates from *signals* produced by *electrical equipment* in the monitoring area. This artifact appears as little "blips" on the monitor tracing. Two types of electrical equipment, *pacemakers and pain control devices* (TENS), may produce these little blips!

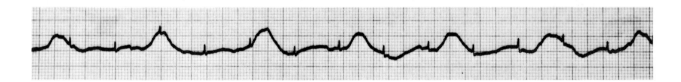

The above tracing demonstrates pacemaker signals, or spikes, produced whenever a patient's pacemaker fires in an attempt to trigger an electrical impulse in the heart. In this particular strip, the only electrical activity one sees originates from the pacemaker. There is no electrical activity arising in the patient's heart and needless to say, *this patient is in trouble*! The *rhythmic motion* (roller coaster) artifact present is probably the result of chest compressions. Pacemaker spikes may have a positive, negative, or biphasic deflection, and their amplitude will vary depending on the lead. Usually, lead II will show a prominent spike. Without going any further into pacemaker mechanics, you can learn to recognize pacemaker spikes when they appear on a tracing.

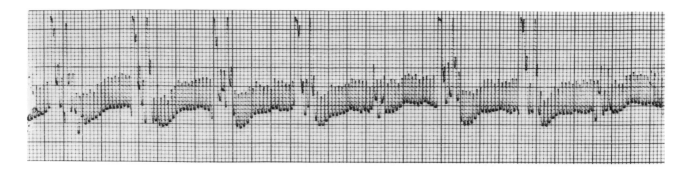

When this patient was admitted to a monitored stepdown unit, the artifact present on his tracings caused quite an uproar until the staff became aware that the patient had a *TENS* unit. *TENS* stands for a *transcutaneous electrical nerve stimulator*. People who suffer from some types of chronic pain may experience pain reduction or elimination by wearing this electrical device. Whenever this TENS unit was turned on, the monitor tracing looked like the one above. In order to obtain a meaningful 12 lead EKG and monitor tracing, the TENS unit had to be turned off.

How about a simple practice exercise?

Practice Exercise 4

1. Little "blips" or spikes occuring on a monitor tracing usually originate from adjacent electrical equipment. Two of the *most*-frequent electrical equipment culprits are _____ and _____ .

2. Pacemaker spikes may be nearly invisible or they may have a larger amplitude than the patient's QRS complexes. This variation in amplitude often depends on the _____ .

For **Feedback 4,** refer to page 189.

| **Input 5: "Off the Monitor"** |

The following tracing (page 183) is from a patient who is "off the monitor." The straight line, indicating the absence of rhythm, may be mistaken for asystole. If you have experience with monitors, you already know that the most common cause of an "asystole-appearing" tracing is a loose electrode. Rarely do patients go directly from a normal rhythm to the complete absence of any rhythm! Reattaching the wire or electrode will restore the normal rhythm to the scope.

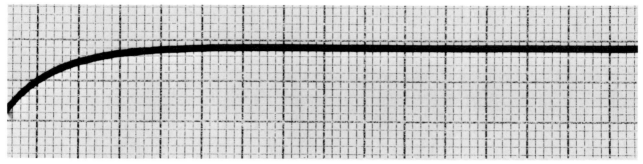

"Off the monitor"

At this point, however, I am reminded of a little lady who, in fact, did go into asystole (the absence of rhythm) from her normal rhythm. The "rescue squad" went to her room immediately to reattach the electrode and found themselves calling a code. Here the maxim is, *"look at the patient—immediately."*

In most monitoring systems, all of the electrodes must be attached to the patient in order for a tracing to be present. If the wires come loose at either end, if an electrode patch comes loose, or if a wire is broken internally, the tracing will disappear.

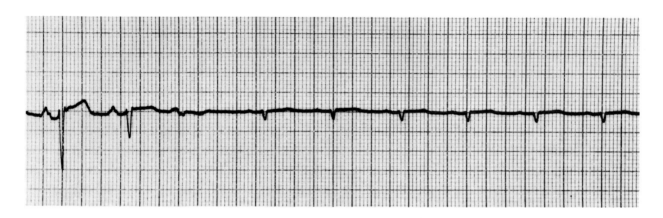

In the above strip, the amplitude setting is decreased and the tracing nearly disappears. The monitor can then no longer "see" the QRS complexes and a rate alarm may be activated.

When your patient looks like this . . .

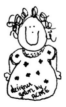

and her tracing looks like this . . .

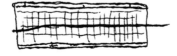

there are several steps you may take to solve the problem.

STEPS FOR CORRECTING "OFF THE MONITOR"

1. Reattach any disconnected wires.
2. Check to see that the cable is attached to the monitor.
3. Check electrode patches for intactness and replace any loose patches, making certain that an ample amount of gel is present.
4. Check the wires with a lead tester for breakage and replace if necessary.
5. Check for a defective cable by replacing the cable.
6. Check the amplitude setting to see if the amplitude is set correctly.

Sometimes the patient intermittently goes "off the monitor" and the tracing looks like this!

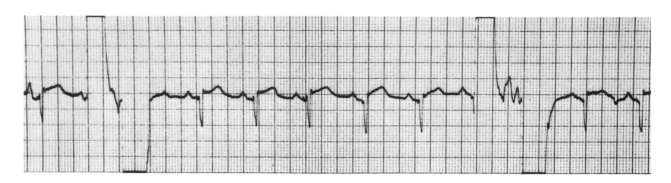

This type of tracing is produced by intermittent interruption of the continuous path from the patient to the monitor. It may be remedied by all the same actions that one might take if the patient were completely "off the monitor."

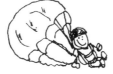

Practice Exercise 5

GO FOR IT!

1. Describe what has happened in this tracing:

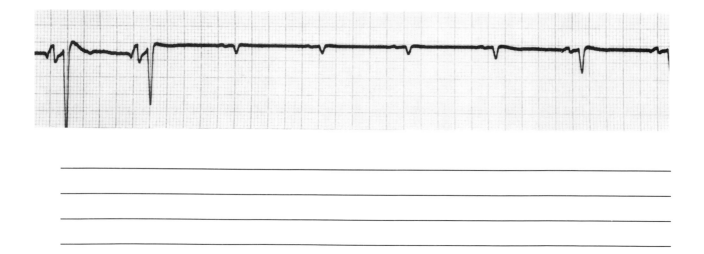

_____

_____

_____

_____

2. Name at least three steps you can take when a patient's tracing looks like the above strip to make it appear like this:

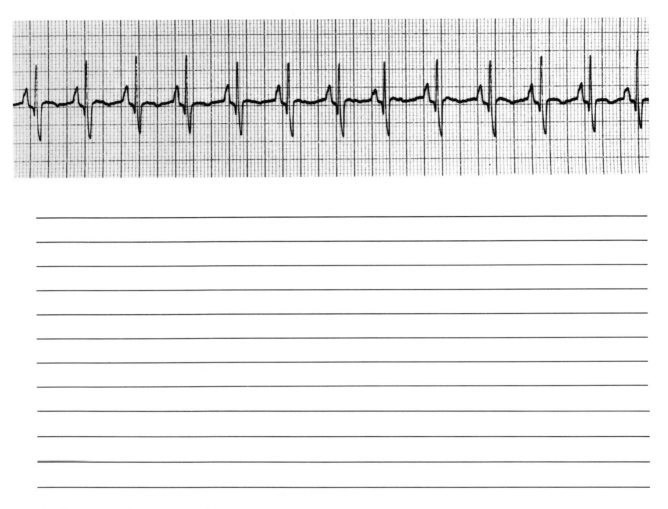

_____

_____

_____

_____

_____

_____

_____

_____

_____

_____

_____

_____

For **Feedback 5,** refer to page 189.

Input 6: Problems Associated with Artifact

There are *three* main problems which may be associated with artifact. The *first* is that artifact may *mimic* atrial or ventricular dysrhythmias and cause treatment to be initiated unnecessarily. (Even if you do not treat the patient, it may cause you unnecessary worry.) With a little practice you will be able to look at a tracing and recognize that something is "wrong with the picture," not your patient's heart!

Here is a list of *clues* that may help you in *determining* the presence of artifact.

CLUES FOR IDENTIFYING ARTIFACT

1. Baselines should be fine, narrow lines.
2. QRS complexes <u>must</u> be followed by T waves. Whenever ventricular depolarization occurs, ventricular repolarization must follow. Also, there cannot be T waves which are not preceded by QRS complexes. If you see a T wave in the middle of nowhere or a QRS complex not followed by a T wave, chances are this is artifact.
3. A change in supraventricular rhythm, e.g., atrial flutter to sinus rhythm or vice versa, is usually accompanied by a change in ventricular rate.
4. Cells in the heart cannot be depolarized by two impulses simultaneously. They must repolarize after the first impulse before they can be depolarized by a second. If you see portions of your patient's QRS complexes superimposed on a run of "ventricular tachycardia," the "V tach" is probably artifact. Whew!
5. P waves should have an established rhythm and a logical configuration. P waves do not usually appear out of nowhere, except sometimes in digitalis toxicity or sick sinus syndrome. If P waves occur early in the cardiac cycle, there should be a pause before the next P wave is seen.
6. Patients rarely go from a normal rhythm to a straight line rhythm. *Usually,* they are off the monitor because of a disconnected electrode or patch. However, ALWAYS check the patient!

If you are still uncertain after considering all of these points, get a second opinion, and remember—look at the patient!

The *second* problem associated with artifact is that it may *mask* underlying dysrhythmias which deserve or warrant treatment. With experience, you will be able to determine the cause of the artifact and then procede with appropriate measures to reduce or eliminate it. For troubleshooting steps, refer back to the specific type of artifact covered in this chapter.

The *third* problem relating to artifact is that it is *time consuming*! Time is spent recognizing and attempting to eliminate confusing artifact! If a computerized monitoring system with storage capacity is in use, it requires additional time to go back and change the computer analysis of the rhythm. Computers really are not very smart . . . they tend to call any large shift in baseline a P.V.C.!

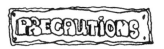

One may take a few simple precautions to prevent or reduce artifact and the problems it causes. The *first* is assuring the presence of conductive gel. (If electrode gel is partially dry, problems with 60-cycle interference and motion artifact will be magnified and intermittent loss of tracing may occur. Completely dry gel will result in the *absence* of any tracing.) To prevent drying, store the electrodes in their original foil package until ready for use. Keep the package tightly closed and avoid storing the container in warm areas. Use the electrodes prior to the expiration date on the package and check each one for adequate gel before applying it to the patient.

The *second precaution* to help prevent artifact is correct skin preparation. Smith ("Rx for EKG Monitoring Artifact," <u>Critical Care Nurse</u>, 1984) recommended a technique which involves removing the outer layer of epidermis, scratching the second layer, and defatting the skin. Removing the outer layer and scratching the second layer can most effectively be accomplished by five to ten strokes with 320–400 grit fine sandpaper (HONEST!). This type of sandpaper is found on the backside of some electrodes. Packaged electrode gels containing gritty materials may also be used. Fine sandpaper or electrode gels produce minimal skin damage or irritation. Vigorous rubbing with a gauze pad or abrading with a rough surface are accepted techniques, but they generally produce more reddening of the skin and do not succeed in scratching the second layer of epidermis. Also, remember that you only have to prep the skin where the gel portion of the electrode is to be applied.

To defat the skin, that is, to remove oils, rub with an alcohol gauze pad. Avoid using acetone which is more irritating, produces less contact, and is a fire hazard!

We will probably have to cope with the various kinds of artifact as long as we monitor patients' cardiac rhythms. The ability to recognize and eliminate artifact is a skill which will help you to monitor your patients safely, effectively, and efficiently.

Before moving on to practice exercise 6, you will need to know that *recognizing artifact is a function of experience*! I do not expect you to remember all the details in this section. However, a periodic review of this material may be helpful. (Personal note from the management!)

Practice Exercise 6

1. QRS complexes must be followed by _____ , and T waves must be preceded by

   _____ .

2. When you see QRS complexes superimposed on a "run of ventricular tachycardia," the "V tach" is

   probably_____ .

3. Describe three methods for storing electrodes to prevent drying of the gel.

   a. _____

   b. _____

   c. _____

4. _____ is the best compound for defatting the skin.

For **Feedback 6,** refer to page 189.

Feedback 1

You probably have answered all the practice exercises correctly. If so . . . **HOORAY!** ☺

1. "Glitches" or "noise" on the monitor tracing is known as <u>artifact</u>, or electrical interference.

2. False. (The presence of artifact is *NOT* a signal that there is a disturbance in the hearts' electrical activity.)

3. False. (The presence of artifact is *NOT* an indication that an electrical device in proximity to the patient is malfunctioning.)

4. To monitor a patient's rhythm effectively, you will need to be able to <u>recognize</u> artifact when it appears, <u>distinguish</u> it from the patient's rhythm, and take appropriate steps to <u>minimize</u> it.

Feedback 2

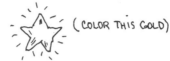 (COLOR THIS GOLD)

You are quickly becoming an expert!

1. Sixty-cycle interference is characterized by a <u>wide</u>, <u>fuzzy</u> baseline.

2. Any of these are acceptable answers:
   a. Make certain that the EKG cable is not draped across, or parallel to, other cables such as call-light, electric bed, or transducer cables.
   b. Make certain that the EKG cable is not touching the metal parts of other electrical equipment.
   c. If possible, try momentarily pulling the plug of any other electrical equipment in contact with the patient to see if the artifact disappears.
   d. Tighten any loose connections in the monitoring system.
   e. Apply new electrode patches using correct skin preparation.
   f. Check for the presence of sufficient gel on the electrode patches.
   g. Replace any defective wires.
   h. Try a different monitor cable.

Feedback 3

You are becoming more skillful at coping with artifact! . . .

1. Motion artifact usually results from electrical signals produced by the <u>skin</u>.

2. This is a little more difficult.
   a. The beginning of the strip shows motion artifact that is fairly obvious and does not look like ventricular tachycardia. This gives you a clue that the patient is moving.
   b. During the portion that looks like "V tach," you can still walk the normal QRS complexes through, and in most cases you can see portions of the normal QRS.
   c. A QRS complex occurs immediately after the cessation of "V tach." There is usually a pause before a normal QRS appears.

3. Any of the following responses are correct. ☺
   a. Check with the patient to see if you can help reduce excessive patient motion.
   b. Make certain all the electrode patches are secure and that sufficient gel is present.
   c. Secure loose wires.
   d. Replace defective wires.
   e. The wandering baseline could be due to respirations. Try changing the location of the positive electrode slightly or try switching to a lead I.
   (Perhaps you can think of others that I neglected to mention.)

Feedback 4

You're doing super!

1. Little "blips" or spikes occurring on a monitor tracing usually originate from electrical equipment. Two of the *most* frequent electrical equipment culprits are <u>pacemakers</u> and <u>pain control devices</u>.

2. The variation in amplitude often depends on the <u>lead</u>.

Feedback 5

You know almost everything there is to know about artifact!

1. Someone has decreased and then increased the amplitude setting. (Sometimes your *tricky* cohorts may try to fool you.)

2. Any three of these actions can be considered:
   a. Make certain that all patches and wires are intact.
   b. Make certain that the monitor cable is plugged in.
   c. Check for defective wires and replace if necessary.
   d. Check for a defective cable by replacing the cable.

Feedback 6

You are truly an expert! (If you have not *absolutely* mastered this material, do not panic.) You may wish to refer back to this chapter for future help when problems with artifact develop.

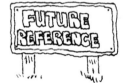

1. QRS complexes must be followed by <u>T waves</u>.

2. T waves must be preceded by <u>QRS complexes</u>.

3. When you see QRS complexes superimposed on a "run of ventricular tachycardia," the "V tach" is probably <u>artifact</u>.

4. Methods for storing electrodes to prevent drying of the gel include:
   a. Keep the electrodes in their original foil package.
   b. Close the package tightly.
   c. Avoid storing in warm areas.
   d. Use the electrodes prior to their expiration date.

5. <u>Alcohol</u> is the best compound for defatting the skin.

NOTES

Section VII
Cardioversion and Defibrillation

OBJECTIVES

When you have completed Section VII, you will be able to describe or identify

1. refractory and vulnerable periods in the cardiac cycle
2. synchronized precordial shock or cardioversion
3. nonsynchronized precordial shock or defibrillation

In previous sections, reference was made to *precordial shock* as a treatment for uncontrolled rapid dysrhythmias producing hemodynamic imbalance. To appreciate precordial shock treatment, one must have an understanding of the cardiac cycle.

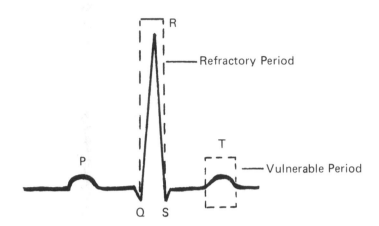

Each cardiac cycle has a *vulnerable period,* essentially the T wave. During this brief period, any electrical stimulus (a shock from an electrical appliance, lightening, a ventricular premature beat, etc.) that occurs during this vulnerable period *may* induce ventricular fibrillation. The vulnerable period is *extremely* sensitive to any electrical stimulation. Likewise, delivering precordial shock during this vulnerable period may cause the nonfibrillating patient to fibrillate!! Since Russian roulette is hardly a therapeutic measure, a method for administering precordial shock that *eliminates* the possibility of the electrical impulse falling during the vulnerable period must be used. Simply, this is *synchronized cardioversion.* Looking at the above illustrated cardiac cycle, you will notice that the QRS is labeled *REFRACTORY.* Refractory simply indicates that the ventricles are in the process of depolarizing; therefore, they are *immune* or *refractory* to any additional electrical stimulation. The QRS, the refractory period, is then a nonvulnerable period in the cardiac cycle. Any electrical stimulus occurring during this refractory period will *not* cause the heart muscle to fibrillate.

Logically then, if precordial shock is to be administered, the electrical energy should be released during the nonvulnerable or refractory period. This is accomplished by synchronizing the defibrillator unit with the patient's heart rhythm. By connecting a cable from any EKG recording device (EKG machine, or monitor) to the defibrillator unit, and setting the synchronize button, the defibrillator unit will be able to sense the tall R wave of the QRS cycle.

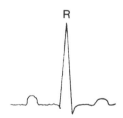

In other words, the defibrillator unit will recognize the R wave of every QRS complex. The defibrillator unit will have an indicator (usually a blinking light signal) that will let you know it is sensing the R wave appropriately. Each time the light blinks, it's saying "I see an R wave, I see an R wave" . . . etc.

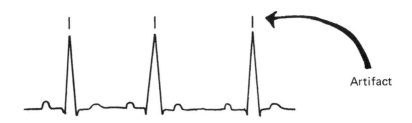

Artifact

In addition, the monitoring device will show an artifact above each R wave. The artifact also indicates that the defibrillator unit is reading or sensing the R wave of each QRS complex. Now, no matter when in the cardiac cycle the buttons for releasing the electrical energy are pressed, the defibrillator unit will not deliver the energy until it senses the R wave! Neat, huh? The synchronized defibrillator does *all* the work.

In essence then, this synchronization prevents the electrical shock from occurring during the vulnerable period (T wave).

The following rhythm strip illustrates a fast supraventricular tachyarrhythmia. Because the patient's clinical condition is deteriorating, the rhythm must be terminated as rapidly as possible. Though the location of T waves or vulnerable periods are uncertain, we *know* that each time the heart muscle depolarizes, there is a rest or recovery period (T wave).

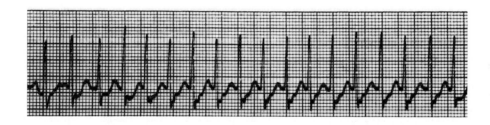

The fastest and most effective way for terminating such a rhythm is synchronized cardioversion. In this instance, we must first synchronize the defibrillator unit with the patient's heart rhythm—because the accidental induction of ventricular fibrillation is non-therapeutic!! Delivering synchronized precordial shock to the patient's chest wall causes all the myocardial cells to depolarize or discharge at once. This momentarily stops all myocardial activity. Hopefully, the patient's sinus pacemaker will then resume as the controlling pacemaker, restoring a normal rhythm! Of course, the patient may need ectopic-suppressing drugs to prevent any abnormal rhythm from breaking through again.

Usually, a *minimal* current setting is all that is required to disrupt a rapid supraventricular rhythm. Commonly, the current setting ranges from 10–250 watt/seconds. However, it is good to remember that the current setting will vary with patient size and the dysrhythmia being treated, considering whether or not the patient has been receiving digitalis or other drugs.

There are two types of precordial shock, *synchronized* and *nonsynchronized*. Synchronized precordial shock is most usually referred to as *CARDIOVERSION*. Nonsynchronized precordial shock is referred to as *DEFIBRILLATION*.

Before, we indicated that there *must* be a QRS complex in order to deliver a synchronized precordial shock. When QRS complexes are *absent*, *defibrillation* or *nonsynchronized* precordial shock is used.

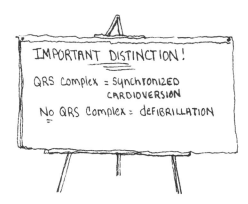

Both synchronized cardioversion and defibrillation work on the same principle. Electrical energy of brief duration is delivered through the chest wall. This shock causes depolarization (release of energy) of all myocardial cells which halts the chaotic or ectopic activity. At this point, all seasoned "rhythm-watchers" say a silent prayer that the "good ol' sinus node" will resume control of the heart rhythm.

Now, look at this rhythm.

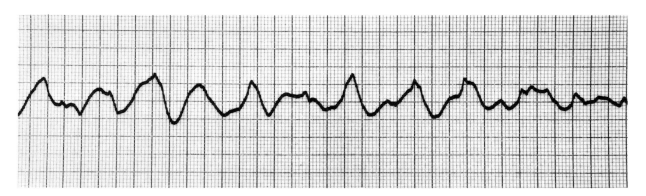

This is a coarse ventricular fibrillation. (It looks like atrial fibrillation *without* any QRS's!) To interrupt this chaotic ectopic activity, precordial shock must be instituted. . . .

. . . but which kind?

synchronized, or nonsynchronized?
cardioversion, or defibrillation?

AH-HA! Since there are no QRS's, it's *impossible* to use synchronized precordial shock! As a matter of fact, if you set or programmed the defibrillator unit to deliver synchronized shock, the machine would *NEVER* release the energy through the paddles. It would hold the engergy until it "sensed" an *R wave* . . . which would never appear!

So, in this strip, because there are no QRS complexes, nonsynchronized precordial shock or defibrillation would be used. Thus, the energy is delivered through the paddles at any point during the chaotic rhythm, as soon as the "energy delivery" buttons are pressed.

When nonsynchronized precordial shock or defibrillation is performed, a high current setting is used—usually between 200 and 400 watt/seconds of energy (depending upon the patient's size and chest wall thickness).

Practice Exercise 1

Let's see how much you remember!

Here is a QRS complex. Label the refractory and vulnerable periods.

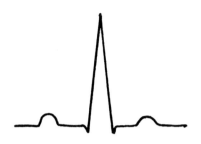

Refractory means that _____

_____

_____

Vulnerable implies that _____

_____

_____

_____

_____

In synchronized precordial shock, or _____ the defibrillator unit will deliver its

energy *only* on _____ of the EKG cycle.

When defibrillation or nonsynchronized precordial shock is used, the defibrillator unit will deliver its

energy _____

_____

_____

_____

_____

Here is the rhythm strip of a little lady experiencing severe chest pain and a falling blood pressure.

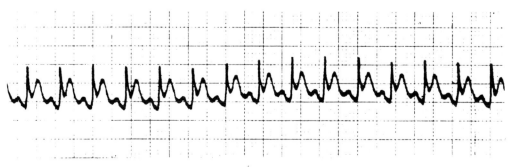

1. This rhythm is an _____ . Because her clinical condition is deteriorating rapidly, it has been decided to administer precordial shock to terminate the ectopic rhythm.

   (circle one) Cardioversion / defibrillation would be used because _____

   _____

   _____

   _____

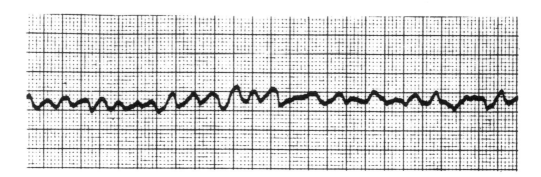

2. The rhythm strip above is that of a code arrest victim. _____ precordial shock would be administered because there are no _____ complexes!

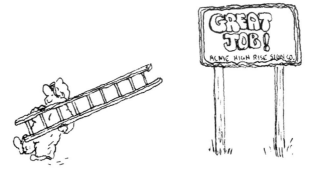

For **Feedback 1,** see next page.

Feedback 1

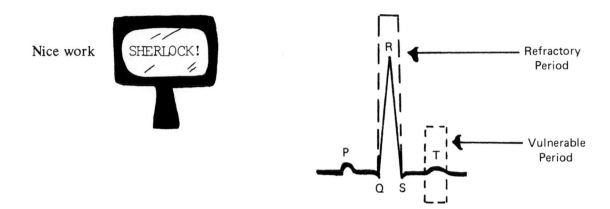

Nice work SHERLOCK!

Refractory Period

Vulnerable Period

Refractory means that <u>this phase in the cardiac cycle (the QRS) is immune to any additional electrical stimulation.</u>

Vulnerable implies that <u>this phase in the cardiac cycle (the T wave) is extremely sensitive to any electrical stimulation. Electrical stimulation during the vulnerable period may induce ventricular fibrillation.</u>

In synchronized precordial shock, or <u>CARDIOVERSION</u>, the defibrillator unit will deliver its energy <u>only</u> on the <u>R WAVE</u> of the EKG cycle.

When defibrillation or nonsynchronized precordial shock is used, the defibrillator unit will deliver its energy <u>as soon as the energy delivery buttons are pressed, anywhere in the chaotic rhythm.</u>

1. This rhythm is <u>atrial tachycardia</u>. (For a quick review of atrial tachycardia, see page 00.)

    <u>Cardioversion</u> would be used because <u>there are QRS complexes and because we don't want to risk the chance of having the patient fibrillate.</u>

    MAKING A PATIENT FIBRILLATE IS NOT A THERAPEUTIC MEASURE!

    (a thought for the day)

2. <u>Nonsynchronized</u> precordial shock or defibrillation would be administered because there are no <u>QRS</u> complexes.

NOTES

Section VIII
Pacemaker Basics

OBJECTIVES

When you have completed Section VIII, you will be able to describe or identify

1. the anatomy and physiology of temporary and permanent pacemakers
2. indications for pacemaker support
3. pacemaker induced heart rhythms
4. pacemaker sensing and capture
5. pacemaker programming

Text by

DEANNA M. CULBERSON

Section VIII is included to provide a basic overview of temporary and permanent pacemakers. Like other technology, pacemakers continue to evolve into smaller and more sophisticated devices. However, their basic intent never changes!

Input 1: Pacemaker Anatomy and Physiology

Pacemakers have "been around" since the 1930s and have been an accepted modality for the treatment of bradyarrhythmias since 1952. A pacemaker is a therapeutic intervention utilized to bolster an inadequate heart rate, or initiate an atrial and/or ventricular response in the absence of normal pacemakers.

PURPOSES FOR PACEMAKER INSERTION

- to increase slow or inadequate ventricular heart rates

- to stimulate atrial activity in the absence of a sinus pacemaker

- to stimulate ventricular activity in the absence of a ventricular or higher order pacemaker

---

Temporary pacemakers utilize an external generator (power source) connected to a pacing wire.

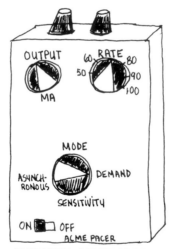

EXTERNAL GENERATOR

OUTPUT or MA — The Impulse Strength Emitted from
  the Generator

RATE = Setting Determines the Timing of Impulses, or the
  Number of Impulses Emitted Per Minute

MODE / SENSITIVITY = Determines Sensitivity to the Patient's
  Own Rhythm

The pacing wire is introduced into a central vein and advanced through the right atrium (RA) into the right ventricle (RV).

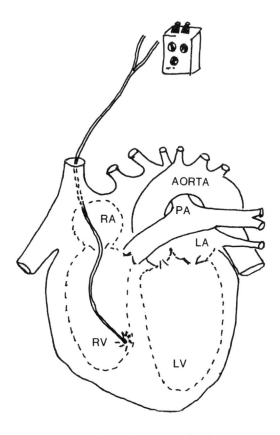

Right Ventricular Pacing

The pacing wire comes into contact with the right ventricular muscle wall. A generated and timed (rate) electrical impulse then causes the ventricular muscle cells to depolarize from the point of stimulus.

It should be noted that patient movement or careless caregiving can dislodge the temporary pacing wire from the right ventricular muscle wall. This results in a failure of the generated impulse to initiate depolarization.

Owing to the location of impulse origination (outside the normal conduction pathway), cells depolarize in a slow and abnormal pattern. Thus, ventricular pacemakers produce widened QRS complexes.

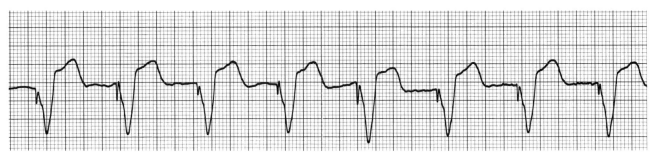

Ventricular pacemakers produce wide QRS complexes. A pacemaker spike precedes each QRS.

Temporary pacemakers are introduced to support short-term, inadequate heart rate pathology or in crisis, or anticipated crisis, situations.

ANTICIPATED SHORT-TERM INADEQUATE HEART RATE PATHOLOGY

- Second degree heart blocks related to acute myocardial infarction
- Drug-induced bradyarrhythmias

CRISIS INTERVENTION

- Third degree heart block
- Symptomatic bradycardia
- Post cardiac surgery

A decision to implant a permanent pacemaker is usually based on permanent or long-term pathology.

EXAMPLES OF LONG-TERM PATHOLOGY

- Sick sinus syndrome
- Third degree heart block
- Sensitive carotid sinus syndrome

Permanent pacemaker function is similar to that of a temporary pacemaker with two notable differences. A permanent pacemaker generator is surgically implanted beneath the skin, and the pacing wire is secured to the right ventricle or the right atrium and right ventricle. Permanent pacemakers have either one (right ventricular) or two (right atrial, right ventricular) pacing wires or leads allowing one or two cardiac chamber muscles to be artificially stimulated.

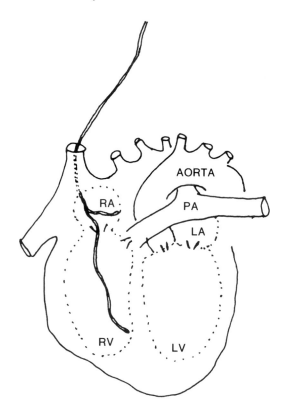

PERMANENT PACEMAKER WITH TWO PACING WIRES.
(RIGHT ATRIUM / RIGHT VENTRICLE)

IN BOTH TEMPORARY AND PERMANENTLY IMPLANTED PACEMAKERS, THE PACEMAKER WIRE(S) IS PLACED IN THE RIGHT HEART MUSCLE WALL.

TEMPORARY PACEMAKER LEAD PLACEMENT

- RIGHT VENTRICULAR MUSCLE WALL

PERMANENT PACEMAKER LEAD PLACEMENT

- RIGHT VENTRICULAR MUSCLE WALL (ONE LEAD VARIETY)
  OR
- RIGHT ATRIAL AND RIGHT VENTRICULAR MUSCLE WALL (TWO LEAD VARIETY)

PACEMAKER STIMULATION INDUCES CELL DEPOLARIZATION IN THE PACED CHAMBER(S). THAT WAVE OF DEPOLARIZATION THEN SPREADS OUTWARD, ACTIVATING ALL MYOCARDIAL MUSCLE CELLS . . . MORE OR LESS OF A DOMINO EFFECT!

Permanent pacemakers must be manually programmed for both rate and function to achieve the desired therapeutic effect. A three letter code guides that manual programming. A function code letter [A], [V], [O], or [D] is selected from each of the vertical, numbered columns.

1	2	3
Chamber Paced	Chamber Sensed	How Pulse Generator Responds
[A] = Atrium	[A] = Atrium	[O] = Not Applicable
[V] = Ventricle	[V] = Ventricle	[I] = Inhibited (Demand)
[D] = Dual (Atrium and Ventricle)	[O] = Not Applicable	[T] = Triggered
	[D] = Dual (Atrium and Ventricle)	[D] = Dual (inhibited and triggered)

An *inhibited* or *demand* generator response means that a pacemaker impulse is generated only when the patient's own heart rate falls below the pacemaker set rate. In other words, if the pacemaker does not "sense" atrial or ventricular activation at, or above, the prescribed (set) pacemaker rate, the generator will release a stimulus. If, however, the patient's heart rate is "self-maintained" at a rate greater than the set generator rate, the generator will not initiate an electrical stimulus!

A demand type setting is sometimes referred to as "synchronous" pacing since the pacemaker generated impulse occurs irregularly, on an "as needed" basis only. The pacemaker works in synchrony with the underlying rhythm. **TEAM WORK!**

In contrast, a *triggered* or non-demand setting programs the pacemaker to fire continuously at the fixed or set rate, regardless of any underlying rhythm. Obviously, this setting is used when the patient's own pacemaking capability is limited or absent! A triggered generator response is sometimes referred to as "asynchronous" pacing. You will note on the previous chart (column 2) that the pacemaker generator is programmed to "sense" patient generated heart activity. An A setting indicates that the generator is set to identify patient generated atrial activity and then respond in accord with the programmed column 3 response.

WHEW!

The following example programming sequence might be used for a permanent single lead pacemaker.

1	2	3		
V	V	I :	Paced	= Ventricle
			Sensed	= Ventricle
			Response	= Inhibited

The above pacemaker programming sequence would achieve pacing of the ventricle (column 1) when ventricular contraction is not sensed (column 2). The pacemaker would fire on demand only, in the absence of a sensed ventricular response (column 3).

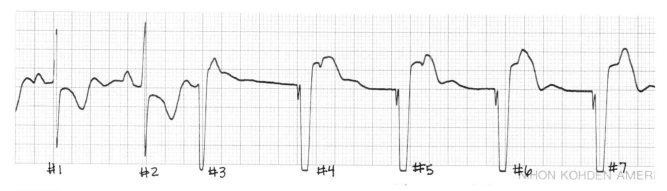

V V I setting. When the pacemaker senses normal heart ventricular activity (beats 1, 2, and 3), it does not discharge a stimulus. When a ventricular beat fails to occur at the expected time (pause following premature beat 3), the pacemaker begins firing. Note the pacemaker spikes occurring before beats 4–7.

Here is another programming example:

1	2	3		
D	D	D :	Paced	= Dual (Atrium and Ventricle)
			Sensed	= Dual (Atrium and Ventricle)
			Response	= Dual (Atrium and Ventricle)

This is an example of an AV (atrial/ventricular) sequential pacemaker. Here the generator paces both the right atrium and the right ventricle, in sequence, and upon demand. In other words, when patient-generated atrial and ventricular activation fails to occur, the pacemaker initiates first an atrial, and then a ventricular (sequenced) stimulus. This dual sensing and pacing requires a two lead pacemaker system! The advantage of an AV sequential pacemaker is that it allows complete atrial emptying and improved ventricular filling (a.k.a. "atrial KICK").

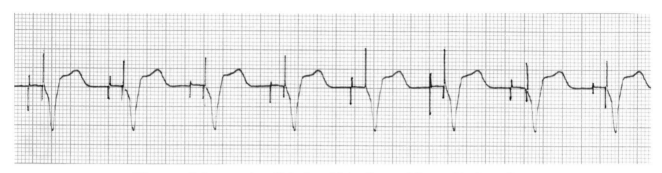

AV sequential pacemaker. Note the atrial spikes and the ventricular spikes.

Practice Exercise 1

1. List two reasons for instituting pacemaker therapy.

   a. _____

   _____

   b. _____

   _____

2. Temporary pacemakers are used to support *anticipated* short-term pathology or to correct crisis situations. List three underlying rhythm disturbances that may warrant temporary pacemaker insertion.

   a. _____

   b. _____

   c. _____

3. Permanent pacemakers differ from temporary pacemakers in two important ways:

   a. _____

   _____

   b. _____

   _____

4. An inhibited or demand pacemaker generator response means that

   _____

   _____

   _____

For **Feedback 1,** refer to page 211.

The pacemaker generator (temporary or permanent) "sends out" a small electrical current intended to stimulate the cells at the point of pacemaker wire or lead contact. In actuality, this generated stimulus creates an irritable focus at the point of muscle contact. This irritation causes cellular depolarization which spreads across the myocardium, outside the normal conduction pathway. Sound familiar?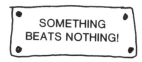

This artificial stimulation is much like a P.V.C. or a P.A.C. You will recall from Section IV that a P.V.C. results from an irritable focus within the ventricles. The wave of ventricular cell depolarization produced by the P.V.C. is slow and anomolous, producing a widened and distorted QRS! In the case of a P.A.C., an irritable focus within the atria causes anomolous atrial depolarization, changing the appearance of the P wave.

The *logical* question to ask is, "Why would one want to artificially create irritable foci in the atria and/or ventricles"? The answer is simple. When there is no rhythm, or an ineffective underlying rhythm, something (artificial ectopic-type activity) beats nothing!!!!

> **SOMETHING BEATS NOTHING!**

When assessing a pacemaker rhythm strip, one must know the pacemaker programming sequence:

- Rate
- Chamber(s) paced
- Response (demand or asynchronous)

The rhythm strip is then evaluated to determine performance in accord with that programming.

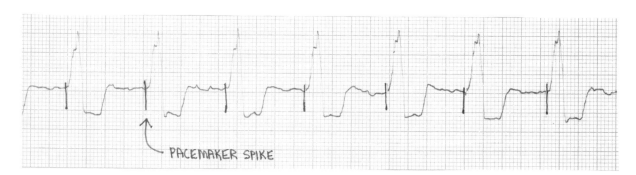

PACEMAKER SPIKE

The above figure demonstrates a ventricular demand pacemaker. The patient's underlying heart rate fell below the pacemaker generator set rate, resulting in a pacemaker induced rhythm. The firing of the pacemaker is evidenced by a prominent spike preceding the QRS. The pacemaker is said to *capture* if the pacemaker spike produces the desired end result (the QRS).

The next strip demonstrates a ventricular pacemaker (demand) competing with the patient's own rhythm. Only when the patient's underlying rhythm slows below the generator set rate does the pacemaker "kick in." The pacemaker spike precedes the pacemaker generated QRS. Nifty!

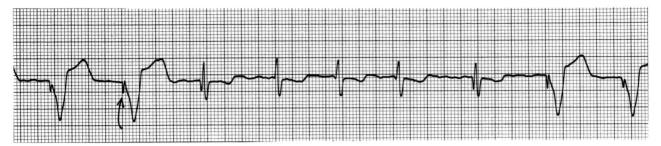

Note the pacemaker spikes preceding each pacemaker induced beat

The following strip is interesting! The first four beats demonstrate a sinus rhythm. Beat 5 is a premature beat of questionable origin that interrupts the underlying rhythm. You will remember that a pause follows a premature beat allowing the sinus pacemaker to reset. However, this patient has a pacemaker programmed on a [V] [V] [I] setting. Since the pacemaker does not sense a ventricular response at the expected time, the pacemaker generator begins pacing. Obviously, the sinus pacemaker failed to resume control of the rhythm!

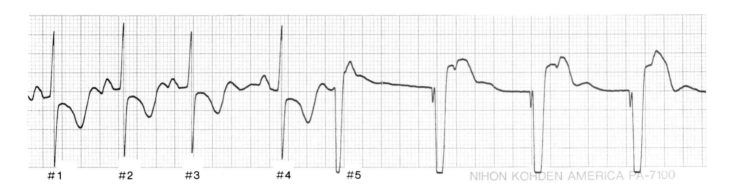

#1   #2   #3   #4   #5   NIHON KOHDEN AMERICA PA-7100

A dual lead AV sequential pacemaker stimulates and activates the atria and ventricles, in sequence. Depending on the program setting, the pacemaker will fire continuously (triggered) or on demand. Atrial pacing will appear on the EKG as a prominent spike preceding the P wave. The "paced" P wave appears similar to a "non-paced" P wave. Following atrial activation, the generator will initiate ventricular stimulation producing a prominent spike prior to the QRS. The pacemaker induced QRS will be wide owing to the anomolous path of ventricular depolarization.

DUAL LEAD AV SEQUENTIAL PACING

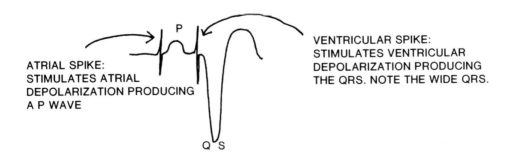

ATRIAL SPIKE:
STIMULATES ATRIAL
DEPOLARIZATION PRODUCING
A P WAVE

VENTRICULAR SPIKE:
STIMULATES VENTRICULAR
DEPOLARIZATION PRODUCING
THE QRS. NOTE THE WIDE QRS.

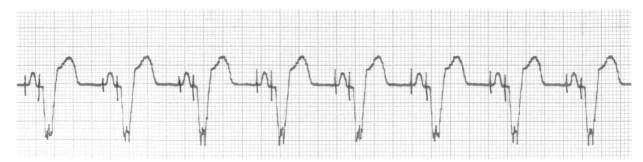

AV sequential pacemaker

When a pacemaker is programmed in an AV sequential mode, one must observe the EKG for the presence of both atrial and ventricular pacemaker spikes and capture. The interval between the atrial and ventricular spikes simulates a P-R interval.

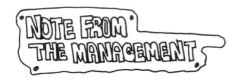

Most implanted pacemakers are of the AV sequential variety (dual lead) and are programmed on a D D D setting. However, when implanted in patients with chronic atrial fibrillation, AV sequential pacemakers are programmed to a V V I setting. Owing to the chronicity of the atrial pathology, the "atrial fib" patient usually does not benefit from the pacemaker induced atrial kick (atrial pacing).

Practice Exercise 2

1. When assessing a pacemaker rhythm strip, one must know the pacemaker programming sequence which includes _____ , _____ , and _____

   _____ .

2. Draw a cardiac cycle demonstrating dual lead AV sequential pacing.

For **Feedback 2,** refer to page 211.

Input 3: Determining Pacemaker Rate

Determining pacemaker rate on an EKG strip is a function of measuring the interval (small squares) between two consecutively paced beats. The trusty rate guide on page 39 can then be consulted, or one can divide 1500 (the number of small squares in one minute) by the number of small squares between the two consecutive paced beats. In the following strip, the pacemaker rate (ventricular rate) is 71 per minute!

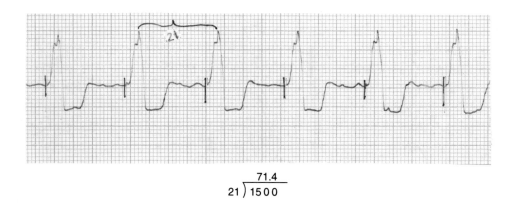

$$\begin{array}{r} 71.4 \\ 21\overline{)1500} \end{array}$$

Practice Exercise 3

1. Calculate the heart rate in the following AV sequential pacemaker rhythm.

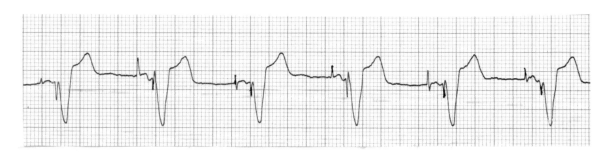

Atrial rate = _____ .
Ventricular rate = _____ .

For **Feedback 3,** refer to page 211.

Input 4: More about Capture

Earlier, the term *capture* was introduced. Capture is the term used to connote muscle depolarization occurring secondary to a pacemaker stimulus. Capture occurs when a pacemaker spike is followed by the appropriate cardiac complex (P wave or QRS). *Non-capture* is present when a pacemaker spike fails to produce the desired effect (atrial depolarization or ventricular depolarization). Non-capture may result from: pacemaker malfunction; failure of the generator; lead placement in electrically inactive scar tissue; or, drifting of the lead wire(s) away from the muscle wall. When non-capture occurs, any of the following *medical* actions may be appropriate.

METHODS FOR "FIXING" PACEMAKER NON-CAPTURE

• Increase energy output of generator

• Change power source

• Reposition the pacer wire (medical intervention)

The degree of medical emergency resulting from sustained non-capture is dependent upon the presence of a life sustaining underlying rhythm.

The following strip demonstrates pacemaker malfunction.

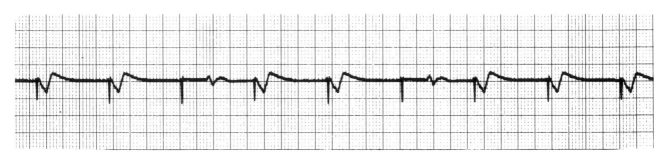

A quick "eyeball" analysis reveals pacemaker spikes occurring regularly throughout in the tracing. The pacemaker is not sensing the underlying rhythm and pacemaker spikes fail to capture. (This patient was scheduled for a "pacemaker replacement"!)

Practice Exercise 4

1. Pacemaker capture means _____

_____

_____ .

2. Pacemaker non-capture *may* be corrected by any of these three methods:

    a. _____

    b. _____

    c. _____

For **Feedback 4,** refer to page 212.

In summary, the indications for the various types and modes of pacing vary greatly depending upon the type and severity of the underlying dysrhythmia, the etiology of the dysrhythmia, and the extent of hemodynamic embarrassment.

This section was intended to be an introduction to pacemakers and a future reference!

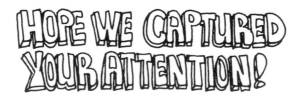

Feedback 1

1. Pacemaker therapy may be instituted for any of the following reasons:
    a. to increase slow or inadequate ventricular heart rates.
    b. to stimulate atrial activity in the absence of a sinus pacemaker.
    c. to stimulate ventricular activity in the absence of a ventricular or higher order pacemaker.

2. Any of the following rhythm disturbances may warrant temporary pacemaker insertion:
    a. second degree AV block associated with acute myocardial infarction.
    b. bradyarrhythmias associated with drug therapy.
    c. third degree AV (complete) block.
    d. symptomatic bradycardia.

3. Permanent pacemakers differ from temporary pacemakers in two important ways:
    a. a permanent pacemaker generator is surgically implanted beneath the skin.
    b. the permanent pacemaker wire(s) is *secured* to the right ventricle or the right ventricle and right atrium.

4. An inhibited or demand pacemaker generator response means that <u>a pacemaker impulse is generated only when the heart rate falls below the pacemaker set rate.</u>

Feedback 2

1. When assessing a pacemaker rhythm strip, one must know the pacemaker programming sequence which includes *rate, chamber(s) paced,* and *response (demand or asynchronous).*

2. Your diagram should look something like this!

DUAL LEAD AV SEQUENTIAL PACING

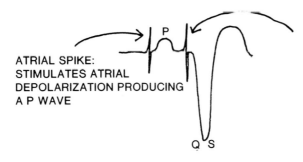

ATRIAL SPIKE: STIMULATES ATRIAL DEPOLARIZATION PRODUCING A P WAVE

VENTRICULAR SPIKE: STIMULATES VENTRICULAR DEPOLARIZATION PRODUCING THE QRS. NOTE THE WIDE QRS.

Feedback 3

1. The AV sequential paced heart rate is 60 per minute.
        Atrial rate = *60*
        Ventricular rate = *60*

Feedback 4

1. Pacemaker capture means that muscle depolarization is caused by the pacemaker stimulus. On the EKG strip, capture occurs when a pacemaker spike is followed by the appropriate cardiac complex (P wave or QRS).

2. Pacemaker non-capture *may* be corrected by
   a. increasing the energy output of the pacemaker generator.
   b. changing the generator (power source).
   c. repositioning the pacer wire.

Bonus Points

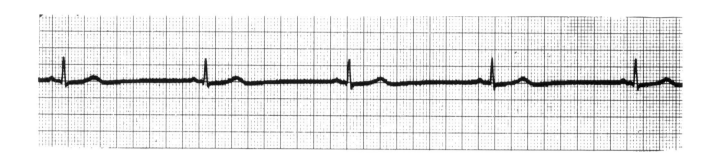

IF YOU THINK THE ABOVE SYMPTOMATIC PATIENT MAY NEED A PACEMAKER... YOU'RE DOING GREAT!

Section IX
Electrolyte Changes

OBJECTIVES

When you have completed Section IX, you will be able to describe or identify EKG manifestations associated with

1. hypokalemia
2. hyperkalemia
3. hypocalcemia
4. hypercalcemia

Section IX deals with certain electrolyte imbalances as reflected on the EKG. Even though that sounds about as intriguing as the "Biological Considerations of the Rattus and Related Genera," there *really* are some unique and interesting things you should know. 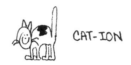 HONEST!

I am making the assumption that you have a good understanding of electrolytes . . . but if you don't, I will include a *brief* overview.

Remember **IONS?** They are the electrically charged particles contained in the various fluid compartments of the body—the intracellular fluid (ICF) compartment and the extracellular fluid (ECF) compartment. If your long-term memory is functioning today, you'll recall that the ECF includes *both* the fluid in the blood vessels (intravascular fluid) and the fluid located between the cells (interstitial fluid).

Anyway, *anions* are negatively charged particles—like bicarbonate (HCO_3^-) and chloride (Cl^-).

Cations are positively charged particles—like potassium (K^+), sodium (Na^+) and calcium (Ca^{++}).

CAT-ION

And electrolytes are combinations of anions and cations in solution!

Just thought you might want to know that!

It's kinda neat to consider what happens to all the ions or charges in the process of heart contraction and relaxation and in the process of depolarization and repolarization.

All cells in the body, including the myocardial cells, have a charge which is a result of all the ions (cations and anions) in the body. These ions are found both inside and outside of the cells—some in greater concentrations than others.

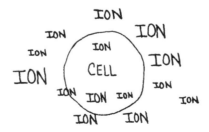

When a cell is at rest (polarized), the inside of the cell has a net negative charge, while the cell membrane has a net positive charge. Sodium (Na$^+$) tends to be mainly outside the cell, and potassium (K$^+$) tends to be mainly inside the cell during this polarized state.

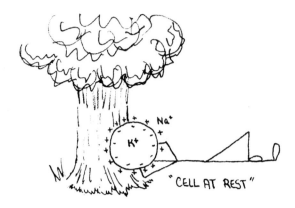

"CELL AT REST"

When a cell is stimulated, the Na$^+$ rushes into the cell, while K$^+$ moves out. Sodium and Potassium basically change places for awhile.

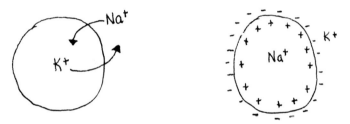

This movement of K$^+$ and Na$^+$ upsets the charge on the inside of the cell—giving it a net positive charge. This reversal of charges is *depolarization*. This depolarization causes calcium to move into the cell. Calcium then causes the mechanical activity of *CONTRACTION*. Neat, huh? Following depolarization, the ions move back to their "resting state" or repolarized positions in order to receive the next impulse.

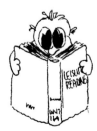

Though this is fairly dry material for leisure reading, it's easy to understand how electrolyte imbalances might affect the depolarization, repolarization, and contractility of the myocardial cells.

Let's look at potassium (K$^+$) for instance, the major intracellular cation. A normal serum potassium ranges between 3.6–5.2 mEq. per liter.

HYPOKALEMIA

Hypokalemia is the term used to describe a serum potassium level below 3.6 mEq/liter. Because the potassium ions play an important role in the repolarization activities of myocardial cells, certain changes occur in the EKG pattern when the potassium level is unbalanced.

For instance, *hypokalemia* may cause any or all of the following EKG changes.

A. *Depressed ST segment*

B. *Prominent U wave**

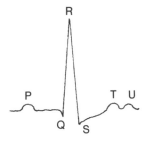

C. *Prolonged QT or QU interval*

The QT interval is measured from the beginning of the QRS complex to the end of the T wave. This QT interval simply represents the total time of depolarization and repolarization.

The appearance of the U wave superimposed upon or near the T wave gives the appearance of a prolonged QT interval. In effect, it is the U wave that makes the interval prolonged.

Just for the record, QT intervals vary with age, sex and heart rate . . . in any event, a normal QT interval should not be greater than half of the R-R interval.

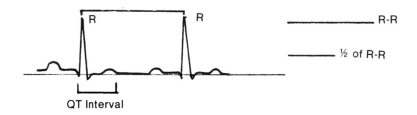

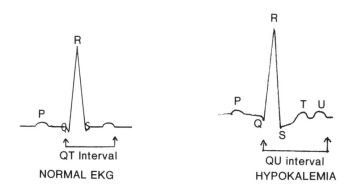

NORMAL EKG   HYPOKALEMIA

---

*The U wave is thought to represent the prolonged repolarization of the Purkinje fibers.

Sometimes it's difficult to tell where a T wave stops and where the U wave begins. It may help to view those leads where the T waves tend to be flat.

Here's an EKG demonstrating hypokalemia.

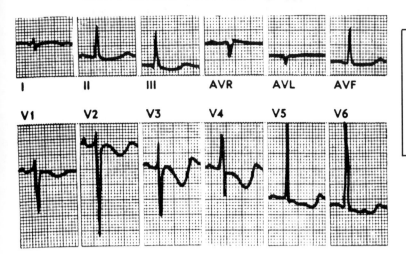

I   II   III   AVR   AVL   AVF

V1   V2   V3   V4   V5   V6

Hypokalemia may be associated with any of the following conditions or therapies:
- starvation
- vomiting
- diarrhea
- diuretic therapy
- intermittant gastric suction
- excessive digitalis therapy
- excessive use of steroids
- excessive use of corticotropins

Because hypokalemia *increases electrical instability,* the following dysrhythmias may be associated with low serum potassium levels.

P.V.C.'s
ATRIAL TACHYCARDIA
JUNCTIONAL TACHYCARDIA
VENTRICULAR TACHYCARDIA
VENTRICULAR FIBRILLATION

If this is *confusing, just remember that potassium mainly affects the repolarization* period of cardiac activity. Since the T wave represents repolarization, *look for EKG changes near the T wave.* Probably the most common EKG feature associated with hypokalemia is the prominent *U wave.*

HERE'S A POEM FOR U ...

Roses are Red
Violets are Blue
Potassiums that are *Low*
Will give you a U (wave)!

Of course, the other side of the coin is *HYPERKALEMIA,* a serum potassium level greater than 5.2 mEq. per liter.

And you guessed it . . . hyperkalemia causes EKG changes too!

The most characteristic EKG features associated with hyperkalemia are:

1. Tall, peaked, narrow, tent-like T waves that are symmetrical.

2. Usually the height or amplitude of the R wave is diminished.
3. The P waves tend to be small or have low amplitude.
4. As the hyperkalemia becomes more severe, the QRS becomes wide (intraventricular block).

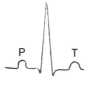

Normal

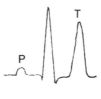

Hyperkalemia
(Mild)

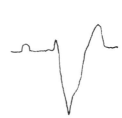

Hyperkalemia
(Severe)

Here's a rather impressive rhythm strip demonstrating a serum potassium level of about 7.0 mEq. per liter.

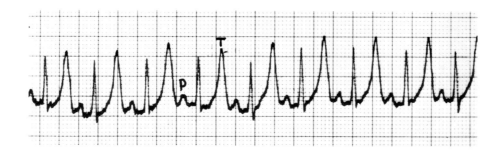

IMPORTANT NOTICE

YOU CAN NEVER DIAGNOSE HYPERKALEMIA FROM AN EKG—YOU CAN ONLY *SUSPECT* IT. HYPERKALEMIA MUST BE CONFIRMED BY A SERUM POTASSIUM LEVEL.

Hyperkalemia *may* be associated with any of the following clinical conditions or therapies:

- burns
- crushing injuries
- adrenal insufficiency
- oliguria
- kidney damage
- infusions of excessive amounts of potassium solutions

Hyperkalemia *depresses* the normal electrical activity of the myocardial cells and may result in any of the following dysrhythmias.

SINUS BRADYCARDIA   IDIOVENTRICULAR RHYTHM
SINUS ARRHYTHMIA   VENTRICULAR TACHYCARDIA
FIRST DEGREE AV BLOCK   VENTRICULAR FIBRILLATION
JUNCTIONAL RHYTHM   ASYSTOLE (the absence of rhythm)

HINT: Tall, peaked (tent-like), symmetrical T waves should lead you to suspect *hyperkalemia*.

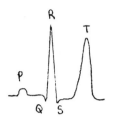

REMEMBER

HYPOKALEMIA	HYPERKALEMIA
$K^+ \downarrow 3.6$ mEq./L.	$K^+ \uparrow 5.2$ mEq./L.
Depressed ST segment	Tall, peaked T waves
Prominent U wave	Small P waves
Prolonged (QU interval)	Wide QRS when severe

. . . I suppose we should try a bit of practice. . . . RIGHT?

Practice Exercise 1

1. Postassium plays an important role in the (circle one) repolarization / depolarization activity of the myocardial cells.

2. During a normal cardiac cycle, the _____ wave represents repolarization activity.

3. This one is easy!
   Match the terms with the appropriate pictures.

   Hypokalemia

   Normal Conduction

   Hyperkalemia

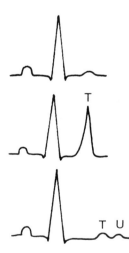

4.

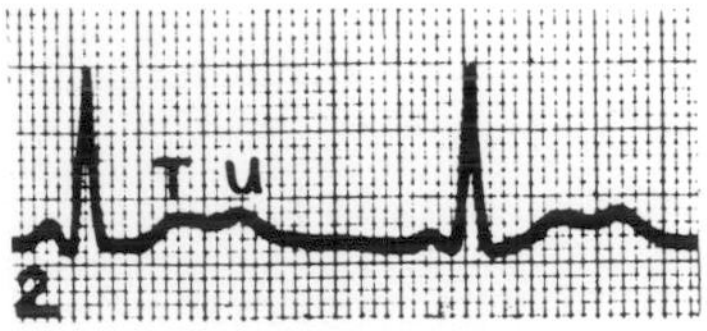

Briefly describe what you see and any appropriate actions.

_____

_____

_____

_____

_____

5.

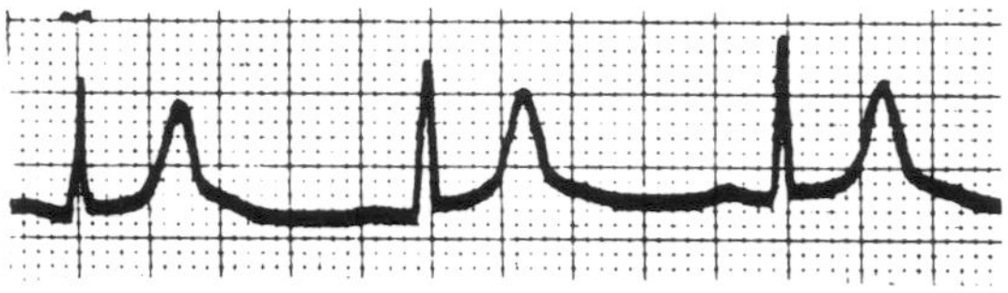

How about this strip? What actions would you take?

_____

_____

_____

_____

_____

_____

For **Feedback 1,** refer to page 224.

Input 2: Calcium

That brings us to Calcium. Remember calcium? That's the cation (—ION) that moves into the cells following depolarization, causing mechanical activity or contraction. In other words, calcium (Ca^{++}) is a cardiac _STIMULANT_ whose main function is _CONTRACTILITY._

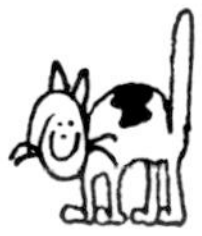

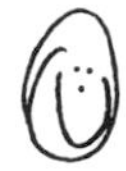

Normal serum calcium levels range between 9–11 mg.%.

HYPOCALCEMIA

Hypocalcemia refers to any serum calcium level below 9 mg.% and causes _decreased contractility of the heart._

EKG changes associated with hypocalcemia are seen in the ST segment of the cardiac cycle.

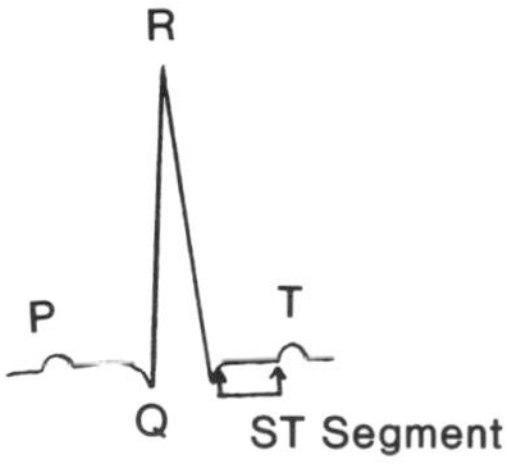

220

A low serum calcium will cause a *lengthening* or prolongation of the ST segment (without changing the appearance of the QRS or the T wave . . . that's because calcium does its work **between** depolarization and repolarization).

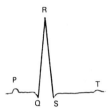

In a hypocalcemic state, the ST segment appears flat (*isoelectric*) and *prolonged*. If you remember the discussion about QT intervals, you will notice that the *QT interval is prolonged*. The other significant feature is that the T waves are usually low or squatty. (I'm not certain that squatty is a real word . . . but you get the idea!)

Here are pertinent EKG leads demonstrating hypocalcemia.

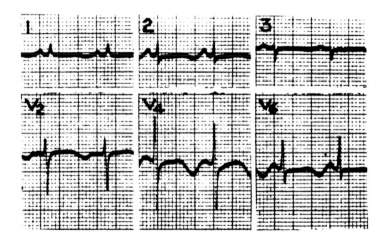

IMPORTANT NOTICE

HYPERCALCEMIA

Hypercalcemia, on the other hand, refers to a serum calcium level greater than 11 mg.%.

A high serum calcium will cause *increased contractility of the heart.*

Hypercalcemia causes EKG changes opposite to those of hypocalcemia (brilliant deduction, right 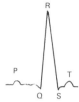 ?).

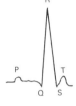

As seen above, hypercalcemia causes shortening of the ST segment (without changing the appearance of the QRS or T wave . . . that's because calcium does its work *between* depolarization and repolarization).

As a matter of fact, the ST segment is *usually* absent! One usually sees an abruptly ascending T wave, just following the QRS.

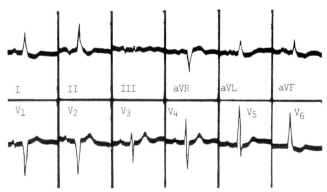

ALWAYS REMEMBER TO WATCH FOR HYPERCALCEMIA WHEN THE PATIENT IS ACIDOTIC.

Here's a patient who has a high serum calcium level.

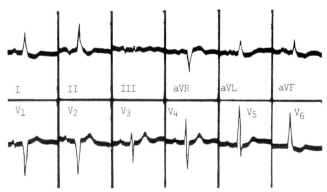

IMPORTANT NOTICE

YOU CAN NEVER DIAGNOSE HYPERCALCEMIA FROM AN EKG—YOU CAN ONLY *SUSPECT* IT. HYPERCALCEMIA MUST BE CONFIRMED BY A SERUM CALCIUM LEVEL!

REMEMBER

HYPOCALCEMIA	HYPERCALCEMIA
Ca^{++} ↓ 9 mg.%	Ca^{++} ↑ 11 mg.%
↓ contractility	↑ contractility
long ST segment	short ST segment

Practice Exercise 2

SURPRISE . . . IT'S PRACTICE TIME AGAIN!

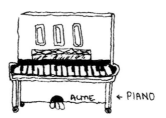

1. Calcium is a cardiac _____ , so its main function is CONTRACTILITY.

2. Hypocalcemia refers to a serum calcium level (circle one) above / below 9 mg.%.

3. Hypocalcemia can be suspected when one sees a _____ ST segment.

4. Draw a cardiac cycle (PQRST) that demonstrates a low calcium effect.

5. Hypercalcemia refers to a serum calcium level above _____ mg.%.

6. Hypercalcemia can be suspected when one sees a _____ ST segment.

7. Draw a cardiac cycle (PQRST) that demonstrates a high calcium effect.

8. Hypocalcemia causes _____ cardiac contractility.

9. Hypercalcemia causes _____ cardiac contractility.

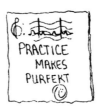

For **Feedback 2,** refer to page 224.

Feedback 1

How did you do? If your answers are similar to mine, you deserve a banana! (Bananas are packed full of potassium. 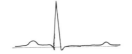)

1. Potassium plays an important role in the (repolarization) / depolarization activity of the myocardial cells.

2. During a normal cardiac cycle, the <u>T</u> wave represents repolarization activity.

3. If your matching does <u>not</u> match mine, the Great Banana suggests that you reread Input 1.

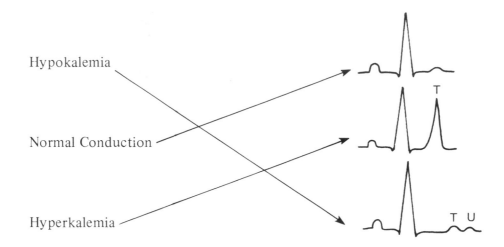

4. This appears to be a sinus bradycardia with a rate between 50–60 beats per minute. The ST segment is slightly depressed and there is a prominent U wave. I suspect hypokalemia, but would need to verify with a serum potassium level.

5. This appears to be a borderline sinus bradycardia with a heart rate of 60. The P waves are small. The T waves are tall and peaked (tent-like). I suspect hyperkalemia, but would need to verify with a serum potassium level.

Feedback 2

YOU'RE DOING SUPER...

. . . ESPECIALLY IF YOU ANSWERED ALL THE QUESTIONS CORRECTLY

1. Calcium is a cardiac <u>STIMULANT</u>, so its main function is CONTRACTILITY.

2. Hypocalcemia refers to a serum calcium level (below) 9 mg.%.

3. Hypocalcemia can be suspected when one sees a <u>lengthened or prolonged</u> ST segment.

4.

5. Hypercalcemia refers to a serum calcium level above <u>11</u> mg.%.

6. Hypercalcemia can be suspected when one sees a <u>shortened</u> ST segment.

7.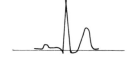

8. Hypocalcemia causes <u>decreased</u> cardiac contractility.

9. Hypercalcemia causes <u>increased</u> cardiac contractility.

NOTES

Section X
Ischemia, Injury, and Infarct

OBJECTIVES

When you have completed Section X, you will be able to describe or identify

1. the normal 12 lead EKG
2. the orientation of EKG leads to the left ventricular surfaces
3. EKG changes associated with ischemia
4. muscle layers in the heart
5. criteria for diagnosing myocardial infarction
6. current injury pattern in leads overlying an infarct
7. the hallmark of myocardial infarction or necrosis
8. anteroseptal wall myocardial infarction
9. inferior wall myocardial infarction
10. criteria suggesting a posterior wall myocardial infarction
11. cardiac enzymes and isoenzymes

Whew!!

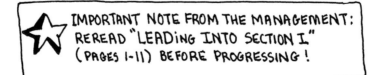
IMPORTANT NOTE FROM THE MANAGEMENT:
REREAD "LEADING INTO SECTION I"
(PAGES 1-11) BEFORE PROGRESSING!

You are making great progress! Just think, the end of this book is almost in sight!

You may not remember, but in the very beginning we talked about leads. Just to refresh your memory, here is a *quickie* summary.

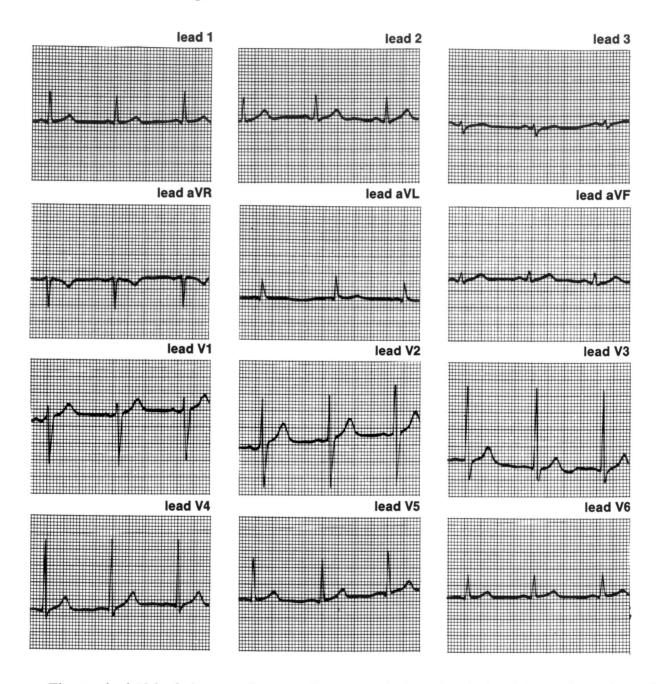

The standard 12 lead electrocardiogram allows one to look at electrical activity on the surfaces of the heart—or to look at the electrical activity from various angles or from various points of reference.

The left ventricle is the most important chamber of the heart in that it functions as "The Pump" or as the driving force for systemic circulation. So . . . because the left ventricle is such an important structure, the 12 leads are designed to look at the various surfaces of the left ventricle! Good thinking, right?!

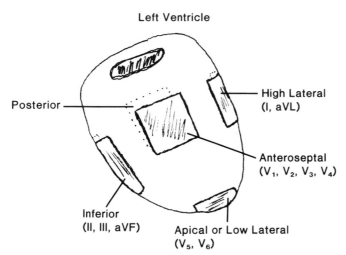

Leads I and aVL look at the lateral surface of the left ventricle (high lateral).

Leads II, III, and aVF look at the inferior or diaphragmatic surface of the left ventricle.

Leads V_1, V_2, V_3, and V_4 look at the antero-septal surface of the left ventricle.

Leads V_5 and V_6 look at the apical surface of the left ventricle (low lateral).

You will remember that there are no leads designated to look directly at the posterior surface of the left ventricle.

Up until now, this "lead business" may have seemed to be of little importance to you . . . BUT your thinking is about to be transformed!

Serious coronary artery disease is reflected on the EKG by ischemic changes, patterns of current injury, and actual myocardial infarction or cellular death. That of course, is nothing new . . . but depending upon the extent of the cardiac embarrassment and the location of the insult, the patient's hospital course and prognosis can be anticipated. And you know what tells us the location of the insult?????? . . . THE LEADS! HURRAY FOR LEADS!

Before going further, let's review the myocardial blood supply.

The heart muscle is supplied by two main coronary arteries—the right coronary artery (RCA) and the left coronary artery (LCA). Please see the diagram at the top of page 229. Both the RCA and the LCA arise from the base of the aorta, traveling on the outer surface of the heart muscle. Small branches of these major arteries penetrate into the deeper muscle layers, thus nourishing the inner muscle with an adequate blood supply. You'll notice that the Left Coronary Artery divides into the Left Anterior Descending artery (LAD) and the Left Circumflex artery. Though not all individuals are exactly alike, in the majority of people, these vessels supply the following portions of the heart muscle.

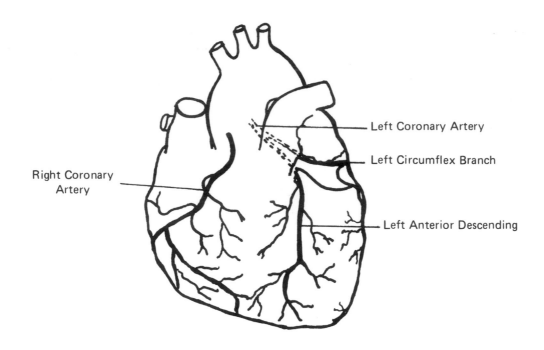

Right Coronary
Artery

Left Coronary Artery

Left Circumflex Branch

Left Anterior Descending

ARTERY	TISSUE SUPPLIED
Left Anterior Descending (LAD)	Anterior surface of the left ventricle Anterior surface of the septum The middle portion of the anterior surface of the right ventricle The lower portion of the posterior surface of the right ventricle
Right Coronary Artery (RCA)	The remainder of the right ventricle The upper portion of the posterior wall of the left ventricle (The SA node is supplied by the RCA in approximately 75% of the population, and the AV node is supplied by a branch of the RCA in about 90% of the population.)
Left Circumflex	Lateral wall of the left ventricle Lower half of the posterior wall of the left ventricle

P.S. I do not expect you to memorize all of this!

So, by knowing which vessels supply certain portions of the left ventricle and by viewing the leads that reflect the electrical activity of the various surfaces of the left ventricle, one can assess ischemia, tissue injury, and muscle infarction in a noninvasive manner. (If that doesn't make sense to you, it will as we go along . . . honest!!)

First, let's talk about myocardial ischemia . . . sometimes referred to as angina or coronary insufficiency. Basically, *ischemia* is the change that results in the myocardial cells from a *temporary, insufficient* blood supply. Most usually ischemia is due to atherosclerosis of the coronary arteries. Atherosclerosis is characterized by narrowing of the lumen of the coronary arteries due to atheroma deposits, fibrosis, and calcification in the intima of the artery.

Let's say that this is the lumen of a healthy coronary artery . . .

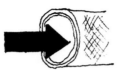

and this is a coronary artery with severe atherosclerotic changes . . .

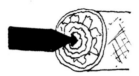

and this is a little lady with atherosclerotic disease.

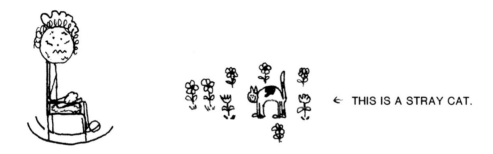

← THIS IS A STRAY CAT.

When the little lady rocks peacefully in her rocking chair she feels fine . . . because at rest her myocardial cells are receiving an adequate blood supply. However, when she chases the stray cat out of her garden, she experiences severe chest pain. Temporarily, the blood supply through her atherosclerotic vessels is inadequate to meet tissue needs. When she sits down to rest again, the pain subsides. This is *ischemia*. Typically, myocardial ischemia or coronary insufficiency is precipitated by exertion and relieved by rest.

The oxygen requirements of the myocardium are approximately three times that of other body tissue. Normally, in a resting state, the myocardium extracts 70–75% of the oxygen from the blood flowing through the coronary arteries. When the oxygen demand increases with exertion, the myocardium cannot increase its oxygen extraction rate significantly. Rather, increased oxygen is realized through increased perfusion! Healthy coronary arteries dilate in response to increased myocardial oxygen demand and can increase perfusion five times that of normal. In the presence of coronary artery disease, the ability to increase blood perfusion is limited. A coronary artery can be as much as 80% obstructed before mechanical hindrance to blood flow results in symptoms (e.g., chest pain)!

If, when our little lady friend was having pain, we had run a 12 lead EKG . . . we would have noticed several things.

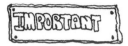 Myocardial ischemia presents on the EKG as ST segment and T wave changes *IN LEADS LOOKING AT THE ISCHEMIC SURFACE*. Frequently, the T waves are inverted or upside down and tend to have an arrow appearance . . .

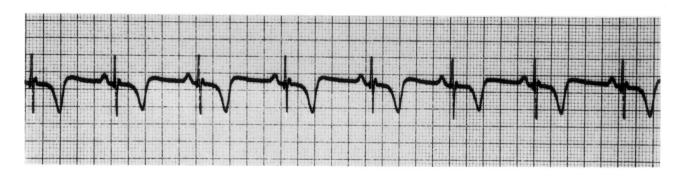

. . . or T waves may be seen as slightly flat or depressed.

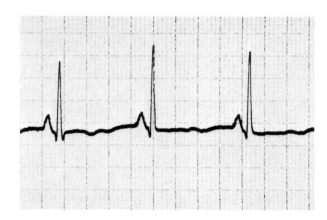

Because the precordial leads (V_1-V_6) are nearest to the ventricles, the T wave changes may be most obvious in these leads.

Coronary insufficiency or ischemia may also be reflected on EKG by ST segment changes. Instead of having a smooth joining of the ST segment and the T wave, there may be sharp angle at

the ST-T junction . . . like so . . .

ST-T junction

. . . or the ST segment actually may be depressed.

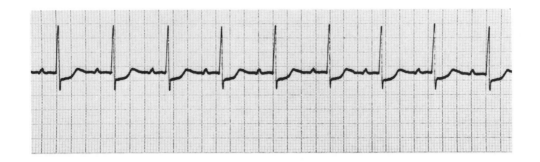

IF YOU THINK THAT THESE ST-T WAVE CHANGES RESEMBLE THOSE CHANGES SEEN WITH CERTAIN ELECTROLYTE AND DRUG EFFECTS, YOU ARE RIGHT!! THAT'S PRECISELY WHY ONE NEVER DIAGNOSES ANY CONDITION BASED SOLELY ON EKG FINDINGS!

. . . *Okay, now back to our little lady chasing the stray cat out of her garden!*
Here is a 12 lead EKG taken while she was experiencing chest pain.

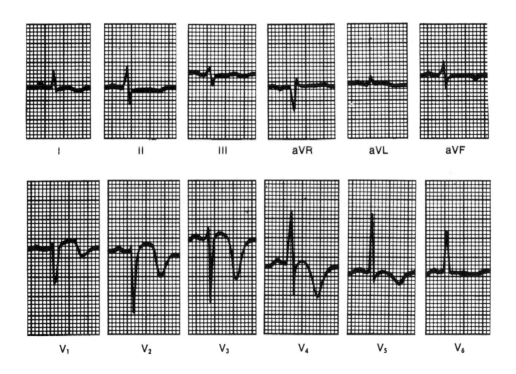

Notice the ST-T wave changes! For a comparison, review the "healthy" 12 lead EKG on page 227.

REMEMBER:

> Lead I and aVL look at the high lateral surface of the left ventricle (LV);
>
> Leads II, III, and aVF look at the inferior surface of the LV;
>
> Leads V_1, V_2, V_3, and V_4 look at the anteroseptal surface of the LV,
>
> and
>
> Leads V_5 and V_6 look at the apical or low lateral surface of the LV.

It's safe to say that our little rocking chair friend has generalized ST-T wave changes throughout, and that her myocardial blood flow may be severely compromised!

Practice Exercise 1

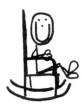

Are you ready for some practice?

We'll keep it simple since this material has a tendency to be somewhat difficult!

1. (Answer yes or no.) The end of this book is in sight. _____

2. The 12 lead EKG allows one to look at the electrical activity of the heart from various _____

_____

3. The most important chamber of the heart is the left ventricle because _____

_____

_____

4. Match the leads with the correct surfaces of the left ventricle.

Leads I and aVL	Lateral surface of the LV
Leads II, III, and aVF	Apical surface of the LV
Leads V_1, V_2, V_3, and V_4	Inferior surface of the LV
Leads V_5 and V_6	Anteroseptal surface of the LV

5. By definition, *ischemia* is the myocardial change that results from _____ blood supply.

6. Myocardial ischemia presents on the EKG as _____ and _____ changes in leads looking at the ischemic surface.

7. Here is a 12 lead EKG. Describe the ischemic ST-T wave changes that you see.

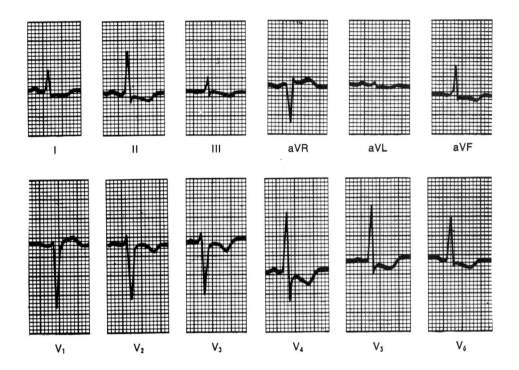

_____

_____

_____

_____

_____

_____

_____

_____

_____

_____

_____

For **Feedback 1,** refer to page 261.

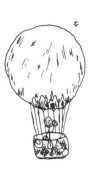

Onward and upward!

Before getting into the subject of myocardial infarction, we should perhaps review the muscle layers of the heart.

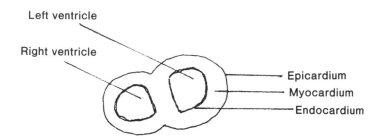

Left ventricle

Right ventricle

Epicardium
Myocardium
Endocardium

The endocardium is the muscle lining on the inside of the heart, while the epicardium is the outer muscle covering. The muscle layer between the endocardium and the epicardium is the myocardium.

Myocardial infarction is the term used to describe actual necrosis and death of part of the heart muscle resulting from an insufficient blood supply to keep the muscle viable. In other words, the heart muscle is deprived of an adequate blood supply over a period of time, thus causing *cellular destruction* and *death*.

A myocardial infarction may be limited to any one of the muscle layers, or may extend through the three muscle layers. When the infarct extends across the entire muscle wall it is known as a *transmural* infarction.

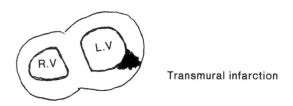

R.V   L.V

Transmural infarction

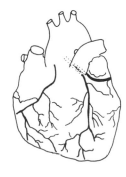

Because the two large coronary arteries (LCA and RCA) supplying the heart muscle run along the epicardium, the inner muscle layers are more prone to injury in the face of coronary artery disease. The inner muscle layers receive their blood supply from small branches of the LCA and RCA that penetrate into the muscle. If these small branches are occluded, muscle destruction is inevitable. In fact, infarction may result from incomplete occlusion of a coronary artery . . . if the blood supply is significantly limited to a portion of the heart muscle!

. . . Then, on the other hand, if the coronary artery disease is slow progressing, sufficient collateral circulation may develop to supply the heart muscle with adequate blood and oxygen. In this case, complete occlusion of a coronary artery *could* occur without muscle destruction. Complicated, right!

Before talking about the EKG findings associated with myocardial infarction, you must first memorize the following:

Ready?

> ### THE DIAGNOSIS OF MYOCARDIAL INFARCTION
> ### IS **NEVER** BASED SOLELY ON EKG FINDINGS.

The diagnosis of a myocardial infarction is BASED ON:

1. POSITIVE PATIENT HISTORY (chest pain, radiating pain, indigestion, jaw pain, elbow pain, sweating, nausea, vomiting, etc.)
2. ↑ SERUM ENZYMES (indicating cellular membrane destruction . . . we will discuss enzymes later (☺))

3. POSITIVE EKG FINDINGS

P.S. It probably should be said that the EKG may remain normal in myocardial infarction . . . or show nonspecific changes that are not diagnostic. *Usually,* however, the following electrocardiographic findings are associated with transmural myocardial infarction.

Usually, the first electrocardiographic finding of myocardial infarction is *ST segment elevation* in the leads overlying the area of injury. ST segment elevation represents *current injury.* ST elevation simply means that the ST segment rises above the isoelectric line.

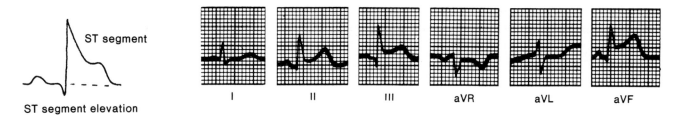

ST segment

ST segment elevation

I   II   III   aVR   aVL   aVF

If monitoring were initiated at the onset of myocardial infarction, tall, peaked, "tent-like" T waves would be evident in leads overlying the infarct. It has been suggested that this is a result of intracellular potassium leaking into the extracellular space from the damaged muscle cells. Within several hours post infarct, however, the tall peaked T waves evolve and are replaced by ST elevation in leads overlying the infarct!

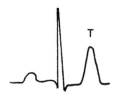

T

Tall peaked T waves may be obvious at the
outset of myocardial cellular damage.

236

What do I mean by the *leads overlying the infarct?*
Remember this little chart?

Leads I and aVL look at the lateral surface of the LV (high lateral).

Leads II, III, and aVF look at the inferior surface of the LV.

Leads V_1, V_2, V_3, V_4 look at the anteroseptal surface of the LV.

Leads V_5 and V_6 look at the apical surface of the LV (low lateral).

Well, if ST elevation is seen in leads I and aVL, I can assume there is current injury of the lateral wall of the left ventricle . . . or, if ST elevation is seen in leads II, III, and aVF, I can assume there is injury of the inferior wall of the left ventricle, etc. (I say I can *assume* there is injury because there are other conditions which result in ST elevation!)

THAT'S FAIRLY EASY, HUH?

So, ST elevation will be observed in the leads overlying the injured myocardial surface. Additionally, *reciprocal ST segment depression* will occur in the leads oriented toward the *uninjured* myocardial surfaces. Look at the illustration on the previous page. Notice the slight ST segment depression in leads I and aVL.

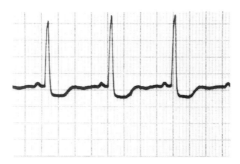

ST segment depression

The EKG *hallmark* of myocardial necrosis in *upright leads* (leads I, II, III, aVL, aVF, V_5, and V_6) is the pathologic *Q wave,* found in the leads oriented toward the necrotic area. To qualify as abnormal, Q waves must be wide and deep in appearance, measuring at least **0.04 seconds in width** (one small EKG square) and measuring **deeper than ¼ of the R wave amplitude.** You will note there is a loss of R wave amplitude as well.

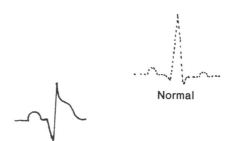

Normal

Pathologic Q Wave

The appearance of the pathologic Q waves follows the appearance of the ST-T wave changes discussed previously. So, it could be said that the appearance of the Q wave is an evolutionary phase in the acute myocardial infarct process.

(P.S. *Small* Q waves, nonpathologic, may normally be seen in leads I, II, V_4, and V_5.)

The EKG *hallmark* of myocardial necrosis in *negative leads* (V_1, V_2, V_3, and V_4) is the loss of the positive R wave (loss of R wave progression) found in leads oriented toward the necrotic area.

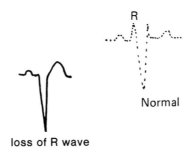

Normal

loss of R wave

The loss of the R wave in negatively oriented leads follows the appearance of the ST-T wave changes (just as the pathologic Q wave appears in upright leads following the appearance of ST-T wave changes). The loss of R waves is an evolutionary phase in the acute myocardial infarct process.

Understanding pathologic Q waves or the loss of R waves requires knowing a little bit about normal or healthy depolarization first!

Depolarization of the ventricles begins in the left side of the interventricular septum . . . and spreads to the right, through the septum.

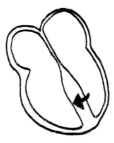

Next, depolarization spreads outward through the free walls of both the left and right ventricles at the same time.

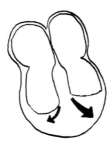

Because the left ventricle has greater muscle mass, the left ventricular forces are greater than the right ventricular forces. Thus, the general direction of ventricular depolarization is leftward.

$$\longleftarrow \; + \; \longrightarrow \; = \; \longrightarrow$$
R   L   L

In summary, depolarization can be thought of as first, a left to right activation of the septum, followed by a large force of activation moving from right to left through the free wall of the left ventricle.

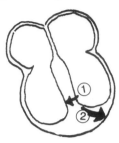

Let's explore the spread of the depolarization movement, using the precordial leads V_6 and V_1 as examples. (Remember, the V leads . . . V_1, V_2, V_3, V_4, V_5, and V_6 . . . are all positive leads.)

Now, if this is the left ventricle . . .

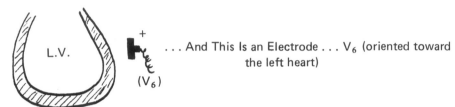

. . . the electrode will first see the left to right depolarization of the septum. Since the depolarization wave is moving away from the positive electrode, the first part of the QRS deflection will be negative. (All V leads are positive leads . . . remember?)

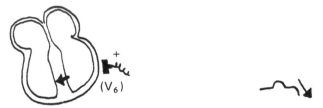

Next, the large force of depolarization moves from right to left through the free wall of the left ventricle (toward the positive electrode), so a large upward deflection is seen on EKG.

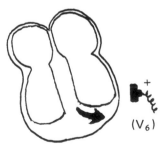

Thus, the entire picture of ventricular depolarization will look like this . . .

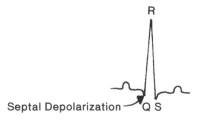

in a lead oriented toward the left ventricle (like V_6).

Now, let's look at the depolarization process from a lead oriented toward the right ventricle (like V_1). Remember, all V leads are positive leads!

The first phase of ventricular depolarization is always septal activation, and you'll remember that the interventricular septum is activated from left to right. That means that the initial depolarization force is moving toward the positive electrode.

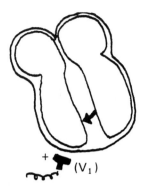

> ANYTIME THAT THE DEPOLARIZATION FORCE MOVES TOWARD A POSITIVE ELECTRODE, THE EKG DEFLECTION WILL BE POSITIVE.

So, the initial part of the QRS deflection seen in this lead (V_1) is positive.

Next, the wave of depolarization moves from right to left through the free wall of the left ventricle (away from the positive electrode).

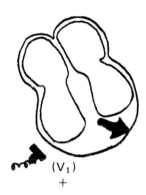

> ANYTIME THAT THE DEPOLARIZATION FORCE MOVES AWAY FROM A POSITIVE ELECTRODE, THE EKG DEFLECTION WILL BE NEGATIVE.

So, the entire picture of ventricular depolarization as seen from a right chest electrode looks like this (lead V_1 or V_2).

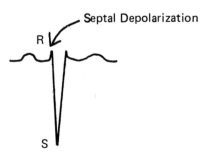

Here are leads V_1 through V_6 as recorded from a healthy individual.

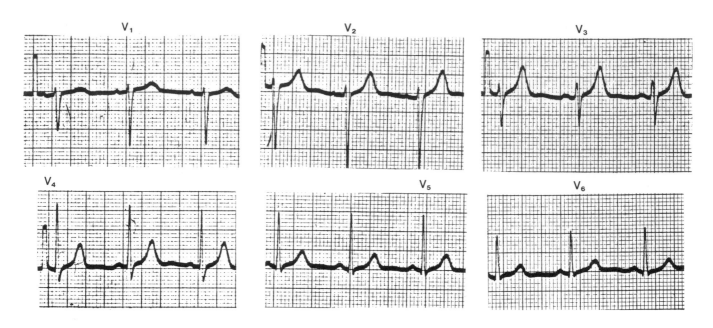

Knowing how the forces of depolarization move through the ventricular muscle, it's easy to understand why each of the V leads appear as they do!

Notice how the R waves gets progressively larger in each lead until the complexes are upright in leads V_4, V_5, and V_6. This is known as *normal R wave progression.*

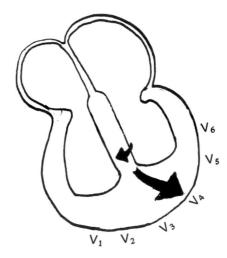

Leads V_1 and V_2 are oriented toward the right heart, while leads V_3 and V_4 are oriented toward the septum. Since the septal force of depolarization moves toward the right, these leads usually record a small initial R wave (positive wave). The remainder of the QRS complex in leads V_1, V_2, V_3, and V_4 is negative, because the major ventricular depolarization force is moving away from those electrodes.

Leads V_5 and V_6 are oriented toward the left heart. Since the septal force of depolarization moves away from these electrodes, a small negative Q wave is the first EKG deflection seen. The remainder of the QRS complex in these leads is positive, as the major ventricular wave of depolarization is moving toward the left chest electrodes.

Sounds relatively simple . . . right?

Pathologic Q waves (in positive leads) and loss of R waves (in negative leads) represent *ELEC-TRICAL DEATH*! In other words, the area of muscle represented by the leads showing abnormal Q waves or loss of R waves has lost its ability to transmit electrical impulses.

That is sometimes a difficult idea to grasp . . . so we'll use the ol' window analogy. Tissue that is dead cannot repolarize or depolarize . . . it is electrically inactive. If all the muscle layers are involved in the infarct (transmural infarct), then electrically speaking, there is a "hole" or a "window" in the muscle.

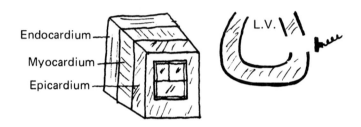

So guess what happens!

Okay . . . this is you 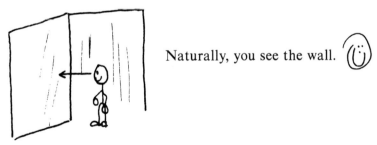 (I hope I drew your nose right).

If you are standing in a room looking at a wall . . . what will you see?

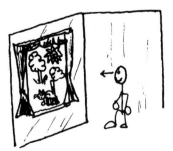
Naturally, you see the wall.

But, if instead of a solid wall, there is a window . . . what will you see?

Naturally, you will see through the window, viewing the activity outside or beyond the window.

Well, that's what happens in the case of an electrical "hole," or "window" too! If an electrode is placed over this window (over the electrically dead muscle tissue), the electrode will see the healthy electrical activity beyond the window!

Here are the precordial (chest leads) of a normal healthy individual.

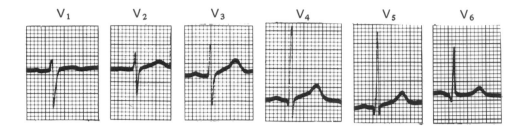

As an example of what I mean . . .

. . . when a transmural infarct occurs in the anteroseptal wall of the left ventricle, the necrotic region becomes a window. Since leads V_1-V_4 view the anteroseptal region of the left ventricle, they will look through the window at distant heart activity.

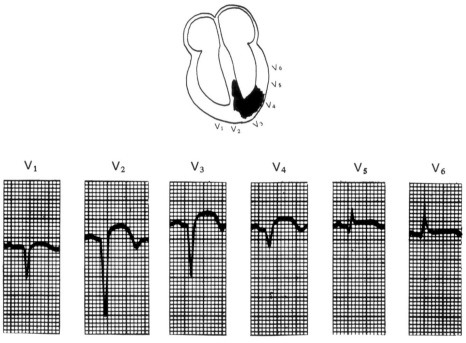

Anteroseptal Wall Infarction: Note the loss of R wave in leads V_1, V_2, V_3, and V_4 and the ST segment elevation in those same leads.

Remember, necrotic tissue has no ability to transmit electrical impulses! So, in this case, leads V_1-V_4 record the forces of depolarization moving away from the electrodes. You'll remember that when the waves of depolarization move away from the positive electrode, the wave deflections (QRS's) are all negatively deflected. The positive R forces in these leads are completely lost. Thus, there are no initial positive R forces. The first deflection is a downward wave ⌢↘, a Q wave. When the deflection is negative (without an R wave), the complex is referred to as a QS—as opposed to a QRS.

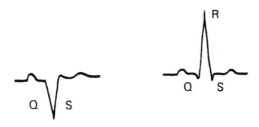

Are you thoroughly confused yet? . . . and if so, that means you are progressing in a normal fashion! Trust me!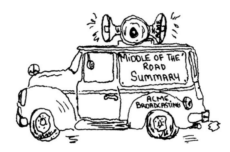

Let's summarize before going further!

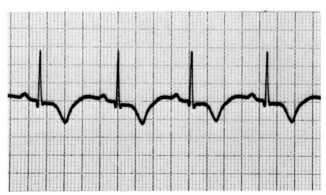

1. The right and left coronary arteries and their branches supply the heart muscle with nutrients.
2. If the blood supply to a portion of the heart muscle is only temporarily interrupted, ischemic changes can be seen in those leads that look at the ischemic heart surface.
3. Ischemic changes include inverted or upside down T waves and ST depression as noted in the following strip.

Pronounced inverted T waves

4. When a coronary artery or a branch of an artery becomes occluded, myocardial tissue damage will usually ensue.

5. Myocardial injury is seen on the EKG as ST segment elevation in the leads overlying the injured tissue.

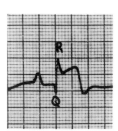
ST elevation in an upright lead

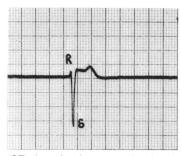
ST elevation in a negative lead

6. As the myocardial infarct evolves, abnormal Q waves become evident in upright leads overlying the infarct. (Q waves represent ELECTRICAL DEATH in upright leads!)

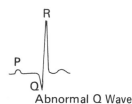
Abnormal Q Wave

7. When an infarct occurs in areas of the heart seen by the right precordial leads (V_1, V_2, V_3, and V_4), the R force is lost, so that only a QS configuration is seen.

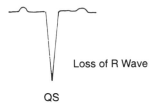
Loss of R Wave

QS

BASICALLY, THAT'S ALL I HAVE SAID THUS FAR. . . .

WHEW! (I'm just long-winded!!)

Before looking at some actual electrocardiograms, there is another phase of myocardial infarct evolution to consider. As the infarct begins to resolve, the abnormal ST segments gradually return to the baseline. In this stage, the T waves will commonly be inverted, denoting *resolution*.

Evolutionary Phases of Myocardial Infarction

Current Injury

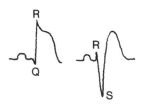
ST segment elevation

Cellular Necrosis

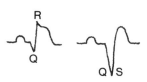
The appearance of the pathologic Q wave or the loss of R wave.

Resolution

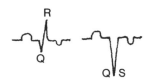
T wave inversion

The only residual (long-term) evidence (seen on EKG) of the infarct will be the persistent Q waves or the absence of R waves. *Almost* all patients retain the Q waves in the leads representing the infarcted muscle tissue.

. . . So when a patient comes back to see you—a hundred years from now . . . you can very intelligently ask him . . . "When was it you had your heart attack?" (You will know he had one sometime back because you will be able to see the pathologic Q waves or the absence of R waves on his EKG!)

Now we're going to look at some actual EKG's . . . and here's a **Summary Chart** to help you.

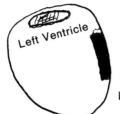

Leads I, aVL

LATERAL WALL INFARCTION (HIGH LATERAL) = pathologic Q waves in leads I and aVL (a lateral wall infarction is caused by an occlusion of the Circumflex Branch of the Left Coronary Artery).

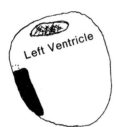

Leads
II, III, aVF

INFERIOR WALL INFARCTION = pathologic Q waves in leads II, III, and aVF (an inferior wall infarction is usually caused by occlusion of the Right Coronary Artery).

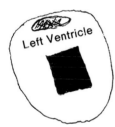

Leads
V_1, V_2, V_3, V_4

ANTEROSEPTAL WALL INFARCTION = loss of positive R forces (QS deflections only) in leads V_1, V_2, V_3, and V_4 (an anteroseptal wall infarction is caused by occlusion of the Anterior Descending branch of the Left Coronary Artery).

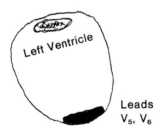

Leads
V_5, V_6

APICAL INFARCTION (LOW LATERAL) = pathologic Q waves in leads V_5 and V_6 (an apical infarct may be caused by occlusion of the Anterior Descending Artery, the Posterior Descending Artery, or the marginal branch of the Right Coronary Artery).

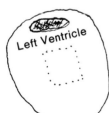

Leads
V_1, V_2 (reciprocal changes)

POSTERIOR WALL INFARCTION = large R waves in leads V_1 and V_2, tall and wide symmetrical T waves in leads V_1 and V_2, possibly Q waves in lead V_6 (a posterior infarct is usually caused by an occlusion of the Right Coronary Artery or one of its branches).

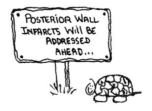

246

THERE IS ONLY ONE MORE THING TO REMEMBER. *IGNORE* lead aVR when looking for infarcts . . . Q waves in this lead are *not* significant. (Rather than being oriented to the left ventricular surface, lead aVR is oriented to the cavity of the left ventricle).

If you need to compare the following electrocardiograms to a normal EKG, look back to page 227.

Okay! Here is a patient that has been experiencing severe chest pain for 24 hours. He has had nausea and vomiting since the onset of chest pain.

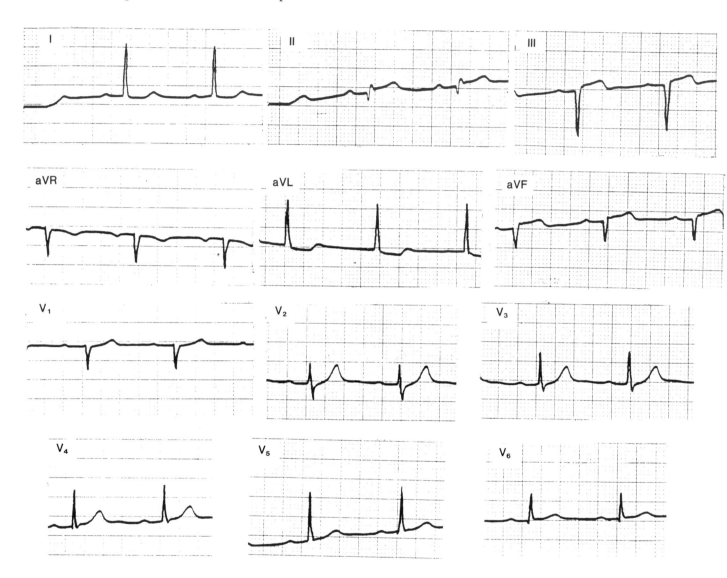

Observe each lead . . . look for any ST elevation (indicating current injury), and look for pathologic Q waves or loss of R waves (indicating necrosis).

How about me helping you 😊 ?

Lead I looks okay to me—there is a normal P, QRS, and T wave. The ST segment is "just a tad" below the isoelectric line.

Except . . . you know what . . . the P-R interval measures 6 small squares or 0.24 seconds! That is grounds for a first degree heart block!

In *Lead II,* I see several abnormalities . . . there is a prominent Q wave and the ST segment is elevated above the isoelectric line.

Lead III also has a large Q wave and ST elevation. You'll remember that *lead aVR* is the lead we are going to *ignore!*

Lead aVL shows slight ST segment depression—dipping below the isoelectric line.

Lead aVF also has a large Q wave and slight ST elevation.

All the V leads (V₁-V₆) look fairly normal.

So, in summary, there are pathologic Q waves and ST elevation in leads II, III, and aVF and slight ST depression in leads I and aVL.

What does all of that mean?

Left Ventricle

Well, look back to the summary chart on page 246. Elevated serum enzymes and pathologic Q waves in leads II, III, and aVF mean that there is an INFERIOR WALL MYOCARDIAL INFARCTION or inferior wall necrosis. The ST elevation implies current tissue injury. The slight ST depression noted in leads I and aVL is simply the reciprocal changes that appear in leads oriented toward the opposite uninjured myocardial surfaces.

Because the inferior wall of the left ventricle borders the diaphragm, it is easy to understand why the patient may be troubled with persistent hiccoughs, nausea, and/or vomiting.

Further, because it is usually the Right Coronary Artery which is occluded with an inferior wall infarction, and because the Right Coronary Artery feeds both the SA node and the AV node, one can anticipate an array of dysrhythmias!

As a matter of fact, that is no doubt why this patient has a first degree heart block! And you know what else—this patient later developed Wenckebach! Remember Wenckebach? If not, review page 140.

What do you think? Is looking at infarcts tough business?

Let's try another one!

*These are EKG calibrations!

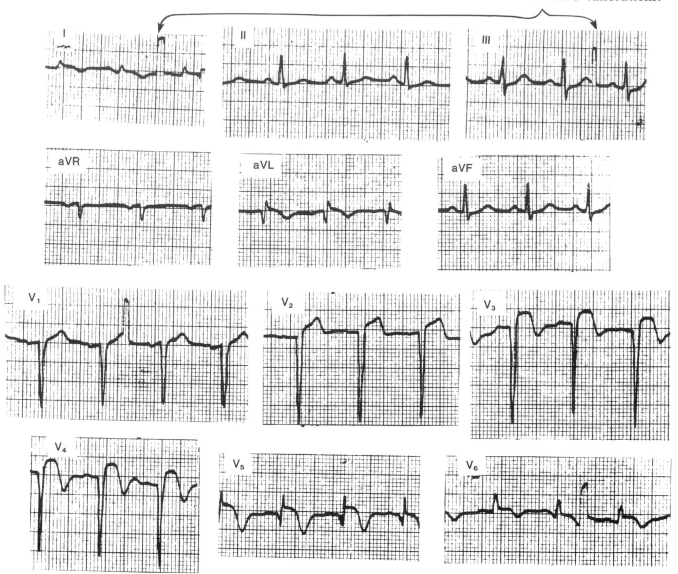

*To make certain that the EKG machine is properly calibrated, a standardized 1 millivolt pulse (10 vertical boxes) is periodically introduced into the tracing.

Remember, look at each lead!

Lead I looks rather "squatty" (low voltage) and the T waves are inverted. There is probably an initial Q wave, but it's difficult to tell for certain. There may also be slight ST elevation.

Leads II, III, and aVF appear normal, though there is slight ST sagging in leads *III* and *aVF*.

Lead aVL demonstrates very pronounced Q waves and inverted T waves. Further, there is slight ST elevation.

249

Lead aVF appears normal.

Leads V_1-V_4 show no R waves, only abnormal negative QS deflections. In addition, there is pronounced ST elevation.

Lead V_5 shows abnormal Q waves, ST elevation, and deeply inverted T waves. Also the R waves are greatly diminished in size.

Lead V_6 shows diminished R waves, a slightly elevated ST segment and inverted T waves.

This one is tough! 😖 Look back to the cheat chart (page 246) if you need to! Sometimes, if there is a lot of pathology, I do things in reverse order. For instance, *leads II, III, and aVF* are normal, so I presume that the inferior wall of the left ventricle is uninvolved.

You will remember that *leads I and aVL* represent the high lateral wall of the left ventricle. Since there are Q waves in both of these leads, I know that suggests high lateral wall myocardial infarction. Because there is slight ST elevation in both of these leads, I am assuming this injury is current. The inverted T waves tell me there is ischemia of the lateral wall as well. So, the Q waves in leads I and aVL probably represent a high lateral wall infarction. Does that make sense? Hope so!

Current injury and infarction in upright leads look like this:

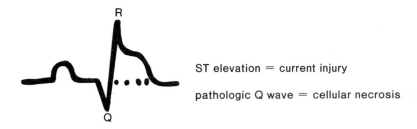

ST elevation = current injury

pathologic Q wave = cellular necrosis

Now, leads V_1-V_4 showed ST elevation and diminished or nonexistent R waves. Looking back at the chart on page 246, I see that leads V_1-V_4 reflect the electrical activity of the anteroseptal wall of the left ventricle. From the above changes in leads V_1-V_4, the patient's history of crushing chest pain and the elevated serum enzymes, I can assume the patient has an anteroseptal infarction. That means there is probably occlusion of the Left Anterior Descending coronary artery.

But wait! We're not done yet! 🙂

Lead V_5 showed abnormal Q waves; lead V_5 and V_6 showed ST elevation and inverted T waves. So, the Q waves represent necrosis, the ST elevations represent current injury, and the inverted T waves represent ischemia. The following day, a prominent Q wave was evident in V_6, as well. Since leads V_5 and V_6 represent the apical area or the low lateral region of the left ventricle, it would appear that the patient infarcted the apical region of the left ventricle as well as the anteroseptal and lateral surfaces!

Ugh! Also, one should bear in mind that the more "lethal" types of dysrhythmias . . . Mobitz II and complete heart block . . . are associated with anterior wall myocardial infarction.

Are you beginning to get the hang of what we're doing? GOOD!  Identifying infarct patterns is a matter of looking at each lead *very carefully* to determine any abnormal changes.

It is not always easy to determine the actual areas of infarct on EKG. There are many other complicating factors that may distort the EKG patterns, such as dysrhythmias, electrolyte imbalances, drug effects, and so forth. That is why the diagnosis of myocardial infarction is never based on the EKG findings alone! Also, if only a portion of the heart muscle wall is infarcted (rather than the entire muscle thickness—transmural), the EKG changes will be much more subtle.

The patient suspected of having an acute myocardial infarction (A.M.I.) or the patient actually having an A.M.I. must be monitored closely and continuously. The cells in the injured area of the heart muscle are ELECTRICALLY UNSTABLE. You will recall from Section IV, ischemic tissue is thought to release a *substance* which is capable of increasing the automaticity of the Purkinje fibers, resulting in electrical instability. This electrical instability may predispose the patient to *lethal* ventricular dysrhythmias. So, be on the lookout for P.V.C.'s! You will remember that most physicians institute lidocaine therapy prophylactically in the face of an acute myocardial infarction.

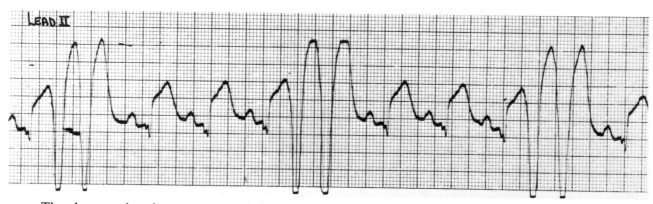

The above patient has an acute inferior wall myocardial infarction. Notice the extreme ST elevation and the prominent Q waves in lead II. This same pattern is evident in leads III and aVF, as well. P.V.C.'s are falling on the downstroke of the vulnerable T waves and are occurring in couplets. This patient is at high risk for ventricular tachycardia or ventricular fibrillation. Lidocaine therapy is the treatment of choice.

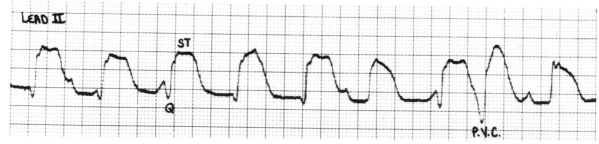

This strip (above) was recorded at the outset of an acute inferior wall myocardial infarction. Note the extreme ST elevation and the pathologic Q waves. Near the end of the strip, a P.V.C. falls near the vulnerable T wave, warning of increasing ventricular irritability. This patient, too, has an acute inferior wall myocardial infarction.

Decreased cardiac contractility occurs secondary to myocardial muscle injury.

WATCH THE ACUTE MYOCARDIAL INFARCT PATIENT
CLOSELY FOR SIGNS OF HEART
FAILURE AND SHOCK-LIKE SYMPTOMS.

The objects of treatment for acute myocardial infarction are to prevent further extension of the infarct and to restore hemodynamic equilibrium. In an uncomplicated infarct, this may include monitoring, rest, supportive therapy (e.g., oxygen, pain medication) and the control of related dysrhythmias. The treatment of a complicated infarct may include the above; plus, management of severe dysrhythmias with drug therapy, pacemakers, or electric shock; counterpulsation; Swan-Ganz pressure monitoring, etc. Principally, it is the degree of left ventricular muscle mass involvement, and secondarily, the occurrence of lethal dysrhythmias, that determine patient prognosis.

At the outset of acute myocardial infarction, thrombolytic drug therapy ("clot busters") may be used in an attempt to restore the patency of the blocked coronary artery. Please see the discussion on thrombolytic drug therapy, Section XII, page 312.

Let's try some practice before discussing posterior wall myocardial infarction!

Practice Exercise 2

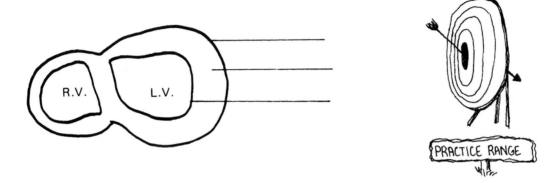

1. Above is a cross section view of the heart. Label the three muscle layers.

2. When an infarction involves the entire muscle wall (all three layers), it is known as a _____ infarction.

3. The diagnosis of myocardial infarction is based upon three criteria. List them!

   a. _____

   b. _____

   c. _____

4. Usually the first electrocardiographic finding of myocardial infarction is _____ , which represents "current injury" in the leads overlying the infarct. Draw a complex showing a current injury pattern.

(Circle the correct word.)

5. Reciprocal ST (elevation / depression) will occur in the leads oriented toward the uninjured myocardial surfaces.

6. The hallmark of myocardial infarction or necrosis is the _____ wave in upright

   leads and the _____ in negatively deflected leads.

7. To be pathologic, abnormal Q waves must meet two criteria: (fill in)

   a. The Q waves must measure at least _____ seconds in width or duration.

   b. The Q waves must be deeper than _____ the R wave amplitude.

8. Okay . . . here we go!

   This patient was admitted to the hospital with crushing chest pain radiating to his left elbow. Leads I, II, III, aVR, aVL, and aVF were essentially normal. Here are the precordial leads from his admission EKG. Study them closely, describe what you see, and make an interpretation using the chart on page 000.

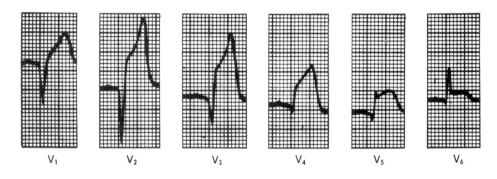

| V_1 | V_2 | V_3 | V_4 | V_5 | V_6 |

_____

_____

_____

_____

_____

_____

_____

_____

_____

_____

9. Here is another patient! This particular patient had indigestion-type pain, nausea, vomiting, and elevated serum enzymes. Study the leads on the next page carefully, describe what you see, and make an interpretation using the chart on page 246.

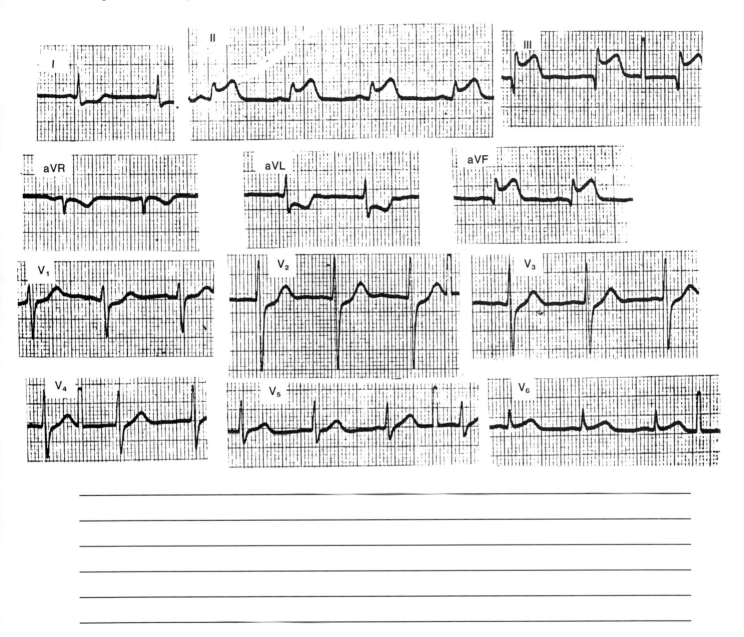

_____

_____

_____

_____

_____

_____

10. Below and continuing on the next page, are five examples (A-E) of various EKG lead patterns. On the following page are five descriptions of EKG patterns. Study the EKG patterns closely! Then write the letter of the example EKG pattern next to the phrase that correctly identifies the strip. (See phrases on page 255.)

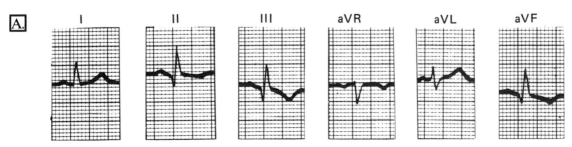

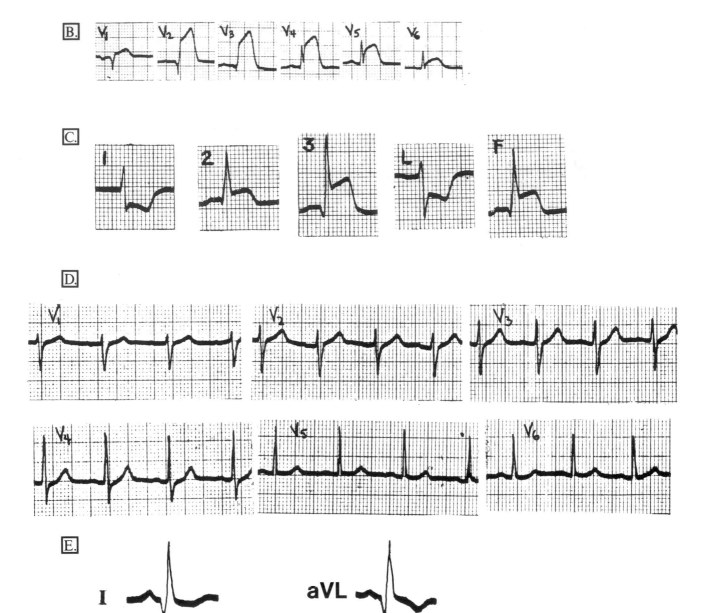

(letter)

_____ Prominent Q waves in leads II, III, and aVF. Inverted T waves in leads II, III, and aVF. Probable old inferior wall infarction with ischemia of the inferior wall.

_____ Marked ST depression and T wave inversion in leads I and aVL. Prominent Q waves and ST elevation in leads II, III, and aVF. Probable acute inferior wall myocardial infarction with reciprocal ST-T wave changes in the lateral leads.

_____ Pathologic Q waves in leads I and aVL. Inverted T waves in lead aVL. Probable old lateral wall infarction. The inverted T waves denote ischemia.

_____ Leads V_1-V_6 appear within normal limits. No pathology evident.

_____ Leads V_1-V_4 show abnormal QS deflections with marked ST elevation. There is marked ST elevation in leads V_5 and V_6. Probable acute anteroseptal wall infarction with injury extending to the apical wall of the left ventricle.

For **Feedback 2,** refer to page 261.

It feels like we've been working on this section forever. . . .

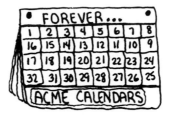

. . . so, we will make this exercise on POSTERIOR WALL MYOCARDIAL INFARCTS brief!

You'll remember that there are no leads that look directly at the posterior wall of the left ventricle. That presents somewhat of a problem! The only way that one can detect injury and infarction on the posterior surface of the heart is by looking at the leads opposite the posterior surface.

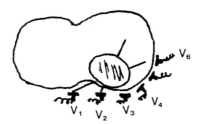

Leads V_1 and V_2 represent the anterior surface of the left ventricle and are opposite to the posterior left ventricular surface.

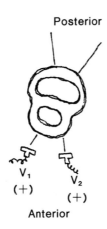

In other words, leads V_1 and V_2 lie opposite to the posterior surface of the heart.

So when looking for a posterior wall infarction, one needs to look at leads V_1 and V_2!

ELECTROCARDIOGRAPHIC FINDINGS ASSOCIATED WITH POSTERIOR WALL IN-FARCTIONS APPEAR <u>THE OPPOSITE</u> OF ELECTROCARDIOGRAPHIC FINDINGS ASSOCIATED WITH ANTERIOR WALL INFARCTIONS AS SEEN IN LEADS V_1 and V_2. So all you really have to remember is what an anterior wall infact looks like!

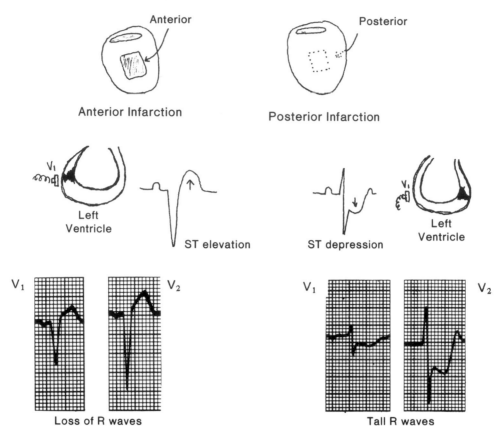

With an acute posterior wall myocardial infarction, one will see *tall R waves in leads V_1 and V_2* (instead of loss of R waves), *slight ST depression in leads V_1 and V_2* (rather than ST elevation), and tall, upright, symmetrical T waves.

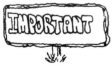

The other thing you should keep in mind is that a posterior wall infarct is usually due to occlusion of the Right Coronary Artery, or one of its branches. It is not uncommon, then, for concurrent injury to occur in both the inferior and posterior walls of the left ventricle.

P.S. WATCH OUT FOR DYSRHYTHMIAS!

As you might suspect, the posterior wall infarct patient may present with back pain, and sometimes this pain is mistaken for "renal pathology."

> . . . BEWARE OF THE PATIENT THAT PRESENTS WITH BACK PAIN. . . .
> (A WARNING FROM THE MANAGEMENT.)

Since this exercise is BRIEF, let's try some practice!

Practice Exercise 3

1. Leads _____ and _____ lie opposite the posterior surface of the left ventricle.

2. When looking at leads V_1 and V_2, the three EKG criteria arousing suspicion of a posterior wall infarction are:

   a. _____

   b. _____

   c. _____

3. This patient was admitted to the hospital with crushing chest pain radiating into his back. He was diaphoretic and nauseated. Look at each lead closely and describe what you see. Refer back to the chart on page 246 to help you with your interpretation.

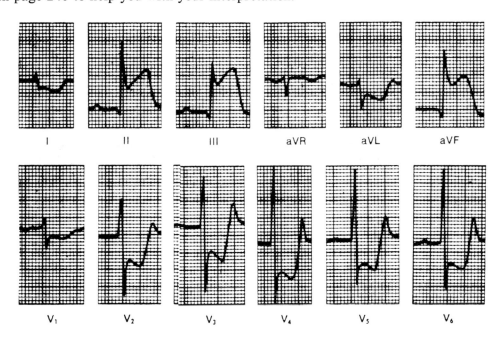

| I | II | III | aVR | aVL | aVF |

| V_1 | V_2 | V_3 | V_4 | V_5 | V_6 |

_____

_____

_____

_____

_____

_____

_____

_____

_____

_____

For **Feedback 3,** refer to page 263.

IMPORTANT NOTES ABOUT CARDIAC ENZYMES

I thought it would be helpful to provide you with some basic information about cardiac enzymes. You will recall that the diagnosis of acute myocardial infarction is based upon three things: (1) a positive patient history, (2) positive cardiac enzymes, (3) specific EKG changes.

Basically enzymes are proteins that serve to catalyze various chemical reactions in the body. Each organ and tissue group tends to have both dominant and less dominant enzymes. In effect, when tissues or organs are damaged, they tend to leak their specific enzymes which can be detected via blood sampling.

It is also important to know that certain enzymes exist in slightly different molecular forms called isoenzymes which can be identified through electrophoresis.

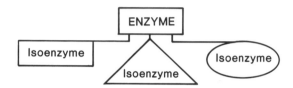

Isoenzymes are more tissue specific than enzymes. (The same enzyme may be found in various organs and tissues; isoenzymes tend to be limited to more specific organs or tissues.) In attempting to identify acute myocardial infarct, we are concerned with three major enzymes (CPK, LDH, SGOT) and three isoenzymes (CPK_2, LDH_1, LDH_2). We will address each of those enzymes and isenzymes separately.

CPK

CPK (creatine phosphokinase) is an enzyme predominantly found in brain, skeletal, and heart tissue. The CPK enzyme rises within the first eight hours following acute myocardial infarct, peaking within the first 24 hours. (The normal CPK level is 20–230 U/L.) An elevated CPK within the first 24 hours is a fairly sensitive indicator of acute myocardial infarction, but it may also be elevated with neuropathology and skeletal tissue damage.

There are three CPK isoenzymes which provide further diagnostic information: CPK_1 (BB) found in the brain, lungs, bowel, and bladder; CPK_2 (MB) predominantly found in the myocardium; and CPK_3 (MM) found in skeletal and heart muscle.

CPK_2 (MB)

We will concentrate on CPK_2 (MB) since it is specific to the myocardium. CPK_2 (MB) is found in the serum of all acute myocardial infarction patients for 48 hours post infarct. It may also be found in the serum of patients having experienced severe myocardial ischemia without frank infarction. Generally, a CPK_2 (MB) level of less than two percent is considered insignificant; a level of two to four percent is considered borderline; a CPK_2 (MB) level of greater than four percent is considered positive. *However*, depending upon the laboratory method used to determine CPK_2 (MB) levels, percentage limits for both normal and abnormal values may vary.

SGOT

SGOT (serum glutamic oxaloacetic transaminase), also known as SAPT (serum apirate aminotransferase), is the second major enzyme to rise when an acute myocardial infarction has occurred. The SGOT (normal level = 8–33 U/L) rises eight to 12 hours following infarction and reaches a level two to three times the upper limit of normal. An elevated SGOT is thought to have a predictive value near 80 percent. The SGOT begins to return to normal limits on the fourth or fifth day post infarct. As with CPK, an SGOT elevation may be associated with other conditions. Specifically, the SGOT may be elevated with liver disease, liver congestion secondary to heart failure, and pulmonary infarction.

LDH

LDH (lactate dehyrogenase) is the third major enzyme to rise in the face of acute myocardial infarction. LDH is predominantly found in the heart, the skeletal muscle, and the liver. Normal serum levels range between 100–190 U/L. When associated with acute infarction, the LDH rises 12 to 24 hours post infarct, reaching a peak on the third day post infarct. It is important to recognize that an LDH rise may also be associated with liver disease, skeletal muscle disease, pulmonary infarct, etc.

LDH_1, LDH_2

Similar to CPK, there are isoenzymes associated with the LDH enzyme, five to be exact. LDH_1 and LDH_2 are the two isoenzymes that we will be concerned with. Both LDH_1 and LDH_2 are found in the heart, the red cells, and the kidney. Normally, the level of LDH_1 is less than the level of LDH_2. In an acute myocardial infarction, LDH_1 is released from the damaged myocardial cells, thus changing the ratio of LDH_1 to LDH_2. In other words, in the face of acute myocardial infarction, the level of LDH_1 is greater than LDH_2. This reversal may be observed one to three days after acute myocardial infarction.

Summary

Based on the above discussion, it is clear that a rise in a single enzyme or isoenzyme is not necessarily conclusive! *For the best diagnostic picture, all of the previously mentioned enzymes and isoenzymes should be analyzed for a one to three day period following the suspected infarct.* The presence of a significant CPK_2 and a reversed LDH_1 to LDH_2 ratio is considered absolute proof of an acute myocardial infarction!

Again . . . I do not expect you to commit all of this information to memory! Rather, this section can serve as a *future reference*. Since this material is a BONUS, there is no practice exercise!

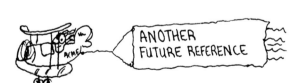

Feedback 1

How did you do? If all your answers are correct, you are entitled to one free stray cat. If you don't believe me, call the animal shelter and ask!

1. YES, YES, YES . . . the end of this book really is in sight . . . honest!

2. The 12 lead EKG allows one to look at the electrical activity of the heart from various <u>angles or from various points of reference</u>.

3. The most important chamber of the heart is the left ventricle because <u>it functions as "The Pump" or the driving force for systemic circulation</u>.

4.

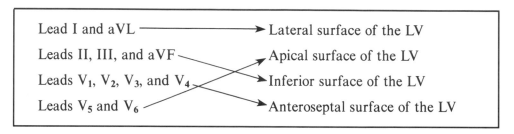

Lead I and aVL ——————→ Lateral surface of the LV

Leads II, III, and aVF ——→ Apical surface of the LV

Leads V_1, V_2, V_3, and V_4 ——→ Inferior surface of the LV

Leads V_5 and V_6 ——→ Anteroseptal surface of the LV

5. By definition, *ischemia* is the myocardial change that results from a <u>temporary, insufficient</u> blood supply.

6. Myocardial ischemia presents on the EKG as <u>ST and T wave</u> changes in the leads looking at the ischemic surfaces.

7. Lead I shows a depressed and flat ST segment and a flattened T wave.
Leads II and III show slight ST depression and inverted T waves.
In lead aVL the ST segment is depressed.
In lead aVF the T wave is inverted.
Leads V_2, V_3, V_4, V_5, and V_6 show ST depression and T wave inversion (generalized ischemic changes).

Feedback 2

Whew! How did you do with this practice section? Sometimes, learning this material is a S-L-O-W process. It may help to read it through several times!

1.

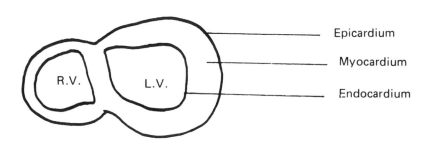

Epicardium

Myocardium

Endocardium

2. When an infarction involves the entire muscle wall (all three layers), it is known as a <u>TRANS-MURAL</u> infarction.

3. The diagnosis of myocardial infarction is based upon three criteria.

    a. <u>Positive patient history</u>.
    b. <u>Elevated serum enzymes</u>.
    c. <u>Specific EKG changes</u>.

4. Usually the first electrocardiographic finding of myocardial infarction is <u>ST ELEVATION</u>, which represents "current injury" in the leads overlying the infarct.

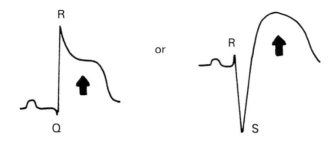

5. Reciprocal ST (elevation / (depression)) will occur in leads oriented toward the uninjured myocardial surfaces.

6. The hallmark of myocardial infarction or necrosis is the <u>ABNORMAL Q</u> wave in upright leads and the <u>LOSS OF R WAVE</u> in negatively deflected leads.

7. To be pathologic, the abnormal Q waves must meet two criteria:

    a. The Q waves must measure at least <u>0.04</u> seconds in width or duration.
    b. The Q waves must be deeper than ¼ the R wave amplitude.

8. INTERPRETATION:
There are abnormal QS patterns and marked ST elevation in leads V_1-V_4. Leads V_5 and V_6 show Q waves and ST elevation. These changes represent probable acute anteroseptal wall myocardial infarction, including infarction of the apical surface of the left ventricle.

9. INTERPRETATION:
Lead I shows depression of the ST segment.
Lead aVL shows ST depression and inverted T waves.
Leads II, III, and aVF demonstrate prominent Q waves and pronounced ST elevation.
Leads V_1-V_6 appear normal.
This EKG represents probable acute inferior wall myocardial infarction with reciprocal ST-T wave changes in the lateral leads.

10. Last, but not least . . .

    <u>A</u> Prominent Q waves in leads II, III, and aVF. Inverted T waves in leads II, III, and aVF. Probable old inferior wall infarction with ischemia of the inferior wall.

    <u>C</u> Marked ST depression and T wave inversion in leads I and aVL. Prominent Q waves and ST elevation in leads II, III, and aVF. Probable acute inferior wall myocardial infarction with reciprocal ST-T wave changes in the lateral leads.

    <u>E</u> Pathologic Q waves in leads I and aVL. Inverted T waves in aVL. Probable old lateral wall infarction. The inverted T waves denote ischemia.

    <u>D</u> Leads V_1-V_6 appear within normal limits. No pathology evident.

    <u>B</u> Leads V_1-V_4 show abnormal QS deflections with marked ST elevation. There is marked ST elevation in leads V_5 and V_6. Probable acute anteroseptal wall infarction with injury extending to the apical wall of the left ventricle.

Feedback 3

IF YOU ANSWERED ALL THREE QUESTIONS CORRECTLY, YOU ARE ENTITLED TO ONE FREE "EKG MERIT BADGE." (Please cut along the dotted lines.)

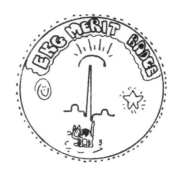

1. Leads V_1 and V_2 lie opposite the posterior surface of the left ventricle.

2. When looking at leads V_1 and V_2, the three EKG criteria arousing suspicion of a posterior wall infarction are:

   a. Tall R wave
   b. Slight ST depression
   c. Tall, upright symmetrical T waves

   P.S. Remember, the diagnosis of acute myocardial infarction is never based on the EKG findings alone.

3. INTERPRETATION:

   Leads I and aVL show significant ST depression.
   Leads II, III, and aVF show prominent Q waves and marked ST elevation.
   Lead V_1 shows a small R wave and ST depression.
   Lead V_2 shows a tall R wave, ST depression, and a tall, upright T wave.
   Leads V_3-V_6 show a fairly normal progression of R waves and severely depressed ST segments.
   The T waves remain upright.

   The pathologic Q waves and ST elevation in leads II, III, and aVF suggest an acute inferior wall myocardial infarction. The ST depression noted in leads I and aVL is simply the reciprocal change occurring in leads oriented toward the uninjured myocardial surface.

   Though by itself, V_1 is only suspicious of a posterior wall myocardial infarction, V_2 confirms any doubts. The ST depression noted in V_3-V_6 is no doubt reciprocal in nature.

   . . . So, there appears to be acute injury and necrosis of both the inferior and posterior surfaces of the left ventricle! UGH!

NOTES

NOTES

SECTION XI
An Introduction to Hemodynamic Monitoring

OBJECTIVES

When you have completed Section XI, you will be able to describe or identify

1. blood flow through the heart, identifying chambers, valves, and major vessels
2. normal right atrial, right ventricular, pulmonary artery, and pulmonary capillary wedge pressure valves
3. typical pressure waveforms associated with right heart chambers and the pulmonary artery
4. relationships among pulmonary artery diastolic pressure, pulmonary capillary wedge pressure, and left ventricular end diastolic pressure
5. causes for abnormal pressures
6. this section as a future reference!!

Text by

DeANNA M. CULBERSON

Like EKG monitoring, hemodynamic monitoring is an important "tool" for assessing the critically ill patient. By definition, hemodynamic monitoring refers to monitoring the *motion* or *mechanics* of blood flow through, in this case, the cardiac chambers and pulmonary vasculature. Thus, the EKG allows the practitioner to access the electrical functioning of the heart, and hemodynamic monitoring provides an avenue for evaluting the mechanical pumping action.

A *transducer* system is utilized to convert the mechanical pumping action into an electrical waveform displayed on a monitor. A transducer is much like a bathroom scale! When weight or pressure is applied to a bathroom scale, the gauge on the scale moves.

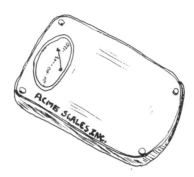

When pressure is applied to a transducer, the resulting waveform rises on the monitor and then falls as pressure is removed. Easy so far, right? As you progress through this section, you will learn that each cardiac chamber presents unique waveform characteristics!

You will recall from Section I, page 22, that monitor paper has both a time and amplitude dimension. Moving across monitor paper denotes time.

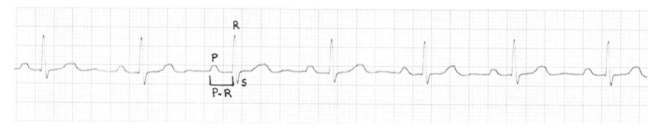

Moving vertically denotes amplitude. Each small square represents 1mm amplitude, and each large square represents 5mm amplitude. As we move forward in the section, waveforms and the pressure they represent will be measured along the amplitude dimension. For example, the pressure waves in this diagram measure $\dfrac{36}{2}$.

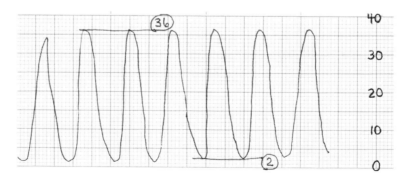

As you can see, some estimation is required since there is ongoing variability in waveforms.

One last introductory note . . . monitors come in a garden variety of sizes, shapes, and capabilities. Multichannel monitoring systems are required to concurrently monitor EKG patterns and hemodynamic parameters. Commonly, multichannel monitoring systems are found in critical care and critical care step down units.

Input 1: Indications for Invasive Hemodynamic Monitoring

The next issue deals with the patient population requiring hemodynamic monitoring. Essentially, all critically ill patients are *hemodynamically* monitored. For example, blood pressure, pulse and respiration monitoring represent *non-invasive* means for evaluating cardiac function and tissue perfusion. Invasive hemodynamic monitoring, however, is usually reserved for the most critically ill and unstable patients. Invasive hemodynamic monitoring requires the insertion of a pulmonary artery catheter (Swan-Ganz catheter), a minor surgical procedure. This patient population may have critical diagnoses (myocardial infarct, chronic pulmonary disease), be undergoing extensive surgical procedures, or have multiple complicating medical problems.

Invasive monitoring provides specific clinical data to guide precise therapeutic intervention. Invasive hemodynamic monitoring allows differentiation between cardiac and pulmonary disease and provides prognostic data regarding the extent of pathology.

THE FUNDAMENTALS

The primary functions of the cardiovascular system are to deliver oxygen and nutrients to the cells and remove wastes.

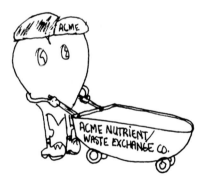

In order to perform this nutrient/waste exchange, the left heart must systemically circulate the oxygenated blood from the pulmonary vasculature throughout the system to the cells. Then, the deoxygenated blood and byproducts are returned to the right heart and lungs.

As can be seen in the following diagram, deoxygenated blood enters the right atrium (RA) via the inferior and superior vena cava. From the right atrium (RA), the blood crosses the tricuspid valve into the right ventricle (RV). Due to its larger muscle mass, the right ventricle (RV) can generate stronger muscle contraction and greater perfusion pressure. The right ventricle (RV) pumps deoxygenated blood across the pulmonic valve into the pulmonary artery (PA). The blood then flows through the pulmonary vascular beds, a passive activity owing to the absence of contracting vessels and valves. Carbon dioxide (CO_2) is exchanged for oxygen (O_2) as the blood flows through the pulmonary vasculature.

The oxygenated blood then returns to the left atrium (LA) via the pulmonary veins. After passing across the mitral valve, the blood begins to fill the left ventricular (LV) chamber. The left ventricle has both the largest and strongest muscle mass of any of the four heart chambers. This muscle mass allows the left ventricle (LV) to generate a pressure of sufficient magnitude to eject the contained blood volume past the aortic valve into the aorta, and out to the vascular beds (systemic circulation).

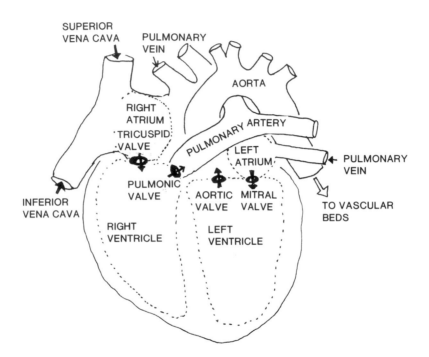

The blood flows from cardiac chamber to chamber in a cyclic manner. The valves (tricuspid, pulmonic, mitral, and aortic) perform gatekeeper functions, keeping the blood flowing in a forward direction. The blood flow cycle can be broken down into two major phases: (1) *systole,* or the contraction/ejection phase; and (2) *diastole,* the relaxation/filling phase. During any given cycle, the pressure and blood volume in each chamber differs. It is this pressure difference that permits the cardiac valves to open and close appropriately.

The following diagram demonstrates ventricular diastole or ventricular filling. The blood volume in the right and left atria has increased which, in turn, has increased the atrial chamber pressures. These mounting pressures force the tricuspid and mitral valves open, allowing the right and left ventricles to fill. The release of pressure in the atrial chambers stimulates the atrial muscle to contract. Atrial muscle contraction immediately follows electrical activation (depolarization) of the atria. The P wave seen on the EKG monitor corresponds with ventricular diastole or filling. You will remember that the P wave represents atrial depolarization.

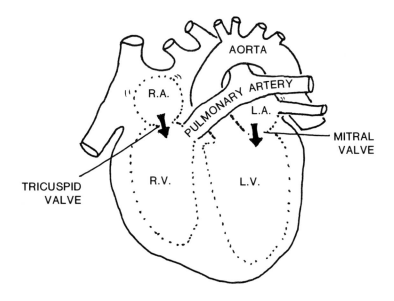

VENTRICULAR FILLING. MOUNTING ATRIAL PRESSURES
FORCE OPEN THE TRICUSPID AND MITRAL VALVES.

Ventricular systole occurs when the pressure and volume in the right and left ventricles exceed atrial pressures. The rising ventricular pressures force the mitral and tricuspid valves closed. The aortic and pulmonic valves are then forced open, allowing blood to flow out of the ventricles.

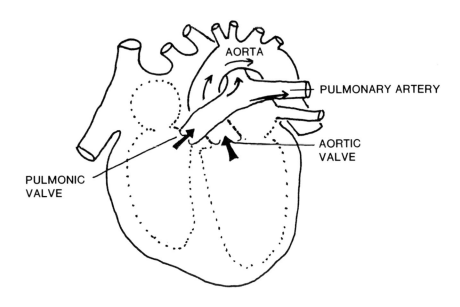

This release of pressure in the ventricular chambers stimulates the ventricular muscles to contract. Ventricular muscle contraction immediately follows electrical activation (depolarization) of the ventricles. Electrical depolarization produces the QRS seen on the EKG monitor!

This systole and diastole business is sometimes confusing! It may be helpful to remember . . .

DIASTOLE = STRETCH AND FILL
SYSTOLE = CONTRACTION AND EJECTION

The following diagram depicts the relationship between diastole and systole and the cardiac cycle. Note the cardiac valve activity in each sequence.

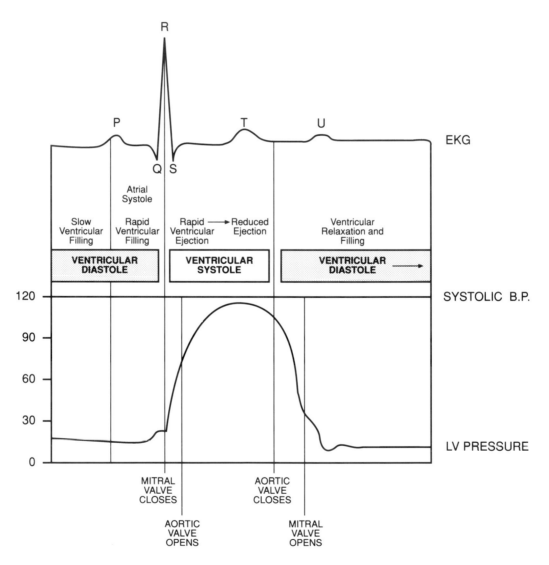

Cardiac cycle demonstrating EKG relationship to ventricular diastole, systole and valve function.

The cycle of increasing and decreasing cardiac pressures was first postulated by Ernest Starling (early 1900s).

Starling's Law
The force of contraction is proportional to the muscle fiber length up to a critical length. When the critical length is exceeded, myocardial contractile force decreases.

To simplify this concept, Starling's Law can be compared to a rubber band stretching. If the rubber band (fiber) is stretched (diastole) a SHORT distance, contraction (systole) is *weak*. If, however, the rubber band is **FULLY** stretched (diastole) to its critical length, contraction (systole) is *forceful* and *efficient*! If a rubber band is repeatedly **OVERSTRETCHED** (diastole), it becomes *weakened* and its contractile force (systole) is *diminished*. And so goes the Starling Theory of rubber bands!

From this point we will now address some practical rubber band and hemodynamic principles! The rubber band length can be compared to mycardial fiber length. *Fiber length* is determined by the amount of *filling pressure*. Filling pressure is the same as *PRELOAD*.

FILLING PRESSURE = PRELOAD

The force of rubber band contraction can be compared to the *myocardial contractile force*. Myocardial force is a measure of cardiac output. If the force of contraction is weak, cardiac output is low or diminished. If the force of contraction is strong, cardiac output is adequate or maximized.

MYOCARDIAL CONTRACTILE FORCE = CARDIAC OUTPUT

STARLING'S LAW viewed the heart as a single pump. Hence, the central venous pressure (CVP) was used as a measure of single pump function. However, the fact that the heart is actually two pumps (right heart and left heart) means that the left sided pump would be in *complete* failure before any change in CVP pressure would be recorded. Conclusion: not good! What was needed was a method to assess left heart preload! (Remember, the CVP measures right heart preload.) What was sought was a method for measuring left atrial pressure! Until the advent of the pulmonary artery catheter, left heart preload measurement would have required open chest surgery!

The introduction of the pulmonary artery (Swan-Ganz) catheter permitted indirect, invasive measurement of left heart pressures. Although the pulmonary artery catheter is placed in the right side of the heart, the opening of the mitral valve allows the tip of the catheter to "view" the left ventricle. Remember, there are no valves between the pulmonary artery and the left atrium!

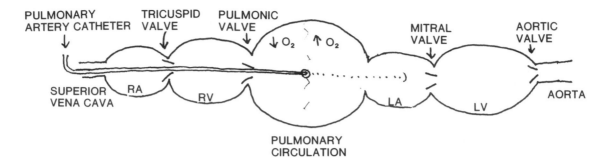

If one thinks of the cardiac circulatory system being laid "end to end", it is easier to understand how a right heart catheter can view the left ventricle.

As we move along this should become more clear.

Practice Exercise 1

1. Invasive hemodynamic monitoring is accomplished via a _____ _____ catheter.

2. The size (mass) and strength of the left ventricle allows oxygenated blood to be ejected past the _____ valve into the _____ , and out to systemic circulation.

3. Correctly label the four cardiac valves.

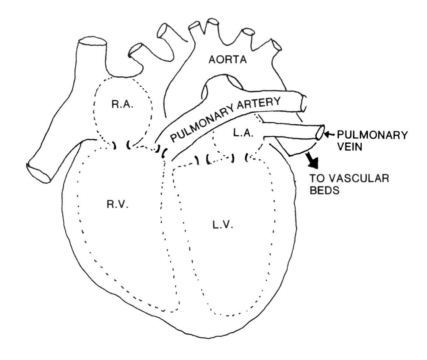

4. The contraction/ejection phase of the blood flow cycle is termed _____; the relaxation/filling phase of the blood flow cycle is known as _____.

5. If a muscle fiber is stretched (diastole) a short distance, contraction (systole) is _____. If a muscle fiber is fully stretched to its critical length, contraction is _____. If a muscle fiber is repeatedly overstretched, contractile force is _____.

6. Starling was a
   ☐ BIRD
   ☐ PLANE
   ☐ LAW MAN
   (sense of humor poll conducted by the management ☺)

7. CVP is a measure of _____ .

8. Cardiac output (CO) is a measure of _____ .

For **Feedback 1,** refer to page 289.

Input 2: The Pulmonary Artery Catheter

The pulmonary artery catheter (Swan-Ganz catheter) is a hollow latex tube with three internal lumens. In addition, a thermistor runs through the length of the catheter. If one were to cut the catheter in half, it would look like the following diagram.

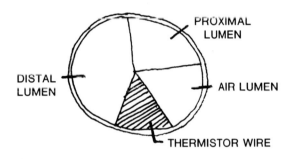

CROSS SECTION: PULMONARY ARTERY CATHETER

The distal catheter lumen opens up at the catheter tip. The proximal catheter lumen opens approximately 30cm from the tip of the catheter. Right atrial pressure is monitored at the proximal lumen opening. The proximal catheter port is utilized for fluid administration.

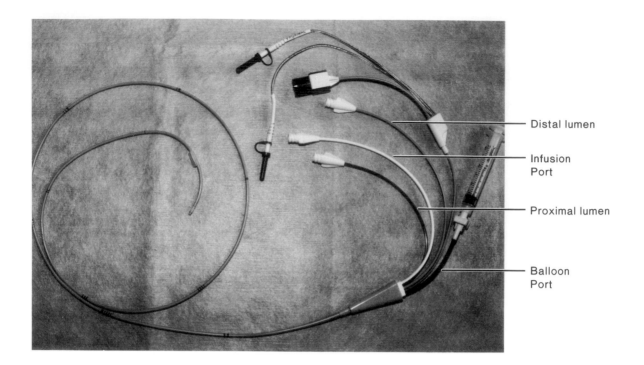

— Distal lumen

— Infusion Port

— Proximal lumen

— Balloon Port

An inflatable latex balloon is located at the tip of the catheter. By injecting air into the "air lumen," the balloon can be inflated. Once the catheter is inserted and the catheter tip is located in the right atrium, the balloon is inflated to allow the catheter to free flow with the blood, from cardiac chamber to chamber, ending in the pulmonary artery. The inflated balloon causes the pulmonary catheter to "wedge" into a small pulmonary vessel facilitating pressure measurement. The thermistor is used to measure the patient's core temperature and to measure cardiac output (when connected to a cardiac output computer).

A NOTE ABOUT
MEASURING CARDIAC OUTPUT

When measuring cardiac output using the thermodilution method, a known volume of fluid (10cc) with a known temperature (iced or room temp.), is injected into the right heart via the proximal lumen of the pulmonary artery catheter. As the fluid mixes with the blood and passes by the thermistor, the computer calculates the cardiac output. Normal cardiac output ranges between 4–7 liters/minute.

To evaluate left heart preload or filling pressure, a pulmonary artery catheter is inserted . . . and wedged into a pulmonary artery branch (wedge position). Readers should remember that the central venous pressure (CVP) is a measure of right heart preload or filling pressure; the pulmonary capillary wedge pressure (PCWP) is a measure of left heart preload or filling pressure. Read ahead to clarify any confusion!

RIGHT HEART PRELOAD = CVP
LEFT HEART PRELOAD = PCWP

Practice Exercise 2

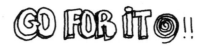

1. The pulmonary artery catheter (Swan-Ganz catheter) has three internal lumens, and a _____ which is used to measure core temperature and _____ .

2. The _____ pulmonary artery catheter port is utilized for fluid administration.

3. _____ atrial pressure is monitored at the proximal lumen opening.

4. An inflated pulmonary artery catheter balloon causes the catheter to _____ into a small pulmonary vessel.

5. Normal cardiac output (CO) ranges between _____ and _____ liters per minute.

6. _____ is a measure of right heart preload or_____ pressure.

7. The pulmonary capillary wedge pressure (PCWP) is a measure of _____ or filling pressure.

For **Feedback 2,** refer to page 290.

Input 3: Pressures and Waveformations

Right Atrium

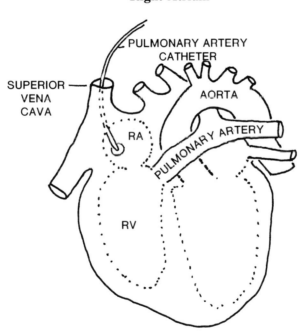

The pulmonary artery catheter
is situated in the right atrium.

The above diagram demonstrates the placement of pulmonary artery catheter in the right atrium. You will recall that blood flow to the right atrium (RA) is passive. Intrathoracic pressure changes occurring secondary to respiration assist blood return to the right heart. Owing to its small muscle mass, the normal right atrial pressure is low. The low pressure produces a low amplitude, oscillating waveform demonstrated in the following diagrams. Because there is minimal difference between right atrial systolic and diastolic pressures, only a mean right atrial (RA) pressure is reported.

RIGHT ATRIAL (RA) PRESSURE WAVEFORM

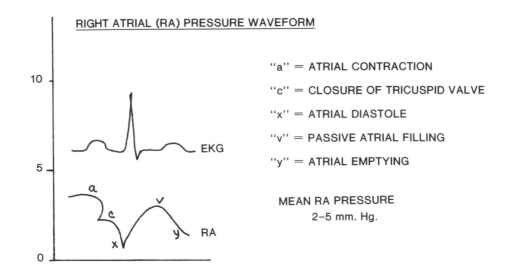

"a" = ATRIAL CONTRACTION

"c" = CLOSURE OF TRICUSPID VALVE

"x" = ATRIAL DIASTOLE

"v" = PASSIVE ATRIAL FILLING

"y" = ATRIAL EMPTYING

MEAN RA PRESSURE
2–5 mm. Hg.

RIGHT ATRIAL (RA) PRESSURE

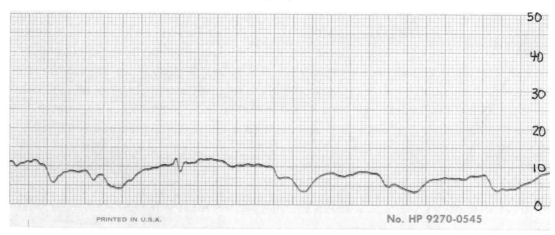

Note the low amplitude, oscillating waveform

NORMAL MEAN RIGHT ATRIAL PRESSURE = 2–5mm Hg.

Low RA pressure may signify hypovolemia or vasodilation. Elevated pressures may signify fluid over-load, RV failure, tricuspid insufficiency or chronic left heart failure.

Right Ventricle

Before you move forward, a bit of review is in order! Earlier in this section, the cardiac valves and their gatekeeper function were discussed. The cardiac valves serve to keep blood flowing in a forward direction. The tricuspid valve (see page 268) is located between the right atrium and the right ventricle. When the tricuspid valve opens, the blood volume in the right atrium (RA) flows into the right ventricle (RV). The right ventricular filling pressure (preload) is a function of right atrial pressure. You will recall from page 270 that filling pressure is the same as diastolic pressure. So, the right ventricular diastolic pressure is equal to the mean right atrial pressure, 2–5mm Hg.

RIGHT VENTRICULAR (RV) DIASTOLIC PRESSURE = 2–5mm Hg.

Secondary to its greater muscle mass, the right ventricle (RV) can generate a greater contractile force and systolic pressure than the right atrium. The systolic or emptying pressure of the right ventricle ranges between 20–30mm Hg.

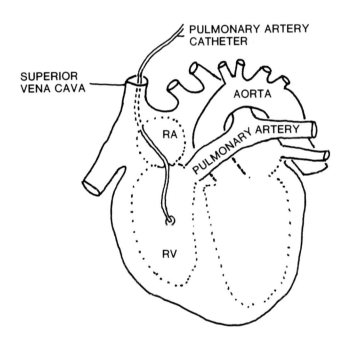

The above diagram demonstrates the placement of a pulmonary artery catheter in the right ventricle. To review:

NORMAL RIGHT VENTRICULAR (RV) PRESSURE = $\dfrac{\text{20–30mm Hg. (systolic)}}{\text{2–5mm Hg. (diastolic)}}$

The following diagrams demonstrate normal right ventricular (RV) waveforms.

RIGHT VENTRICULAR (RV) PRESSURE WAVEFORM

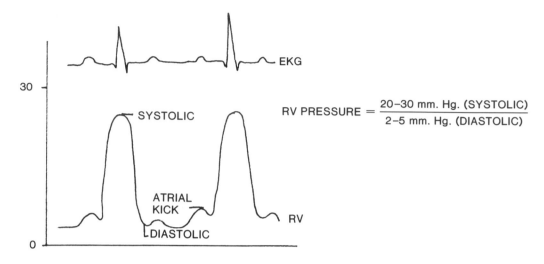

$$\text{RV PRESSURE} = \frac{\text{20–30 mm. Hg. (SYSTOLIC)}}{\text{2–5 mm. Hg. (DIASTOLIC)}}$$

NOTE: THE RV WAVEFORM AND PRESSURE CAN *ONLY* BE RECORDED ON CATHETER INSERTION SINCE THERE IS NO CATHETER OPENING INTO THE RIGHT VENTRICULAR CHAMBER. THIS IS NOT A DESIGN FLAW!! A CATHETER OPENING INTO THE RV COULD INDUCE VENTRICULAR DYSRHYTHMIAS!

RIGHT VENTRICULAR (RV) PRESSURE

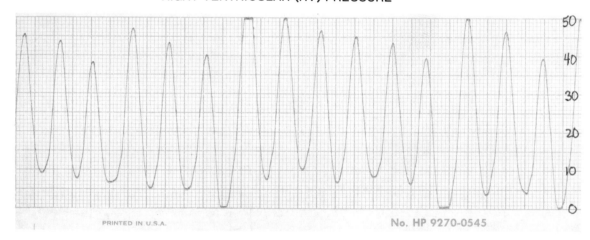

PRINTED IN U.S.A.   No. HP 9270-0545

Low RV pressures indicate hypovolemia or vasodilation. Increased RV pressures may relate to right ventricular failure, pulmonic valve insufficiency, chronic lung disease, chronic left ventricular failure, mechanical ventilation, or cardiac tamponade.

How are you doing thus far! At best, the hemodynamic monitoring concepts should create a stretch in your thinking!

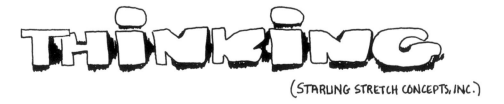

(STARLING STRETCH CONCEPTS, INC.)

Pulmonary Artery

When the pulmonic valve opens secondary to increasing right ventricular pressure, blood and the pulmonary artery catheter move out of the right ventricle into the pulmonary artery (PA). Though the pulmonary artery has no contractile properties, both systolic and diastolic pressures can be measured.

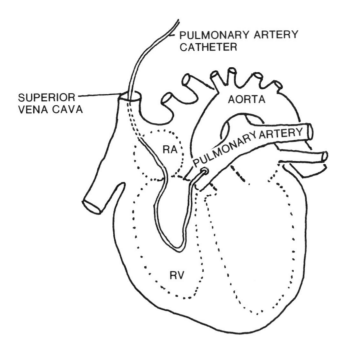

The above diagram demonstrates the pulmonary artery catheter placed in the pulmonary artery. (HOME AT LAST!) Pulmonary artery filling is a function of right ventricular contraction and emptying.

The pressure generated (systolic pressure) by the right ventricle is also the pulmonary artery (PA) systolic pressure!

RV SYSTOLIC PRESSURE = PA SYSTOLIC PRESSURE
20–30mm Hg. 20–30mm Hg.

Let's backtrack a minute. You will remember that the right atrial (RA) pressure was 2–5mm Hg. Right atrial (RA) pressure drives the filling of the right ventricle (RV). As the RV fills, the right ventricular muscle stretches, forcing the pulmonic valve system open. This release of pressure stimulates the RV muscle to contract. As the muscle contracts, it generates a higher pressure, thus allowing complete emptying of the RV chamber. That emptying pressure is 20–30mm Hg. in the healthy heart. When the pulmonic valve opens, the RV pressure is now reflected—ejected—into the pulmonary artery. So the highest or systolic pressure in the pulmonary artery is also 20–30mm Hg.!

PRESSURE POINTS			
	RIGHT ATRIUM (RA)	RIGHT VENTRICLE (RV)	PULMONARY ARTERY (PA)
SYSTOLIC MEAN DIASTOLIC	2–5mm Hg.····	20–30mm Hg.··········20–30mm Hg. ———————— ···2–5mm Hg.	————————

Makes sense, right!

Following pulmonary artery filling, the pulmonic valve closes to keep blood flowing in a forward direction. Valve closure creates a "back slosh" of blood against the valve, producing a distinctive notching in the waveform. This notching is referred to as the *dicrotic notch*. Please see the following diagram.

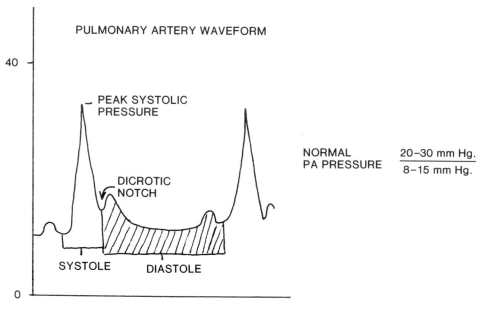

The dicrotic notch is produced by closure of the pulmonic valve.

Low systolic pulmonary artery (PA) pressures would signify hypovolemia and/or vasodilation. Elevated pressures may be associated with a number of causes including pulmonary emboli, mitral insufficiency, left ventricular failure, cardiac tamponade, and mechanical ventilation.

From the pulmonary artery, blood then flows passively through the pulmonary vasculature. Remember, there are no valves or "other blood flow controlling devices" in the pulmonary beds or left atrial juncture! Oxygenation occurs as the blood flows through the pulmonary system. As the blood disperses across the pulmonary vascular beds, the pressure drops to a resting or diastolic level. The resting pulmonary artery (PA) diastolic pressure ranges between 8–15mm Hg.

280

In summary, a normal pulmonary artery pressure (PAP) will reflect the following norms:

PULMONARY ARTERY =	20–30mm Hg. (systolic)
PRESSURE (PAP) =	8–15mm Hg. (diastolic)

The following diagram demonstrates a pulmonary artery catheter moving from the right ventricle into the pulmonary artery. Note that both the RV and PA pressures are elevated.

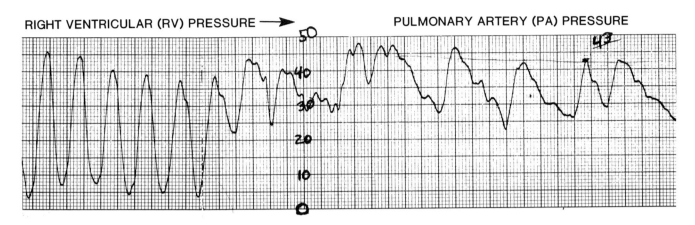

RIGHT VENTRICULAR (RV) PRESSURE ⟶   PULMONARY ARTERY (PA) PRESSURE

The following table may help clarify any confusion relating to the chamber pressures discussed thus far.

PRESSURE POINTS		
	RIGHT ATRIAL (RA) PRESSURE	RIGHT VENTRICLE (RV) PRESSURE	PULMONARY ARTERY (PA) PRESSURE
SYSTOLIC		20–30mm Hg.· · · · · · · · · ·	20–30mm Hg.
MEAN	2–5mm Hg. · · · · · ·	_____	_____
DIASTOLIC	· · · · · · · ·2–5mm Hg.	8–15mm Hg.

As you can see in the above table, a relationship exists between the various chamber and pulmonary artery pressures! (The pressure in any given chamber is reflective of the preceding chamber.)

Left Atrium

Earlier discussion indicated that there are no valves present in either the pulmonary vascular system or the left atrial junction. Thus, blood flows passively from the pulmonary artery into the left atrium (LA).

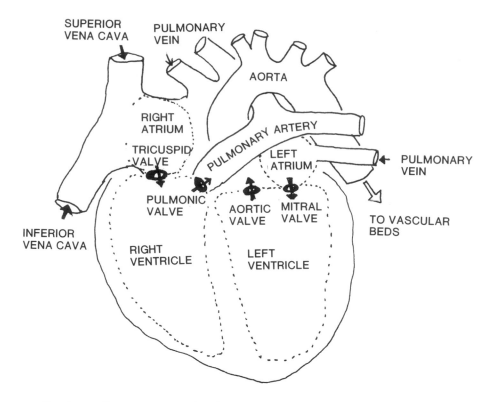

This absence of valves allows pressure in the pulmonary artery (PA) and the left atrium (LA) to equalize. Thus, the pulmonary artery (PA) resting or diastolic pressure equals the mean left atrial pressure. Similar to the discussion on right atrial pressure, a mean left atrial pressure is recorded, since there is a minimal difference between left atrial systolic and diastolic pressures. The following table maps pressure relationships from the right atrium to the left atrium.

	RIGHT ATRIAL (RA) PRESSURE	RIGHT VENTRICLE (RV) PRESSURE	PULMONARY ARTERY (PA) PRESSURE	LEFT ATRIAL (LA) PRESSURE
PRESSURE POINTS (continued)				
SYSTOLIC		20–30mm Hg. · · · · · · · ·	20–30mm Hg.	
MEAN	2–5mm Hg. · ·	————	————	8–15mm Hg.
DIASTOLIC		· · 2–5mm Hg.	8–15mm Hg. · · ·	

Clear as a foggy day, right! Bear in mind that no one masters hemodynamic concepts on the first pass. Mastery is gained through repetition and actual clinical practice.

IMPORTANT DETAIL :

Before going further, it is important to point out that the pulmonary artery catheter cannot be passed beyond the pulmonary artery! Therefore, left atrial and left ventricular pressure measurements cannot be made directly using the pulmonary artery catheter.

READ ON FOR CLARIFICATION ...

Pulmonary Capillary Wedge Pressure (PCWP) vs. Left Atrial Pressure

The notion that a catheter inserted into the right heart can measure left heart functioning is confusing. The secret is the 1.5cc latex balloon at the tip of the pulmonary artery catheter. When inflated with a syringe, the balloon occludes or wedges into a small branch of the pulmonary artery and blocks any interference coming *from the right heart*. In effect, the inflated balloon creates an artificial valve. (Remember

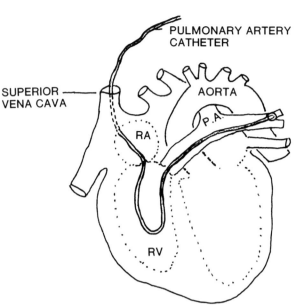

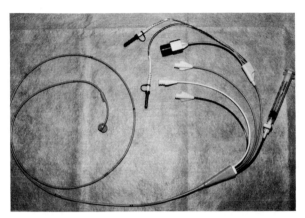

The inflated balloon on the pulmonary catheter is wedged into a small branch of the pulmonary artery.

there are no valves or "blood flow restricting devices" in the pulmonary vascular system or left atrial junction.) This "artificial valve" or blockage allows for a longer look at the resting (filling) pressures of the pulmonary vasculature and the left atrium (LA). Both the pulmonary capillary wedge pressure (PCWP) and the left atrial pressure (LA), will be 8–15 mm.Hg. (mean values).

PRESSURE POINTS (continued)				
RIGHT ATRIAL (RA) PRESSURE	RIGHT VENTRICLE (RV) PRESSURE	PULMONARY ARTERY (PA) PRESSURE	PULMONARY CAPILLARY WEDGE PRESSURE (PCWP)	LEFT ATRIAL (LA) PRESSURE
SYSTOLIC	20–30mm Hg.	20–30mm Hg.		
MEAN 2–5mm Hg.			8–15mm Hg.	8–15mm Hg.
DIASTOLIC	2–5mm Hg.	8–15mm Hg.		

The pulmonary capillary wedge pressure (PCWP) waveformation is presented in the next two diagrams.

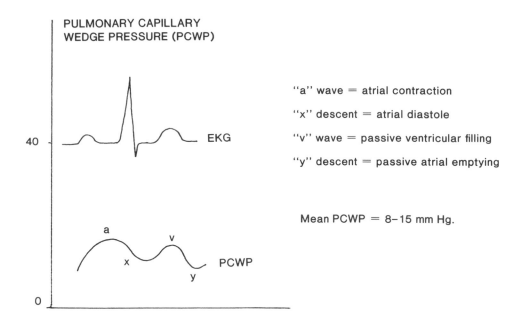

PULMONARY CAPILLARY
WEDGE PRESSURE (PCWP)

40 —

0

EKG

a   v
  x
     y   PCWP

"a" wave = atrial contraction

"x" descent = atrial diastole

"v" wave = passive ventricular filling

"y" descent = passive atrial emptying

Mean PCWP = 8–15 mm Hg.

The PA waveform "flattens out" as the pulmonary artery catheter balloon is inflated and subsequently wedges in the pulmonary artery. The resulting waveform has little systolic-diastolic pressure change. Thus, the PCWP is reported as a mean pressure.

PULMONARY CAPILLARY WEDGE PRESSURE (PCWP)

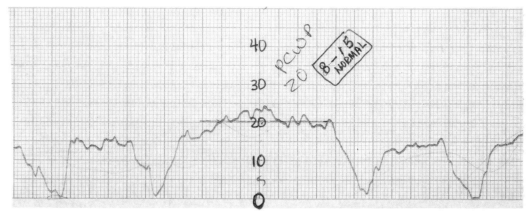

Note the elevated pulmonary capillary wedge pressure (PCWP).

Pulmonary Capillary Wedge Pressure (PCWP) vs. Left Ventricular End Diastolic Pressure (LVEDP)

Finally, the last topic in the hemodynamic monitoring process is to relate previously discussed pressures to left ventricular (LV) function. Given that the left ventricle is the "driver" for systemic circulation, it is the most important cardiac chamber! The left ventricle (LV) has the greatest muscle mass of the four cardiac chambers which supports its pumping function.

On page 277, we presented the concept that the right ventricular (RV) diastolic or filling pressure is equivalent to the mean right atrial (RA) pressure. These pressures are equivalent owing to the *passive* flow of blood from the right atrium to the right ventricle. VOILÀ! The same phenomenon occurs in the left side of the heart!

The left ventricular filling or diastolic pressure should equal the left atrial mean pressure because blood flows passively from the left atrium into the left ventricle. Make sense, right? Thus, at the conclusion of the left ventricular filling phase, the *left ventricular end diastolic pressure* (LVEDP) equals the mean left atrial pressure. WHEW!

Now, have a look at the entirety of pressure relationships.

	RA PRESSURE	RV PRESSURE	PA PRESSURE	PCWP	LA PRESSURE	LVEDP
SYSTOLIC		20–30mm Hg.	20–30mm Hg.			
MEAN*	2–5mm Hg.			8–15mm Hg.	8–15mm Hg.	
DIASTOLIC		2–5mm Hg.	8–15mm Hg.			8–15mm Hg.

PRESSURE POINTS

* mean pressures are reported for the right and left atria and PCWP because minimal differences exist between systolic and diastolic pressures in those chambers/vessels.

Key:
RA = Right Atrium
RV = Right Ventricle
PA = Pulmonary Artery

PCWP = Pulmonary Capillary Wedge Pressure
LA = Left Atrium
LVEDP = Left Ventricular End Diastolic Pressure

So, in reviewing the pressure points, the PA diastolic, PCWP, LA, and LVEDP should be equal pressures. Thus, a catheter placed in the right heart *can* assess left heart function!! Double WHEW!!

The left ventricular end diastolic pressure (LVEDP) is a critical measure of left ventricular function. If the LVEDP rises, it is an indication that left ventricular emptying is incomplete. Incomplete left ventricular emptying may occur secondary to pump failure (left ventricular failure) caused by acute myocardial infarction (muscle injury and necrosis). Incomplete LV emptying may also result from *aortic stenosis*. In aortic stenosis, the aortic valve fails to open completely, thus restricting the free flow of blood out of the left ventricular chamber.

HINT: Aortic stenosis reminds me of a Sunday morning church service finale, where 200 people attempt to exit a single door obstructed by a bastion of hand shakers! The hand shakers create congestion and crowd backup. This "obstructed emptying" causes tension (pressure) to rise!

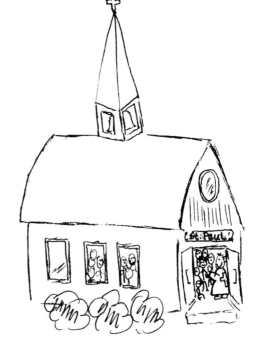

A decrease in the pulmonary capillary wedge pressure (PCWP) or the left ventricular end diastolic pressure (LVEDP) is often attributable to hypovolemia, dehydration, or extreme vasodilation.

The following diagram provides "basic" guidelines for the medical management of hemodynamic imbalances. Similar to the interpretation of EKG's, the *single* most important thing to remember is the value of "face to face" patient evaluation. Though hemodynamic pressures for any given patient may deviate from the "textbook parameters," they may, in fact, be normal for that patient!

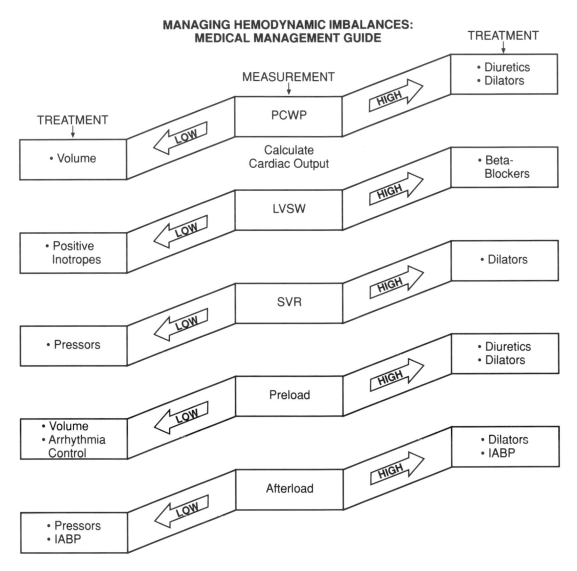

**MANAGING HEMODYNAMIC IMBALANCES:
MEDICAL MANAGEMENT GUIDE**

(Another trusty guide worth remembering, compliments of the management.)

The right heart pressures are but a small portion of the hemodynamic picture. Right heart pressures are used to further calculate cardiac function and vascular stability. The glossary of terms (p. 292) defines other aspects of the hemodynamic profile.

Practice Exercise 3

NOTE: DIFFICULTY AHEAD... BE PREPARED TO STOP FOR REVIEW ☺

1. Owing to its (circle one) small/large muscle mass, the normal right atrial pressure is low/high.

2. Minimal differences between systolic and diastolic pressures are reported as _____ pressures.

3. Mean right atrial pressure normally ranges between _____ and _____ mm Hg.

4. Correctly match right atrial pressure abnormalities with probable pathologies by placing the letter L or H in the spaces provided.

   L = Low right atrial pressure
   H = High right atrial pressure

   _____ Right ventricular failure
   _____ Fluid overload
   _____ Vasodilation
   _____ Tricuspid valve insufficiency
   _____ Chronic left heart failure
   _____ Hypovolemia

   ☺ WHEW !!!

5. Explain why the right ventricular diastolic pressure equals the mean right atrial pressure (to cheat, turn to page 277).

   _____

   _____

   _____

   _____

6. Normal right ventricular (RV) pressure is (circle one).

   2–5 mm. Hg.   20–30 mm. Hg. $\dfrac{20\text{–}30 \text{ mm. Hg.}}{2\text{–}5 \text{ mm. Hg.}}$

7. The dicrotic notch in the pulmonary artery waveform is produced by

   _____

   _____

   _____

☐ CHECK (X) IF YOU ARE ALIVE AND WELL . .
☐ CHECK (X) IF YOU ARE UNCERTAIN! ☺

287

8. Correctly match systolic pulmonary artery pressure abnormalities with suspect pathologies by placing the letter L or H in the spaces provided.

L = Low systolic PA pressures   ____ Pulmonary emboli
H = High systolic PA pressures   ____ Hypovolemia
                                         ____ Mechanical ventilation
                                         ____ Left ventricular failure
                                         ____ Vasodilation

9. Normal pulmonary artery pressure (PAP) is ____ mm Hg.
                                             8–15mm Hg.

10. The pulmonary artery (PA) resting or diastolic pressure equals the mean left atrial (LA) pressure because there are no _____ in the pulmonary vascular system or left atrial junction. The absence of _____ allows the pressures to equalize.

11. If the diastolic PA pressure is 10mm.Hg., the mean LA pressure will be _____ mm Hg.

12. The pulmonary artery catheter cannot be passed beyond the _____ !

BREAK TIME... PLEASE RETURN IN 15 mm Hg. ☺

· · · · · · · · · · · · · ·

☐ I RETURNED ON TIME
☐ I WAS TARDY

13. Left ventricular filling or end diastolic pressure equals the left atrial mean pressure because _____

_____

_____

14. Correctly match left ventricular end diastolic pressure (LVEDP) abnormalities with associated pathologies by placing the letter H (high) or L (low) in the spaces provided.

H = elevated LVEDP (>15mm Hg.)   ____ Hypovolemia
L = low LVEDP (<8mm Hg.)   ____ Aortic stenosis
                                         ____ Incomplete LV emptying
                                         ____ Left Ventricular failure
                                         ____ Dehydration

15. In the spaces provided, write the words represented by the following abbreviations. *Then,* note normal pressures for the various hemodynamic measures!

Pressures

RA = _____

RV = _____

PA = _____

PCWP = _____

LA = _____

LVEDP = _____

BRAVO!

For **Feedback 3,** refer to page 290.

Feedback 1

GREAT JOB!

1. Invasive hemodynamic monitoring is accomplished via a <u>pulmonary artery</u> catheter.

2. The size (mass) and strength of the left ventricle allows oxygenated blood to be ejected past the <u>aortic</u> valve into the <u>aorta,</u> and out to systemic circulation.

3.

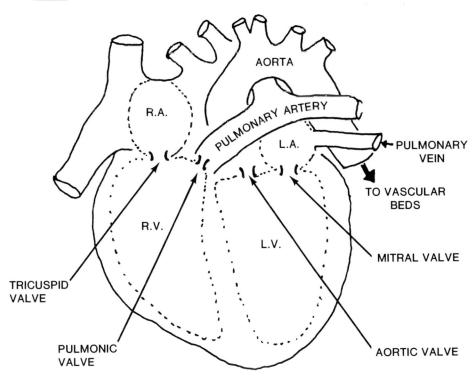

4. The contraction/ejection phase of the blood flow cycle is termed systole; the relaxation/filling phase of the blood flow cycle is known as diastole.

5. If a muscle fiber is stretched (diastole) a short distance, contraction (systole) is weak. If a muscle fiber is fully stretched to its critical length, contraction is forceful. If a muscle fiber is repeatedly over-stretched, contractile force is diminished.

6. Starling was a ☐ BIRD
                   ☐ PLANE
                   ☒ LAW MAN

7. CVP is a measure of right atrial pressure or right heart preload.

8. Cardiac output (CO) is a measure of myocardial contractile force.

Feedback 2

1. The pulmonary artery catheter (Swan-Ganz catheter) has three internal lumens, and a thermistor which is used to measure core temperature and cardiac output.

2. The proximal pulmonary artery catheter port is utilized for fluid administration.

3. Right atrial pressure is monitored at the proximal lumen opening.

4. An inflated pulmonary artery catheter balloon causes the catheter to "wedge" into a small pulmonary vessel.

5. Normal cardiac output (CO) ranges between 4 and 7 liters per minute.

6. Central venous pressure (CVP) is a measure of right heart preload or filling pressure.

7. The pulmonary capillary wedge pressure (PCWP) is a measure of left heart preload or filling pressure.

Feedback 3

1. Owing to its small muscle mass, the normal right atrial pressure is low.

2. Minimal differences between systolic and diastolic pressures are reported as mean pressures.

3. Mean right atrial pressure normally ranges between 2 and 5mm Hg.

4. L = Low right atrial pressure
   H = High right atrial pressure

    H   Right ventricular failure
    H   Fluid overload
    L   Vasodilation
    H   Tricuspid valve insufficiency
    H   Chronic left heart failure
    L   Hypovolemia

5. When the tricuspid valve opens, the blood volume in the RA flows passively into the RV. It is the mean right atrial pressure that forces the valve open. That pressure is maintained in the action stage of right atrial ejection and the relaxation stage of RV filling via the open tricuspid valve. WHEW!

6. Normal right ventricular (RV) pressure is

20–30 mm. Hg.
2–5 mm. Hg.

7. The dicrotic notch in the pulmonary artery waveform is produced by <u>the back slosh of blood against the pulmonic valve. The pulmonic valve closes following pulmonary artery filling.</u>

8. L = Low systolic PA pressures
   H = High systolic PA pressures

__H__	Pulmonary emboli
__L__	Hypovolemia
__H__	Mechanical ventilation
__H__	Left ventricular failure
__L__	Vasodilation

9. Normal pulmonary artery pressure (PAP) is $\dfrac{20\text{–}30\text{mm Hg.}}{8\text{–}15\text{mm Hg.}}$

10. The pulmonary artery (PA) resting or diastolic pressure equals the mean left atrial (LA) pressure because there are no <u>valves</u> in the pulmonary vascular system or left atrial junction. The absence of <u>valves</u> allows the pressures to equalize.

11. If the diastolic PA pressure is 10mm. Hg., the mean LA pressure will be <u>10</u>mm. Hg.

12. The pulmonary artery catheter cannot be passed beyond the <u>pulmonary artery</u>!

13. Left ventricular filling or end diastolic pressure equals the left atrial mean pressure because <u>the blood flows passively from the left atrium into the left ventricle via the open mitral valve.</u>

14. Correctly match left ventricular end diastolic pressure (LVEDP) abnormalities with associated pathologies by placing the letter H (high) or L (low) in the spaces provided.

   H = elevated LVEDP (>15mm Hg.)
   L = low LVEDP (<8mm Hg.)

__L__	Hypovolemia
__H__	Aortic stenosis
__H__	Incomplete LV emptying
__H__	Left ventricular failure
__L__	Dehydration

15. In the spaces provided, write the words represented by the following abbreviations. <u>Then</u>, note NORMAL pressures for the various hemodynamic measures!

	Pressures
RA = right atrium	2–5mm Hg.
RV = right ventricle	20–30mm Hg.
	2–5mm Hg.
PA = pulmonary artery	20–30mm Hg.
	8–15mm Hg.
PCWP = pulmonary capillary wedge pressure	8–15mm Hg.
LA = left atrium	8–15mm Hg.
LVEDP = left ventricular end diastolic pressure	8–15mm Hg.

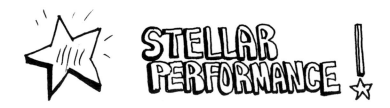

STELLAR PERFORMANCE!

GLOSSARY OF TERMS

Afterload: the aortic pressure that the left ventricle must overcome to eject blood (systole).

Beta Receptors: release epinephrine and norepinephrine leading to increased heart rate and blood pressure. Beta-blockers (Class II antiarrhythmic drugs) slow or block the effects of epinephrine and norepinephrine.

Cardiac Output (CO): 4–7 L./min.—the amount of blood ejected from the ventricle per minute. Changes in cardiac output are associated with stroke volume, heart rate, and contractility.

Inotropes: affect the contractility of the heart muscle and thereby alter cardiac output.

Intra-aortic balloon pump (IABP): a mechanical device used to decrease left ventricular workload and increase coronary perfusion.

Left ventricular stroke work (LVSW): measure of contractility that estimates the amount of energy (calories) used by the left ventricle.

Preload: the filling pressure of the ventricles. Changes in preload are related to blood volume and vascular space.

Pulmonary Vascular Resistance (PVR): blood flow impedance from the pulmonary artery to the left atrium.

Systemic Vascular Resistance (SVR): blood flow impedance from the aortic valve to the right atrium.

NOTES

NOTES

Section XII
Antiarrhythmic and Thrombolytic Medications

OBJECTIVES

When you have completed Section XII, you will be able to describe or identify

1. the autonomic nervous system control of heart rate
2. drug actions in terms of agonists, antagonists, and receptors
3. the body's handling of drugs
4. the four categories of antiarrhythmic drugs
5. general therapeutic and toxic effects of the four antiarrhythmic drug classifications
6. EKG effects associated with antiarrhythmic drugs
7. thrombolytic drug therapy for acute myocardial infarction

Text by

MIKE LUCEY

ANTIARRHYTHMIC AND THROMBOLYTIC MEDICATIONS

Arrhythmias are often "fun" to analyze, but once identified, one needs to consider "what next!" Should the dysrhythmia be treated? If so, how?

These are really "loaded" questions! Recent knowledge explosions have resulted in many exciting (and confusing) issues relating to the treatment of arrhythmias. The introduction of new technologies and drugs, combined with surprising results from clinical trials, have resulted in a whirlwind of change.

(WHIRLWIND) CHANGE

As a result, *today's* drug "treatment of choice" for a certain arrhythmia may soon be replaced by another drug! Change is the only constant in drug therapy, which evolves in accord with clinical research, technology advances, and successful drug salesmen!

A word about drug names: each drug is assigned a generic name which is unique for that chemical substance. Drug manufacturers will attach a "brand" or "trade" name to a drug which is *usually* easier to remember than the generic name. There can be several brands of the same generic drug, which can be confusing. In this section, generic names are mentioned first; brand names, if significant, will follow in parentheses.

Input 1: Autonomic Control of Heart Rate

Let's begin the discussion on cardiac medications by first reviewing "normal body" heart rate controls. Though this may not make sense now, but it will become clear later in the discussion. You have learned that the SA node is the heart's normal pacemaker since it has the most rapid rate of spontaneous depolarization. However, the heart must be able to vary its rate to accommodate changing perfusion demands (stress, varying temperature, activity, and so forth).

The SA node (and other key cardiac tissues) have nerve connections from the autonomic nervous system. These nerves communicate with the SA node by releasing a chemical from the nerve ending called a *neurotransmitter. Norepinephrine* is the neurotransmitter for the *sympathetic* branch of the autonomic nervous system. *Acetylcholine* is the neurotransmitter for the *parasympathetic* branch of the autonomic nervous system. The body has a number of other neurotransmitters with *interesting* names, as well!

Neurotransmitters bind to special proteins called *receptors* that sit on the surface of SA nodal cells. A receptor will bind to *only* one type of neurotransmitter. These receptor types have funny names, too. So, norepinephrine binds to a *beta-adrenergic receptor,* and acetylcholine binds to a *muscarinic receptor.*

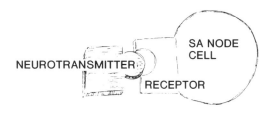

When a rapid heart rate is required under conditions such as exercise, danger, or stress, the sympathetic nerve connections to the heart are stimulated. This stimulation releases norepinephrine near the SA node, some of which will bind to the beta-adrenergic receptors on the SA cells. This binding of norepinephrine causes both the automaticity of the SA node and the frequency of depolarization to increase. The net result is an increase in heart rate to meet perfusion demands.

It is important to note that this sympathetic stimulation can increase the automaticity of other cardiac tissues as well. This can result in ectopic beats and subsequent arrhythmias!

Likewise, if a decrease in heart rate is required, the parasympathetic nerve connections to the heart are stimulated. This stimulation causes acetylcholine release near the SA node. Some acetylcholine binds to muscarinic receptors on the SA cell surfaces. This binding causes a decrease in both the automaticity and frequency of SA node depolarization, and a subsequent decrease in heart rate. If parasympathetic stimulation is too intense, a dangerous bradycardia may occur.

This sequence of *nerve stimulation* → *neurotransmitter release* → *receptor binding* → *cardiac action* is helpful in understanding drug actions.

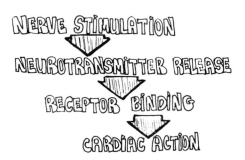

Some drugs are chemically similar to natural neurotransmitters, acting at the same receptors and producing the same effects. Any chemical which acts at a receptor site and produces an effect is called an **agonist.**

So, agonists include both neurotransmitters and any drug which mimics the neurotransmitter by binding to the same receptor site and producing the same effects. **Epinephrine (Adrenaline)** is a drug which acts at the beta-adrenergic receptor site to produce an increased heart rate. Epinephrine mimics the usual neurotransmitter *norepinephrine,* and is therefore an agonist at that receptor. Makes sense, right?

Some drugs can bind to a receptor *without* producing a subsequent effect. In fact, the drug can *prevent* or *reverse* the effects of an agonist. These drugs are called **antagonists** (they "antagonize" the action of agonists).

As you shall later see, the drug **propranolol (Inderal)** is a beta-adrenergic antagonist which prevents or reverses the action of an agonist like norepinephrine or epinephrine. Propranolol produces a decrease in heart rate, and can reduce ectopy caused by excess sympathetic stimulation.

Likewise, **atropine** is an antagonist of acetylcholine at the muscarinic receptors. Since the *agonist* acetylcholine causes a decrease in heart rate, the *antagonist* atropine will cause the opposite effect, an increase in heart rate!

Practice Exercise 1

1. In response to stress, the _____ nerve connections to the SA node are stimulated.

2. Match the neurotransmitter with the correct branch of the autonomic nervous system (ANS) and with its function.

ANS BRANCH	NEUROTRANSMITTER	FUNCTION
Parasympathetic	Norepinephrine	Increased heart rate
Sympathetic	Acetylcholine	Decreased heart rate

3. An agonist is _____

_____ .

4. A drug which binds to a receptor without producing an effect, or prevents or reverses the effects of an agonist, is known as an _____ .

5. Correctly match the drugs with their respective function.

Epinephrine (Adrenaline)	Beta-adrenergic agonist
Propranolol (Inderal)	Beta-adrenergic antagonist
Atropine	Muscarinic antagonist

6. ☐ I would like to be a clinical pharmacist.
   ☐ Antagonist → agonist → agony →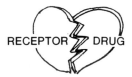

For **Feedback 1,** refer to page 314.

Input 2: Antiarrhythmic Drugs: Actions and Toxicity

Other antiarrhythmic drugs also produce their effects by binding to a receptor (a portion of a cardiac cell) similar to the neurotransmitter binding in the autonomic nerve example. The chemical shape of both the drug and the receptor are such that if they "like" each other, binding takes place!

RECEPTOR DRUG

Again, most receptors for antiarrhythmic drugs are proteins that sit on the surface of the cardiac cell. The receptors are therefore "receptive" to binding with the drug!

A specific receptor will usually bind only to one drug or type of drug. However, a cardiac cell may have many different receptor types on its surface, and may therefore interact with many different types of drugs. Receptors for various drugs can be found in the SA node, the AV node, cardiac muscle cells, and the His-Purkinje system. Once a drug binds to the receptor, chemical changes take place which produce an effect or action.

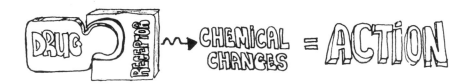

DRUG RECEPTOR ⤳ CHEMICAL CHANGES = ACTION

Antiarrhythmic drugs work by affecting one or more of the following cardiac tissue properties:

1. Automaticity
2. Rate of impulse conduction
3. Duration of the refractory period
   (or the time needed for repolarization)

The particular way in which an antiarrhythmic drug works is called its *mechanism of action.* So, when describing the receptor that a drug binds to and the resulting effect on automaticity, conduction, or the refractory period, you have described the drug's mechanism of action. (Pharmacy talk!)

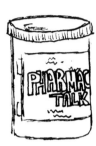

THE BODY'S FOUR PROCESSES FOR DRUG HANDLING

In order for drug therapy to be effective, the drug must travel to its site of action (the receptor on the cardiac cell) in sufficient quantities to produce the desired effect. If an insufficient quantity of drug is present at this site, the treatment will be ineffective. Conversely, if an excessive amount of drug is present, toxicity is likely to occur.

Now, consider the following. What factors determine (1) The administration route most effective for the arrhythmia in question? (2) The dosage? (3) The frequency of administration? These questions have more to do with the way the body handles the drug, than on how the drug affects the body!

There are four basic *pharmacologic processes* governing the body's handling of drugs. Those processes are:

1. Absorption
2. Distribution
3. Metabolism
4. Excretion

Read on for the details!

Absorption

Absorption is the process by which a drug gains access to circulation from the site of administration. Absorption depends on the route of administration. Absorption takes place across the intestinal membrane when the oral route of administration is employed, and across capillary membranes from an intramuscular site of administration. The intravenous route bypasses a "true" absorption step and, therefore, produces more *immediate* effects.

In any form of absorption, the end result is that the drug moves from the site of administration into the bloodstream. Absorption will be slow if there is poor blood flow at the administration site. Not all antiarrhythmic drugs are well absorbed by the oral route. **Bretylium,** for example, is too highly "charged" to cross intestinal membranes.

In a pinch, when an intravenous route is unavailable during cardiac arrest, some antiarrhythmics (**lidocaine, atropine**) can be given through an endotracheal tube. In this instance, absorption takes place across the capillary membrane in the lung tissue.

Distribution

Once the drug is in the bloodstream (following absorption), it is distributed by blood flow throughout the system. Most drugs are distributed widely throughout the body, regardless of the intended site of action. (The body has no way of knowing that the circulating drug is intended to act in the heart!) A drug may concentrate in certain tissues depending on its chemical characteristics.

Highly perfused organs, such as the brain, heart, lungs, kidneys, and liver, are exposed to administered drugs more quickly and in greater amounts than organs with less perfusion. However, these less perfused tissues will eventually take up the drug from the circulation. For instance, the administration of a single intravenous bolus dose of **lidocaine (Xylocaine)** has a rapid antiarrhythmic effect, since cardiac tissue is highly perfused. This effect is short lived, though, since the blood lidocaine concentration rapidly drops. The drop in concentration occurs as other tissues with lower perfusion remove lidocaine from the circulation. The process of distribution steals lidocaine away from its intended site of action. Subsequent lidocaine bolus doses and/or continuous infusion are required to maintain effective blood concentration. Drug distribution during cardiac arrest (asystole or ventricular fibrillation) is impaired since there is no effective blood flow to move the drug from the site of administration to the heart, the intended site of action. During cardiac arrest, blood flow is dependent on the provision of effective CPR.

In a cardiac arrest situation, a delay of one to two minutes should be anticipated following drug administration before the drug reaches the central circulation and heart (American Heart Association). When possible, the *central* venous route is the preferred route for drug administration in order to minimize this time delay. Peak drug concentrations reaching the heart are lower when drugs are administered via a *peripheral* vein. Therefore, saphenous (leg) veins and veins in the hands and wrists are *less* desirable than more proximal veins. Peripheral blood flow is minimal during cardiac arrest, thus inhibiting drug distribution to the intended site of action.

Metabolism

Metabolism of an administered drug is the process by which the drug is chemically altered, usually by the action of enzymes located in various tissues of the body. The liver is the primary location for both enzymes production and drug metabolism.

Chemical alteration yields a product called a *metabolite,* which has different actions and toxicities than its *parent* drug. Most metabolites are *inactive,* meaning they do not possess the antiarrhythmic actions of the administered drug. The metabolism of some drugs, however, such as procainamide, disopyramide, lidocaine, and encainide, results in *active metabolites* which share the antiarrhythmic activity of the parent drug. Most active metabolites have less activity than the parent drug, though in some instances, the metabolite is responsible for most of the drug's action! How is your mental metabolism?

Excretion

Excretion is the process by which drugs and drug metabolites are eliminated from the body. The two major routes for excretion are the urinary tract and the liver, into the bile.

A common measure for describing the rate of drug elimination from the body is called **half-life.** Half-life is the time required to reduce (by metabolism and/or excretion) the amount of drug in the body by one half. The table below reveals a wide range a half-lives for various antiarrhythmic drugs.

HALF LIFE OF VARIOUS ANTIARRHYTHMIC DRUGS	
Drug	**Half-life**
Amiodarone (Cordarone)	25 days
Digoxin (Lanoxin)	39 hours
Disopyramide (Norpace)	6 hours
Esmolol (Brevibloc)	8 minutes

Note the wide *differences* among the above half-life values! Some half-life values are measured in minutes, others in days (almost a month). Given the extended half-life of select drugs, correct dosing is paramount!

The processes of absorption and distribution determine the time to the onset, or beginning, of drug action. A drug must be given by an administration route that results in good absorption at an acceptable rate. What is "acceptable" is determined by the patient's clinical condition.

Metabolism and excretion determine the duration of drug action, since these processes remove the drug from the site of action. Metabolism and excretion also determine the necessary frequency of drug administration and dosage. Therefore, a drug with a rapid rate of metabolism, like **lidocaine,** must be administered frequently to maintain an effective or therapeutic drug level. In clinical practice, lidocaine is administered via continuous infusion to assure the desired therapeutic effects.

SERUM DRUG CONCENTRATIONS AND THE "THERAPEUTIC RANGE"

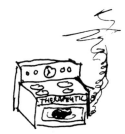

The Therapeutic "Range"
(Pharm Art, Inc.)

Some antiarrhythmic drugs are more effective when the serum drug concentration exceeds a certain minimum value. Likewise, toxicity is more frequent when the serum drug concentration becomes excessive. For some antiarrhythmic drugs, a desirable range of serum concentrations has been established which effectively controls most arrhythmias, and avoids excessive toxicity. This desired range of drug concentrations is called the **therapeutic range.** Drug concentrations below the range are likely to be ineffective. The therapeutic range is intended to be a guideline, and can assist in determining optimal dosage for a particular patient.

For example, the therapeutic range for **quinidine** is 2 to 5 micrograms (mcg.) of drug per ml. of serum. If a patient has poor control of an arrhythmia during quinidine treatment, a measurement of a serum quinidine concentration may provide useful information. If quinidine is absent from the serum, the patient may be noncompliant with regard to drug administration. If the result is only 1–2 mcg./ml., the current dosage may be inadequate and a dosage increase may be required to control the disorder. If the concentration is within the therapeutic range, perhaps quinidine should be replaced with another drug.

Practice Exercise 2

... MORE "PHARMACIST-WANNA-BE" PRACTICE

1. Cardiac cells may interact with or respond to different types of drugs because _____
_____
_____

2. Antiarrhythmic drugs work by affecting one or more of the following cardiac tissue properties:

   a. _____ .

   b. _____ .

   c. _____ .

3. Drug absorption depends on the _____ .

4. The intravenous route of drug administration produces "near-immediate" effects because one of the following processes is bypassed. Check the omitted process.

   ☐ Absorption
   ☐ Distribution
   ☐ Metabolism
   ☐ Excretion

5. A continuous infusion of lidocaine is necessary to maintain an effective blood concentration because _____

   _____

   _____

   _____ .

6. During a code arrest situation, a central venous route of drug administration is recommended because

   _____

   _____

   _____ .

7. The _____ is the primary location for drug metabolism.

8. Drug "half-life" refers to _____

   _____

   _____ .

For **Feedback 2,** refer to page 315.

Input 3: Drug Treatment of Arrhythmias

The decision to begin antiarrhythmic drug therapy can be *tricky.* In life-threatening disorders (ventricular fibrillation or sustained ventricular tachycardia), the proper drug is required immediately since perfusion to vital organs is diminished or absent. The long term treatment of "non-emergent" disorders is less clear.

Accurate diagnosis and careful patient selection is fundamental to antiarrhythmic drug administration since harmful, even fatal, effects can occur from drug use. Some types of dysrhythmias respond well to proper drug treatment, while other rhythm disorders are completely resistant to drug effects.

The presence of physical symptoms, underlying cardiac disease (CHF or a recent MI), resultant undesirable changes (hypotension, reduced cardiac output, changes in heart rate), or high-risk status for a serious event (atrial embolization) will influence the decision to use an antiarrhythmic drug.

If an arrythmia is caused by a correctable condition (electrolyte imbalance, hypoxia, toxicities, is-chemia), treatment should be aimed at correcting the underlying condition. An antiarrhythmic drug may be needed only temporarily until the underlying condition has been resolved.

THE CLASSIFICATION OF ANTIARRHYTHMIC DRUGS

Antiarrhythmic drugs can be classified (or grouped) according to their mechanism of action, EKG effects, and toxicities. By grouping drugs in this manner, one does not need to memorize each drug's effects separately! Rather, one should focus on remembering the drug effects produced by different drug groups. The most common classification system used is the "Harrison modification of the Vaughn Williams system. . .

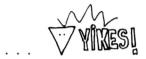

In this system, there are four distinct drug classes: Class I, Class II, Class III, and Class IV.

Class I Drugs

Earlier, you learned that cardiac cell depolarization occurs when sodium cations come "whooshing" into the cell. These sodium ions come through tiny alleys called *sodium channels*. All class I drugs work by binding to the sodium channel (their receptor) slowing the passage of sodium through to the cell. This slowing of sodium passage serves to decrease the rate of depolarization which is important in treating rapid ectopic rhythms. That's it! . . .

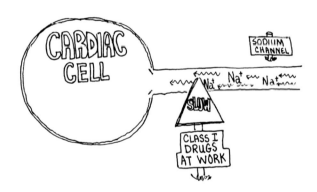

. . . however, there is one *minor* glitch. Research has demonstrated that not all sodium channel blockers (i.e., class I drugs) produce the same electrocardiographic effects. So, to make matters complicated, class I drugs were subdivided into classes IA, IB, and IC. *All the class I drugs decrease automaticity, but the subgroups (IA, IB, IC) have different effects on conduction and repolarization!* Whew! The differences are shown in the following table.

CLASS I DRUGS AND ACTIONS		
Class	**Actions**	**Drugs: Generic name (Trade name)**
IA	• Moderate slowing of conduction • Repolarization prolonged (widened QRS, prolonged QT interval) • Increased P-R interval	Quinidine Procainamide (Pronestyl) Disopyramide (Norpace)
IB	• Little effect on conduction • Repolarization shortened (QT interval may shorten)	Lidocaine (Xylocaine) Mexiletine (Mexetil) Phenytoin (Dilantin) Tocainide (Tonocard)
IC	• Conduction slows significantly • Repolarization: little effect • Marked increase in P-R and QRS duration	Encainide (Enkaid) Flecainide (Tambocor) Propafenone (Rhythmol)

The Class IA antiarrhythmics are called *broad spectrum* drugs because they are used for a *variety* of supraventricular and ventricular arrhythmias, including paroxysmal supraventricular tachycardia, atrial flutter or fibrillation, PVC's, and ventricular tachycardia.

As noted in the above table, both **quinidine** and **pronestyl** are class IA antiarrhythmic agents with similar actions and toxic manifestations. Quinidine and pronestyl *serve to depress or control ectopic activity arising in the atria and the ventricles.* In addition, quinidine and pronestyl cause the refractory period to be prolonged (*PROLONGED QT INTERVAL*). The prolonged QT interval can predispose to the "R on T" phenomenon!

Most of the quinidine effects seen on EKG are related to the slowing of depolarization and repolarization.

Quinidine *will produce a wide P wave that is notched, a slight widening of the QRS complex, a lengthening of the QT interval and a U wave that may be fused with the T wave* . . . something like this (similar to the EKG changes seen with hypokalemia).

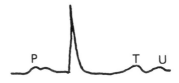

As noted above, Quinidine *accelerates or speeds up conduction across the AV node* when initially given. Therefore, Digoxin is administered prior to Quinidine when treating atrial fibrillation, atrial flutter, and other rapid supraventricular rhythms.

Pronestyl, on the other hand, is somewhat similar to lidocaine . . . except that it has less central nervous system effect. Pronestyl may be used to treat ectopic impulses arising in the atria, the AV junctional tissue, or the ventricles (P.V.C.'s, ventricular tachycardia).

Both quinidine and pronestyl toxicity will cause *widening of the QRS complex*.

Some people say that quinidine toxicity resembles a "roller coaster" pattern. . . .

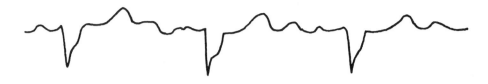

. . . what do you think?

Class IB drugs are used almost exclusively for the treatment of ventricular arrhythmias. Class IC agents are employed only for life-threatening ventricular arrhythmias.

Each of the Class I drugs has its own toxicity profile and systemic effect. The following discussion highlights important adverse reactions for selected Class I drugs.

Class IA Toxicities

Quinidine is fascinating, even if one only considers its toxicity. Almost one-third of patients discontinue taking the drug secondary to gastrointestinal effects: nausea, vomiting, and/or diarrhea. Severe slowing of conduction may occur. If the QRS duration increases by 50 percent or more compared to pretreatment measurements, the dosage should be reduced. Syncope and sudden cardiac death have occurred, which may be related to the drug's prolongation of the Q-T interval which can predispose to the "R on T" phenomenon. Thrombocytopenia with severe bleeding may rarely result.

Disopyramide (Norpace) can reduce the heart muscle contractility and can lead to congestive heart failure (CHF), especially in patients with pre-existing CHF. Its strong anticholinergic effects cause urinary retention, especially in men with prostatism.

Procainamide (Pronestyl, Procan SR) is notorious for causing a syndrome resembling systemic lupus erythrematosis (SLE) in 15–20 percent of patients. It should be noted that rapid IV administration can cause hypotension. Agranulocytosis has a 0.5 percent frequency.

Class IB Toxicities

Lidocaine toxicity presents primarily as neurological effects: drowsiness; agitation; paresthesias; progressive disorientation; convulsions; or, respiratory arrest. However, when discontinued, lidocaine toxicity is short lived secondary to the rapid metabolism.

Another class IB drug, **tocainide** (Tonocard), causes agranulocytosis 0.2 percent of the time. Pneumonitis and pulmonary fibrosis occur rarely.

Class IC/Toxicities

This class of drugs has been associated with *proarrhythmic effects,* which means that the arrhythmia sometimes *worsens* during treatment rather than showing improvement. A proarrhythmic effect has resulted in increased mortality in some studies (CAST Study).

Flecainide can cause CHF.

Class II Drugs # BETA - BLOCKERS

Class II antiarrhythmics are beta-adrenergic antagonists (usually called **beta-blockers**). These agents block (reverse or prevent) the cardiac actions of agonists such as epinephrine (Adrenaline) and norepinephrine (the neurotransmitter), at the beta-adrenergic receptor.

CLASS II DRUGS AND ACTIONS		
Class	**Actions**	**Drugs: Generic Name (Trade Name)**
II	• Blocks beta-receptors • Decreases SA node automaticity • Decreases heart rate • Decreases ectopy secondary to sympathetic overstimulation • Increases duration of AV node refractory period	Propranolol (Inderal) Atenolol (Tenormin) Acebutolol (Sectral) Metoprolol (Lopressor) Esmolol (Brevibloc) Many others

The beta-blockers are frequently administered to control supraventricular tachyarrhythmias such as atrial fibrillation, atrial flutter, or paroxysmal supraventricular tachycardia. Though a beta-blocker will not usually eliminate the supraventricular dysrhythmia, it will decrease the rate of ventricular response by antagonizing sympathetic nerves going to the AV node. This antagonism increases the AV node refractory period, which limits the number of impulses conducted through to the ventricles.

For example, a rapid atrial fibrillation (ventricular rate 130/minute) might be reduced to a controlled rate atrial fibrillation (ventricular rate less than 100/minute); or, a 2:1 atrial flutter might be reduced to a 3:1 atrial flutter. If you need review, see page 66.

Beta-blockers are also used to treat ventricular dysrhythmias caused by either extreme sympathetic nervous system overactivity (from exercise), or excessive amounts of circulating epinephrine (pheochromocytoma).

Clinical trials have demonstrated that the long-term administration of beta-blockers following acute myocardial infarction consistently reduces mortality. The mortality reduction averages around 20 percent compared to control groups.

Class II Toxicities

Beta-blockers can cause bronchospasm in patients with existing respiratory disease (asthma and COPD). They can also precipitate CHF in susceptible individuals. Beta-blockers should *never* be suddenly discontinued in patients with a history of angina pectoris, since anginal attacks, arrhythmias, or acute myocardial infarctions have followed. Fatigue, depression, and sleep disturbances may be associated with the administration of Class II beta-blockers.

Class III Drugs

The Class III drugs are a "mixed bag" of chemical agents which bear little resemblance to one another except for their prolongation of ventricular repolarization.

CLASS III DRUGS AND ACTIONS		
Class	**Actions**	**Drugs**
III	• Prolongs repolarization • Increases refractory period	Amiodarone (Cordarone) Bretylium (Bretylol)

Both amiodarone and bretylium are drugs reserved for *life-threatening* ventricular arrhythmias (ventricular tachycardia or ventricular fibrillation), when other drug therapy has been unsuccessful! Sometimes, amiodarone is used to treat stubborn supraventricular arrhythmias.

Class III Toxicities

Amiodarone is a highly toxic antiarrhythmic agent. A large percentage of patients cannot tolerate this drug. Pulmonary toxicity can be fatal. Corneal microdeposits are very common. The liver is affected frequently. Hypo- and hyper-thyroidism, blue skin discoloration, photosensitivity, and worsening of arrhythmias may also occur.

Hypotension is the primary adverse effect associated with the administration of bretylium.

Class IV Drugs CALCIUM CHANNEL BLOCKERS

Class IV antiarrhythmics are the **calcium channel blockers.** These drugs inhibit the flow of calcium into cardiac cells, thereby decreasing conduction through the AV node and slowing rapid supraventricular rhythms.

CLASS IV DRUGS AND ACTIONS		
Class	**Actions**	**Drugs**
IV	• Blocks calcium channels • Decreases AV node conduction • Increases P-R interval • Decreases ventricular rate in atrial fibrillation	Verapamil (Calan, Isoptin) Diltiazem (Cardizem)

Calcium channel blockers are used *exclusively* for controlling supraventricular arrhythmias (such as PSVT) and for decreasing the ventricular response rate in atrial fibrillation or flutter.

Class IV Toxicities

Intravenous **verapamil** can cause hypotension, AV block, bradycardia, and decreased cardiac output. It is contraindicated in patients with: atrial fibrillation associated with Wolff-Parkinson-White syndrome; sick sinus syndrome; AV block; hypotension; and severe heart failure.

Important Antiarrhythmics Without "Class"

Certain drugs, important in the treatment of dysrhythmias, are not included in the above classification scheme.

As mentioned earlier, **atropine** is an acetylcholine antagonist at the parasympathetic nervous system receptors. Parasympathetic stimulation of the heart has two primary effects: a decrease in the rate of SA node depolarization (with a decrease in heart rate); and slowed conduction through the AV node. Atropine, acting as an antagonist, has the opposite effect. Atropine increases heart rate and improves AV conduction. These effects are useful for the treatment of: AV block; sinus bradycardia with associated symptoms of hypotension or confusion; or junctional escape rhythms.

Caution must be used when atropine is administered to patients with acute myocardial infarction or severe angina pectoris since an increase in heart rate may exacerbate ischemia or extend the area of infarction.

Digoxin is a drug commonly used for treating congestive heart failure. Digoxin increases the force of cardiac muscle contraction and works by inhibiting the "pump" on cardiac cells that keeps potassium in the cell and sodium out.

Further, digoxin slows conduction in the AV node, an action which makes it a useful therapy for rapid supraventricular dysrhythmias.

As you will later note, digitalis is primarily employed to block the conduction of rapid atrial impulses through to the ventricles. Blocking rapid atrial impulses provides the ventricles more filling time, thus improving pump efficiency. (Remember the flushing toilet example on page 58?)

In therapeutic ranges, digoxin produces *characteristic EKG effects* or pattern changes. On EKG, Digoxin effects may include a prolonged P-R interval, a flattened T wave, ST segment depression, and a shortened Q-T interval. The hallmark of digoxin effect is ST segment changes.

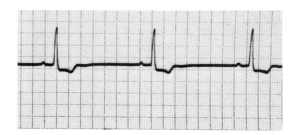

Digoxin produces a gradual downward sloping of the ST segment. This downward sloping of the ST segment may resemble a check mark or, may slope more gradually with a symmetrical appearance—or **SCOOPED** . . . more or less like the hull of a boat!

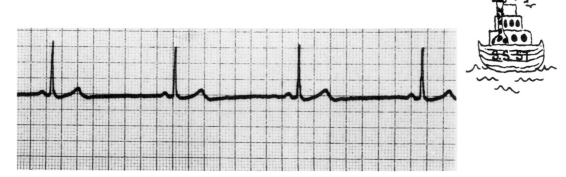

THAT'S PRECISELY WHY EKG INTERPRETATION IS SO DIFFICULT! YOUR BEST BET IS TO DESCRIBE WHAT THE ST SEGMENT LOOKS LIKE. . . .

HINT: It is much easier to determine ST segment appearance when viewing a lead that has no demonstrable S wave!

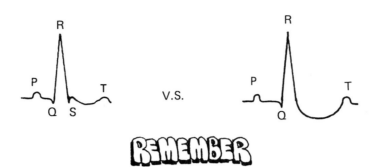

V.S.

REMEMBER

Digoxin induced ST depression is most usually seen in leads that have the *tallest* R waves . . . and this effect is characteristic of digitalis administration (*NOT* TOXICITY)! When characteristic ST segment changes are observed in *most* leads (including leads without tall R waves), digitalis toxicity should be suspected.

Digoxin is eliminated slowly: and the margin between an effective dosage and a toxic dosage is narrow. Here is an EKG demonstrating extreme digitalis effect.

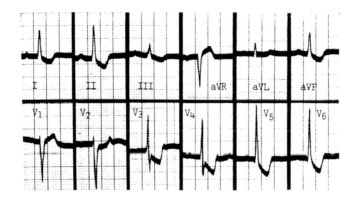

Though this listing is not all-inclusive, these are *some* of the conditions that **predispose** the patient to *digitalis toxicity.*

- age
- renal impairment
- elevated serum Ca^{++}
- liver impairment
- acute hypoxia
- corpulmonale
- hypothyroidism
- low serum K^+ (*adequate potassium serves to buffer the irritating effects of digitalis*)
- recent myocardial infarction

You may not believe this, but . . . it takes approximately twice as much digitalis to induce toxicity when the serum K^+ is 5.0 mEq./L. compared to 3.0 mEq./L!!

P.S. You can always expect renal function to diminish with advancing age!

There are several non-EKG manifestations that are early indications of digitalis intoxication, such as *anorexia, nausea, vomiting, diarrhea, lethargy, confusion, tinnitus* (ringing in the ears) and *distortion in yellow-green color perception . . .* though a patient may exhibit none of these symptoms.

It is rumored that Vincent Van Gogh (the painter) had a heart condition. As was typical for the times (late 1800's), he took digitalis leaf to manage that condition. It is thought that he became digitalis toxic, which might explain his erratic behavior, his use of yellow-greens in his paintings, and why he cut off his off his ear!  Anyway . . . that's the rumor!

Digoxin in excessive amounts retards AV conduction, thus producing the various forms of heart block—sinus block, first degree AV block, second degree AV block, blocked P.A.C.'s, paroxysmal atrial tachycardia with block . . . etc. Ironically, a variety of ectopic rhythms result from digoxin toxicity, as well.

Probably the *most common* dysrhythmias seen as a result of digitalis toxicity include

> P.V.C.'s
> multifocal P.V.C.'s
> bigeminy P.V.C.'s
> trigeminy P.V.C.'s
> ventricular tachycardia
>
> (WARNING)

Unfortunately, digoxin induced ventricular dysrhythmias are rarely responsive to lidocaine therapy. Dilantin may control digitalis-induced ventricular ectopic rhythms.

IMPORTANT Notice

Dilantin, a Class IB drug, depresses ectopic activity in the atria, AV junction and ventricles . . . and shortens ventricular repolarization time.

Practice Exercise 3 — **CLASS ACT PRACTICE** ☆

1. Antiarrhythmic drugs are classified in accord with their

   a. _____

   b. _____

   c. _____

2. Class I drugs work by binding to their receptor, the _____ channel, slowing the passage of _____ through to the cell. Slowing the passage increases/decreases (circle one) the rate of depolarization.

3. There are _____ subgroups of Class I drugs. All class I drugs decrease automaticity; however, the subgroups have differing effects on _____ and _____ .

308

4. Match the Class I subgroups with their appropriate actions. Then, match the example drugs to the appropriate subgroup.

ACTION	CLASS	SAMPLE DRUG
Shortened repolarization	IA	Rhythmol
No repolarization effect	IB	Quinidine
Prolonged repolarization	IC	Lidocaine

5. Class IA antiarrhythmic drugs are broad spectrum and are used to treat both _____ and _____ arrhythmias.

6. Class IB drugs are almost exclusively used to treat _____ arrhythmias.

7. Class _____ drugs are utilized to treat life-threatening ventricular arrhythmias.

8. Check all toxicities that may be related to the administration of lidocaine.

☐ weight gain   ☐ confusion   ☐ convulsions
☐ drowsiness   ☐ disorientation ☐ baldness
☐ agitation   ☐ hives   ☐ numbness

IF YOU ARE EXPERIENCING ANY OF THE
ABOVE SYMPTOMS, YOU MAY TAKE FIVE!!

The Management ☺

9. A proarrhythmic effect means that _____
_____
_____
_____ .

10. Class II antiarrhythmics are called _____ blockers. Class II drugs are frequently administered to control _____ .

11. Calcium channel blockers, Class IV drugs, inhibit the flow of calcium into the cardiac cells and function by _____
_____
_____ .

12. Calcium channel blockers are used exclusively for controlling _____ .

13. Digoxin works by _____
_____
_____
_____ .

309

14. Draw a cardiac cycle (PQRST) demonstrating digitalis effect.

For **Feedback 3,** refer to page 315.

Input 4: Treatment of Specific Rhythm Disorders

ATRIAL FIBRILLATION AND ATRIAL FLUTTER

The primary goal for treating atrial fibrillation and atrial flutter is the reduction of the rapid ventricular rate. If the rapid ventricular rate results in compromised circulation, electrical cardioversion is the treatment of choice. Otherwise, digoxin is usually employed as the drug therapy of choice. Digoxin reduces the ventricular rate by causing a partial AV block. Fewer atrial impulses are then conducted through to the ventricles. Reduction of the ventricular rate does not signify that the arrhythmia has been corrected. Rather, the negative impact on heart function has been reduced.

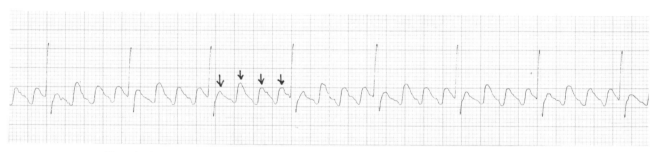

Digoxin therapy successfully reduced a 2:1 atrial flutter to the above 4:1 atrial flutter.
This is a controlled atrial flutter with a ventricular response rate of 68 per minute.

If digoxin is ineffective in reducing a rapid ventricular rate, beta-blockers (class II drugs) or verapamil (a class IV drug) may be used to decrease AV conduction or increase AV block. Digoxin may be useful in combination with propranolol (a beta-blocker) or verapamil.

Once the ventricular rate is controlled (60–100 beats per minute), the atrial abnormality itself is treated with a class IA agent such as quinidine, procainamide (Pronestyl), or disopyramide (Norpace). If this order of treatment is reversed (that is, if quinidine is started before digoxin), an *unexpected* increase in ventricular rate may occur! This occasionally occurs because quinidine can increase AV conduction thereby permitting a greater number of rapid atrial impulses to reach and activate the ventricles. Quinidine may also block the effect of parasympathetic nerves on the AV node, thereby increasing AV conduction! Whew!

A reexamination of older clinical studies has indicated that quinidine may increase mortality in the treatment of atrial fibrillation. Further research is required to clarify this possibility.

VENTRICULAR ECTOPY: PVC'S

Results of recent studies have challenged some earlier ideas regarding drug therapy for PVC's. The most visible study was the Cardiac Arrhythmia Suppression Trial (abbreviated CAST). The CAST studied patients who had arrhythmias (ventricular ectopy) following acute myocardial infarction. Some patients received drug therapy [encainide (Enkaid), flecainide (Tambocor), or moricizine (Ethmozine)], while others received a placebo.

The study found that the mortality, or death rate, was higher in the patient groups receiving drug therapy than in the placebo group! The findings were surprising since drug therapy did suppress ventricular ectopy. However, successful arrythmia treatment did not improve mortality.

As you might guess, these findings have led to a very cautious use of these drugs for treating "post-MI" ventricular dysrhythmias. The study results suggest that *some arrhythmias may be better left untreated.* It was felt that deaths were attributable to drug-induced worsening of the arrhythmia, called a **proarrhythmic effect.** This toxicity is the most feared effect of the antiarrhythmic drugs!

In other studies, beta blockers have been shown to reduce mortality following acute myocardial infarction, even if P.V.C.'s were not a significant problem. Therefore, many patients are given beta-blockers immediately following a myocardial infarction for periods of months or even years. Some patients have conditions which contraindicate the use of beta-blockers, however. Respiratory disease or congestive heart failure are common contraindications to beta-blocker administration. PVC's occurring *during* acute myocardial infarction are usually treated with lidocaine to prevent subsequent ventricular fibrillation! For a quick refresher on P.V.C.'s associated with acute myocardial infarction, see page 251.

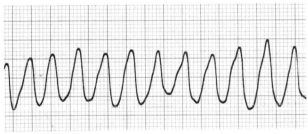

Ventricular tachycardia

SUSTAINED VENTRICULAR TACHYCARDIA

When sustained ventricular tachycardia is accompanied by hemodynamic compromise (hypotension, CHF, angina, or no pulse), cardioversion is the initial treatment of choice. Acute drug treatment includes lidocaine (a class IB drug) as first choice, given initially as bolus IV injections, followed by a continuous lidocaine infusion. Procainamide or bretylium are alternatives if lidocaine is contraindicated or ineffective.

A variety of other drugs can be used orally for the long-term suppression of ventricular tachycardia—the class IA drugs, beta-blockers, amiodarone, or mexiletine.

Lidocaine cannot be administered orally since only one-third of an oral dosage reaches the general circulation. It is well absorbed at the intestine, but all blood returning from the intestine must pass through the liver (the so-called "first pass"). There, the liver promptly metabolizes two-thirds of the lidocaine! A "significant loss of drug, secondary to metabolism during the first pass through the liver (following oral administration)", is termed a first pass effect. Just thought you would like to know that! (Pharmacy trivia!)

VENTRICULAR FIBRILLATION

Prompt defibrillation is the first order treatment for ventricular fibrillation. Drug treatment plays a secondary role to prevent subsequent ventricular irritability. Lidocaine is again the preferred antiarrhythmic agent. Bretylium or procainamide are drug treatment alternatives.

The preferred treatments for severe dysrhythmias requiring emergency treatment (sustained ventricular tachycardia, ventricular fibrillation, PSVT, symptomatic bradycardia, etc.) are outlined in the current *Standards and Guidelines for Cardiopulmonary Resuscitation and Emergency Cardiac Care* published by the American Heart Association. These guidelines are presented in algorithm fashion to guide therapeutic decision making and patient management.

THROMBOLYTIC DRUG TREATMENT FOR ACUTE MYOCARDIAL INFARCTION

A recent and exciting development in the treatment of acute myocardial infarction (AMI) has been the introduction of the thrombolytic agents, or **clot busters**.

The generic and trade names for these agents appear below.

THROMBOLYTIC AGENTS	
Generic Name	**Trade Name**
Streptokinase	Kabikinase, Streptase
Alteplase (TPA)	Activase
Urokinase	Abbokinase
Anistreplase	Eminase

Thrombolytic drugs are proteins which act as enzymes at key points in the blood coagulation system. To understand the role of these agents, one must be familiar with the pathophysiology of an acute myocardial infarction.

The genesis of acute myocardial infarction (AMI) is usually atherosclerotic disease in the coronary arteries. (See page 230 for a quick review.) In atherosclerosis, plaques of fatty-like material adhere to the inside walls of coronary (and other) arteries in the body. Accumulation of plaque limits the amount of blood that can flow through the artery. Reduction in blood flow can result in angina pectoris, heart failure, and arrhythmias.

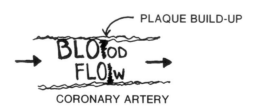

These plaques can also tear or damage the smooth inner lining of a coronary artery, exposing proteins which activate the blood clotting sequence at the site of the injury. Blood clotting involves a series of clotting factors, which are enzymes, acting together to make a fibrin plug. Fibrin is a protein which is made of smaller building blocks called fibrinogen. Thrombin, a clotting enzyme, takes the fibrinogen pieces and assembles them into fibrin.

Usually, fibrin's "job" is to "plug up" sites of bleeding in the circulatory system. However, a fibrin plug in a coronary artery can obstruct or severely minimize vital blood flow. This lack of blood supply to the cardiac muscle results in ischemia, damage, and, if prolonged, death (necrosis) of cardiac muscle. Because necrosis occurs progressively, damaged cardiac muscle can be *saved* if blood flow can soon be restored to the area.

The body has a naturally occurring enzyme, plasmin, which digests fibrin. (If there was no plasmin, fibrin would accumulate throughout the system!) Plasmin comes from the activation of plasminogen. In acute myocardial infarction, if one could activate plasminogen to plasmin, the fibrin clot could be dissolved.

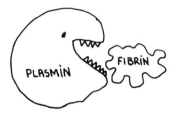

Mechanism of Action

Enter the thrombolytic agents! Thrombolytic drugs act by converting plasminogen to plasmin. The plasmin subsequently *digests* fibrin in the clot occluding the coronary artery. If the clot is dissolved soon enough, the subsequent restoration of blood flow will limit further heart muscle damage. The opening of a previously clotted artery is called **reperfusion.**

The timely reperfusion of an occluded coronary artery results in improved cardiac function and survival. Signs of reperfusion include relief of chest pain, reduction of ST segment elevation, and the onset of arrhythmias called *reperfusion arrhythmias.* Through these arrhythmias may require treatment, they signal restored perfusion. ("Good" arrhythmias!)

Thrombolytic agents should be administered as soon as possible following the onset of acute myocardial infarct symptoms in order to save the greatest amount of heart muscle. Little benefit is anticipated if treatment is initiated 12 or more hours following the onset of pain.

Thrombolytic drugs not only dissolve "bad" clots in coronary arteries, but also dissolve "good" clots plugging up any other area of bleeding. Thus, the major side effect associated with thrombolytic agent administration is bleeding from any site of injury.

Bleeding can range from a minor problem (a little oozing from cuts or IV sites) to serious, life-threatening episodes (intracranial bleeds). Therefore, patients must be *carefully* screened for *predisposing* conditions. Thrombolytic drugs *should be avoided* in patients with a history of recent surgery, childbirth, or trauma. Pregnancy, uncontrolled severe hypertension, recent stroke, and coagulation abnormalities are also contraindications to thrombolytic drug administration.

Reperfusion secondary to thrombolytic drug administration is successful about 35–75 percent of the time, and usually takes 30–60 minutes to occur. Heparin (an anticoagulant) is commonly administered for several days following successful thrombolytic treatment to prevent *reocclusion,* or a repeat thrombus formation in the same artery.

Thrombolytic drugs differ from one another in terms of source of drug, allergenicity, dosage, administration, duration of thrombolytic effect, cost . . . and here's the controversial part . . . efficacy and toxicity. TPA and urokinase are human proteins, and are therefore *less likely* to produce allergies than streptokinase or anistreplase, which are produced by streptococcal bacteria. However, streptokinase is much less expensive than other thrombolytic agents and has been shown to have similar efficacy in large clinical trials.

Thrombolytic agents are usually administered intravenously, though they can be administered directly into the coronary artery during a cardiac catheterization procedure.

This is the conclusion of input 4. Lets try some practice before moving on to smaller things!

PRACTICE EXERCISE 4

1. The primary objective for treating atrial fibrillation is to _____
_____ .

2. In treating atrial fibrillation, digoxin is administered before a class IA antiarrhythmic drug. Explain
why. _____
_____
_____
_____

3. P.V.C.'s occurring during acute myocardial infarction are treated with _____ , a class
_____ drug, to prevent _____
_____ .

4. _____ have been shown to decrease mortality in the post-myocardial infarction period.

5. Thrombolytic drugs are proteins that act by _____
_____
_____ .

6. A reperfusion arrhythmia is _____
_____
_____ .

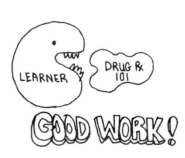

For **Feedback 4,** refer to page 316.

Feedback 1

1. In response to stress, the <u>sympathetic</u> nerve connections to the SA node are stimulated.

2. Parasympathetic ⟶ Norepinephrine⟶Increased heart rate
   Sympathetic ⟶ Acetycholine⟶Decreased heart rate

3. An agonist is <u>any chemical which acts at a receptor site and produces an effect.</u>

4. A drug which binds to a receptor without producing an effect or prevents or reverses the effects of an agonist is known as an <u>antagonist.</u>

5. Epinephrine (Adrenaline)⟶Beta-adrenergic agonist
   Propranolol (Inderal)⟶Beta-adrenergic antagonist
   Atropine⟶Muscarinic antagonist

6. ☐ Antagonist→agonist→agony→

1. Cardiac cells may interact with or respond to different types of drugs because <u>cardiac cells have many different receptor types on the cell surfaces.</u>

2. Antiarrhythmic drugs work by affecting one or more of the following cardiac tissue properties:
   A. <u>automaticity.</u>
   B. <u>rate of impulse conduction.</u>
   C. <u>duration of refractory period.</u>

3. Drug absorption depends on the <u>route of administration.</u>

4. The intravenous route of drug administration produces "near-immediate" effects because one of the following processes is bypassed. Check the omitted process.
   ☒ Absorption

5. A continuous infusion of lidocaine is necessary to maintain an effective blood concentration because <u>lower perfusion tissues remove lidocaine from circulation. The drug distribution steals lidocaine away from its intended site of action.</u>

6. During a code arrest situation, a central venous route of drug administration is recommended because <u>drug distribution delay is minimized. Peak drug concentrations reaching the heart are higher when drugs are administered via a central line.</u>

7. The <u>liver</u> is the primary location for drug metabolism.

8. Drug "half-life" refers to <u>the time required to reduce (by metabolism or excretion) the amount of drug in the body by one half.</u>

1. Antiarrhythmic drugs are classified in accord with their
   a. <u>mechanism of action.</u>
   b. <u>EKG effects.</u>
   c. <u>Toxicities.</u>

2. Class I drugs work by binding to their receptor, the <u>sodium</u> channel, slowing the passage of <u>sodium</u> through to the cell. Slowing the passage decreases the rate of depolarization.

3. There are <u>3</u> subgroups of Class I drugs. All class I drugs decrease automaticity; however, the subgroups have differing effects on <u>conduction</u> and <u>repolarization.</u>

4. **ACTION**   **CLASS**   **SAMPLE DRUG**

Shortened repolarization — IA — Rhythmol

No repolarization effect — IB — Quinidine

Prolonged repolarization — IC — Lidocaine

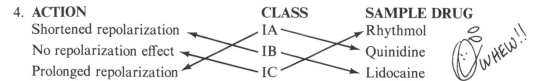

(crossing lines connect the actions to the classes and sample drugs)

OWHEW!!

5. Class IA antiarrhythmic drugs are broad spectrum and are used to treat both <u>supraventricular</u> and <u>ventricular</u> arrhythmias.

6. Class IB drugs are almost exclusively used to treat <u>ventricular</u> arrhythmias.

7. Class <u>IC</u> drugs are utilized to treat life-threatening ventricular arrhythmias.

8. The following toxicities may be related to the administration of lidocaine.
   - ☐ weight gain
   - ☒ drowsiness
   - ☒ agitation
   - ☒ confusion
   - ☒ disorientation
   - ☐ hives
   - ☒ convulsions
   - ☐ baldness
   - ☒ numbness

9. A proarrhythmic effect means that <u>the arrhythmia worsens during treatment rather than showing improvement.</u>

10. Class II antiarrhythmics are called <u>beta</u>-blockers. Class II drugs are frequently administered to control <u>supraventricular tachyarrhythmias.</u>

11. Calcium channel blockers, Class IV drugs, inhibit the flow of calcium into the cardiac cells and function by <u>decreasing conduction through the AV node (thereby slowing supraventricular rhythms).</u>

12. Calcium channel blockers are used exclusively for controlling <u>supraventricular arrhythmias.</u>

13. Digoxin works by <u>increasing the force of muscle contraction and by slowing conduction in the AV node.</u>

14.

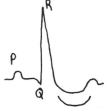

SCOOPED ST SEGMENT DEMONSTRATES DIGITALIS EFFECT

Feedback 4

1. The primary objective for treating atrial fibrillation is to <u>reduce the rapid ventricular rate. (If you need a quick review of atrial fibrillation, turn to page 68).</u>

2. In treating atrial fibrillation, digoxin is administered before a class IA antiarrhythmic drug because <u>class I agents can increase the AV conduction which would increase the ventricular response rate. Since digoxin slows AV conduction, it is started first!</u>

3. P.V.C.'s occurring during acute myocardial infarction are treated with <u>lidocaine</u>, a class <u>IB</u> drug, to prevent <u>ventricular fibrillation.</u>

4. *Beta blockers* have been shown to decrease mortality in the post-myocardial infarction period.

5. Thrombolytic drugs are proteins that act by <u>converting plasminogen to plasmin, which subsequently digests the clot occluding the coronary artery.</u>

6. A reperfusion arrhythmia is <u>a dysrhythmia that presents secondary to restored coronary artery perfusion. Though reperfusion arrhythmias may require treatment, they are GOOD NEWS!</u>

Before moving ahead to Section XIII, begin to

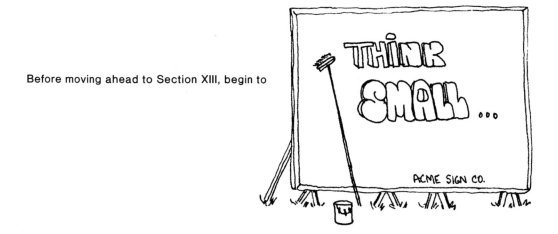

NOTES

Section XIII
Kidstuff

OBJECTIVES

When you have completed Section XIII, you will be able to describe or identify

1. children are not small adults
2. normal heart rate norms for children
3. normal duration of P, P-R, QRS, and QT intervals
4. recognition of the following cardiac dysrhythmias in kids:

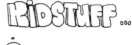
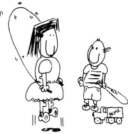

   • sinus arrhythmia
   • sinus bradycardia
   • sinus tachycardia
   • sinus arrest/sinus block
   • sick sinus syndrome
   • atrial tachycardia
   • P.A.C.'s
   • atrial flutter
   • atrial fibrillation
   • wandering atrial pacemaker
   • junctional escape rhythms
   • premature junctional beats
   • junctional tachycardia
   • P.S.V.T.
   • P.V.C.'s
   • ventricular tachycardia
   • ventricular flutter
   • ventricular fibrillation
   • W.P.W. syndrome
   • first degree heart block
   • second degree heart block
   • third degree heart block
   • bundle branch blocks
5. drug and electrolyte manifestations

Text by:

JANE D. WERTH

Back in the days of Michelangelo, painters frequently painted children as little adults—same body shape, same body proportions, and the same skin tone. It didn't work then and it doesn't work now. . . .

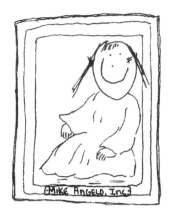

. . . *children are not just adults in miniature*. They have different health care problems and different body function norms . . . so follows the reason for this section. It is important to understand both the similarities and differences between adult and pediatric electrocardiography.

Birth through 18 years of age covers a wide time span! However, for the sake of simplicity we will use the term *pediatrics* to cover this age span in most references. The term *newborn* applies to babies 0–1 month of age, and the term *infant* applies to infants 1 month–one year!

So bearing that in mind, let's start! . . . Just one more thing. . . .

. . . you may find it helpful to read the corresponding "adult" version as you ponder pediatric dysrhythmias . . . that's why the rest of this book is attached!

The stable EKG pattern seen in the normal adult does not completely develop in the child until around the age of ten. Most changes that do occur in pediatric EKG's are due to a shift from right ventricular dominance (seen in the newborn) to left ventricular dominance (seen in the adult).

At birth, the right ventricle is thicker than the left side counterpart. During the first month of life there is a dramatic decrease in right ventricular pressure and a subsequent decrease in right ventricular wall thickness.

Well, if you're still insistent on learning more, let's talk about something a lot more exciting.

In many instances, dysrhythmias in children differ in *cause* and *frequency* from adults. For instance, ventricular dysthythmias are seen less frequently in children owing to the absence of atherosclerotic heart disease.

More commonly seen in children are the EKG dysrhythmias and abnormalities which occur secondary to structural problems in the heart. Now, just take a minute and remember atrial septal defects . . . tetrology of Fallot . . . and patent ductus arteriosus (you may have studied those in Anatomy 101). Basically, many congenital heart defects, like those named above, create artificial openings in heart chambers that can greatly increase chamber pressure gradients. These pressure increases can cause chamber *HYPERTROPHY*. Since congenital heart defects occur in approximately eight to ten of every 1,000 newborns, hypertrophy induced EKG changes are very common.

Let's look at *atrial hypertrophy* for a moment. As you will recall, the P wave represents atrial depolarization. The P wave then reflects depolarization of both the right and left atria. In reality, the P wave can be divided into two components.

Right Atrial Component ↘ P ↙ Left Atrial Component

(Remember, leads II, III, and aVF display the most prominent P waves.) If atrial hypertrophy exists, there is an increase in the *amplitude* or the *duration* of the P wave.

P

amplitude

P

duration

Looking at atrial depolarization in lead II, right atrial hypertrophy is reflected as a prominent P with increased amplitude. (Lead V₁ is included for comparison.)

Right Atrial ↘
← Left Atrial

Lead II

Right Atrial ↘ P
← Left Atrial

Lead V₁

Left atrial hypertrophy may present as a prolonged P wave or a notched P.

Right Atrial ↘ P ↙ Left Atrial

Lead II

Right Atrial ↘
P
← Left Atrial

Lead V₁

If both right and left atrial hypertrophy are present, the P wave may reflect a combination of the above patterns.

Right Atrial ↘ P ← Left Atrial

Lead II

Right Atrial ↘ P
← Left Atrial

Lead V₁

LEADING STATEMENTS

Remember leads? We talked about the limb leads, the augmented leads, and precordial leads in the beginning of the book. Basically, leads view electrical activity from different perspectives or angles. Since ventricular dysrhythmias are less common in children, usually "kids" are monitored on leads which best reflect atrial activity! Commonly then, children will be monitored on leads II, III, and aVF.

Input 1: You Have to Know the Rules to Win the Game

It's an old story . . . unless someone lets you in on the rules, you can make some *bozo* moves whenever you start something new (thought for the day ☺)!

So let's get some ground rules straight before we move on.

Rule #1   Heart rate norms vary in children from year to year (and sometimes month to month). Though the following norms are approximations, most authorities tend to agree with these parameters!

PEDIATRIC HEART RATE NORMS		
Age	**Range**	**Average Rate**
0–1 month	100–180	(160)
2–3 months	110–180	(150)
4–12 months	100–180	(150)
1–3 yrs.	80–180	(130)
4–5 yrs.	70–150	(100)
6–8 yrs.	68–140	(100)
9–11 yrs.	60–125	(88)
12–16 yrs.	50–125	(80)
>16 yrs.	50–90	(70)

As you can see, there is a tremendous variation in the norms (depending on age), but as a general rule . . .

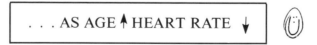

. . . AS AGE ↑ HEART RATE ↓ ☺

In any case, *heart rate must be evaluated in relation to the age of the child and the underlying clinical condition.* Heart rate increases may be related to crying, anxiety, fear, fever, etc. In fact, the heart rate may go up eight to ten beats per minute for each Fahrenheit degree increase in temperature. (*Remember that?*) Decreases in heart rate may be related to sleep, increased vagal tone, abdominal distention, increased intracranial pressure, apnea, and a variety of *other* factors.

Rule #2 Another general rule that can be applied to pediatrics is,

---

AS AGE ↓, THE DURATION OF THE P-R AND QRS
INTERVALS ↑ AND THE DURATION OF THE QT
INTERVAL ↓ .

So . . . let's explore each of those intervals separately. In fact, let's explore all the wave forms!

THE P WAVE

You will recall that the P wave represents atrial excitation spreading from the SA node through the right and left atria. Normally the duration of the P wave is 0.06 ± 0.02 seconds in children.

Remember each small EKG paper square represents 0.04 seconds!

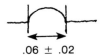

.06 ± .02

The maximum P wave duration is 0.10 seconds in children and 0.08 seconds in infants.
A prolonged P wave may be due to atrial hypertrophy as we discussed on page 000.

THE P-R INTERVAL

You will remember that atrial activation and atrial repolarization are represented on the EKG as a P wave followed by a straight line—this is the P-R interval.

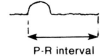

P-R interval

The P-R interval further represents the time for the impulse to pass from the SA node through the AV junction, through the ventricles to the Purkinje fibers. Like the duration of the P wave, the duration of the P-R interval tends to vary with age.

PEDIATRIC P-R INTERVALS	
Age	**Duration of P-R Interval**
0–4 months	0.08–0.12 seconds
4–12 months	0.08–0.13 seconds
1–3 years	0.09–0.16 seconds
4–5 years	0.10–0.16 seconds
6–8 years	0.10–0.18 seconds
9–16 years	0.10–0.20 seconds
>16 years	0.12–0.20 seconds

A prolonged P-R interval ⌐⟷¬ represents increased conduction time and may be seen in conditions such as first degree heart block, myocarditis, excessive vagal stimulation, atrial septal defect, etc.

A shortened P-R interval ↔ P-R may be seen in rhythms with accelerated conduction such as Wolff-Parkinson-White (W.P.W.) Syndrome.

QRS DURATION

Remember, the duration of the QRS indicates the time elapsed during ventricular activation (depolarization . . . you're so smart). Normal pediatric QRS durations are as follows:

KIDS' QRS's	
Age	**QRS Duration**
Premie	0.04 sec.
0–3 years.	0.04–0.08 sec.
4–16 yrs.	0.05–0.09 sec.
>16 years.	0.05–0.10 sec.

When the QRS is greater than the prescribed upper limit, i.e., a *ventricular conduction delay* exists. This conduction delay may be caused by:

- severe hyperkalemia
- quinidine toxicity
- procainamide toxicity
- bundle branch block (remember the skinny vs. the fat QRS??)

QT INTERVAL

The QT interval represents the time for both ventricular depolarization and repolarization.

Just like the adult, the QT interval varies with heart rate and a variety of other things! In the infant, however, the *QT interval varies with age!* From six months of age to adulthood, the normal QT interval should not exceed 0.425 seconds. During the first six months, the QT interval is longer and may measure up to 0.49 seconds.

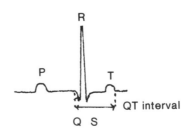

Though *no one sits around measuring QT intervals,* it is probably worthwhile noting that QT interval prolongation is associated with hypocalcemia, myocarditis, and the administration of quinidine. A *short* QT interval may be seen with hypercalemia and digitalis effect.

We're getting near the end of the lineup!

THE ST SEGMENT

The ST segment (straight line between the S and T waves) represents the early phase of ventricular repolarization. Similar to grown-ups, ST segment elevation may be associated with acute pericarditis (inflammation of enveloping membranes of heart) or acute myocardial infarct. ST segment depression is principally associated with hypokalemia or digitalis effect.

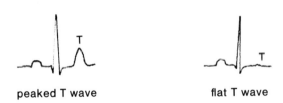

ST segment elevation   ST segment depression

As with adults, it is important to remember that EKG's are not diagnostic, only suggestive! Last, but not least . . .

THE T WAVE

The T wave is the recovery phase (repolarization) after ventricular depolarization. Tall, peaked T waves may be seen in hyperkalemia and ventricular hypertrophy. Flat, low T waves may be seen in newborn infants as a normal phenomenon or associated with hypothyroidism, hypokalemia (there it is again), pericarditis, myocarditis, or digitalis effect.

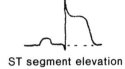

peaked T wave   flat T wave

All these components come together for the *normal EKG lineup:*

- Rate—varies with age.
- Rhythm—regular.
- P waves—each QRS will be preceded by a P wave. All P waves will appear uniform.
- QRS—all QRS complexes will appear uniform in configuration.
- Conduction—each P will be followed by normal QRS.
- T wave—may be flipped (inverted) from birth to adolescence in the right precordial leads V_1, V_2.
- P-R interval and QRS duration normal for age

For those of you who care for the *littlest of lambs,* there are multiple subtle changes in EKG patterns as the infant develops. Some of the major, early observed changes are now discussed.

Rule #3 | Be aware of *subtle* changes.

Premie EKG (birth before 37 weeks gestation):

1. Lower voltage QRS and T in limb leads (I, II, III).
2. Shorter P-R, QRS, QT intervals (have you forgotten what QT intervals are—review page 324).

Normal newborn EKG:

1. Small (short!!) QRS in limb leads (this time you tell me . . . leads _____ , _____ , and _____).
2. T wave in V_1 usually becomes flipped (inverted or negative) by third day and remains flipped until the age of five (this phenomenon occurs because of the changing nature of the developing heart)!

So, we're almost ready to play, *What's My Dysrhythmia*? First, let's review the steps you learned previously for analyzing EKG's—these steps are as appropriate for pediatric rhythms as they are for adult rhythms!

1. Determine the heart rates using methods discussed on page 27 (get your glasses out, you're counting small squares)!

2. Is the rhythm basically regular or irregular??
3. Look at atrial activity (P waves). Is atrial depolarization occurring at an expected rate with a regular rhythm? Are the P waves so rapid that there are more atrial impulses than there are QRS complexes? Is it difficult to distinguish atrial activity?
4. Look at ventricular activity—what are the QRS's doing? Are the QRS's of normal duration? Is there a QRS following each P wave? Are the QRS's occurring regularly (consistent R-R interval)?
5. Try to determine the relationship between atrial activity and ventricular activity. Is each P wave producing a QRS? Is the P-R constant? Are there any dropped beats or pauses?

Remember—*What's in a name*? A dysrhythmia by the *wrong* name may spell defeat! *It is more important to describe what you see than apply a label.* (Unfortunately, people disagree over labels . . . actually, without labels, this is all very logical!)

Practice Exercise 1

1. The heart rate, the duration of P-R, QRS, and QT intervals all vary with _____ .

Circle the correct answer:

2. The heart rate <u>increases/decreases</u> with increasing age.

3. The P-R interval <u>lengthens/shortens</u> with increasing age.

4. The duration of the QRS is <u>longer/shorter</u> with increasing age.

5. The duration of the QT interval <u>increases/decreases</u> with increasing age.

6. What does this picture represent?

R
P   T
Q S

_____

_____

_____

For **Feedback 1,** refer to page 360.

Input 2: Sinus Anomalies

Sinus rhythms are so called because they originate in the sinoatrial node. The SA node is the normal pacemaker of the heart because it has the fastest pacemaking capability or the *highest automaticity*. As with everything in pediatrics, the inherent rate of SA node discharge (thus the rate of conduction or heart rate in a normal heart) varies with age . . . so much for precision! Need a quick rate review? Please turn back to page 322.

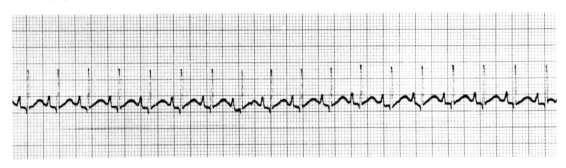

Normal sinus rhythm in a normal newborn. The heart rate is 166 because the baby is crying!

SINUS ARRHYTHMIA

The first dysrhythmia to be considered is *sinus arrhythmia*. Sinus arrhythmia is a slightly irregular rhythm that is initiated by the SA node. Usually the irregularity of the rhythm is due to respiration. The heart rate tends to increase with inspiration and decrease with expiration. Sinus arrhythmia is more pronounced in adolescence than in childhood.

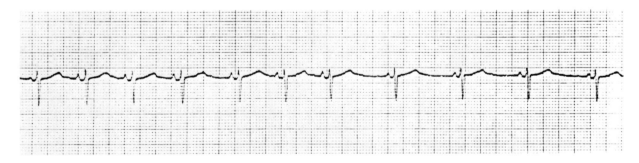

A nonpathologic sinus arrhythmia. Note the irregular P-P interval.

Sinus arrhythmia is a variation of normal and can be differentiated from a truly abnormal arrhythmia by having the child hold his or her breath. In sinus arrhythmia, cessation of breathing will cause the heart rate to remain steady.

Let's look at sinus arrhythmia.

- Rate—variable with age.
- Rhythm—irregular.
- P waves—
  - uniform in appearance
  - irregular P-P interval
  - precede each QRS complex
- P-R interval nonvarying.
- QRS's are all of normal configuration, but the R-R intervals are irregular.

Sinus arrhythmia is a common dysrhythmia that is usually a *variation of normal*. Though no treatment is required, one should be aware that it exists. Just for fun, measure the varying P-P and R-R intervals in this rhythm strip.

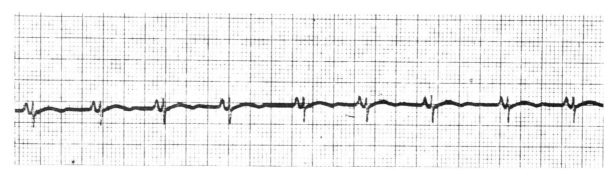

Normal newborn with sinus bradycardia and sinus arrythmia secondary to maternal Inderol treatment for P.A.T.

SINUS BRADYCARDIA

Bradycardia has a few drawbacks . . . remember bradycardia is a term used to describe a rate slower than normal. Of course, the definition of bradycardia varies with age in pediatrics (and you're saying, *"What doesn't?"*). Generally speaking, *sinus bradycardia* is defined as a rate of less than 100 beats/minute in newborns and less than 70 beats/minute in children.

Getting back the shortcomings of bradycardia . . . if sinus bradycardia develops gradually, compensatory cardiac changes (such as increased stroke volume and chamber dilation) may prevent a fall in cardiac output. That's good! Unfortunately, if the bradycardia comes on suddenly, the heart is less likely to compensate and cardiac output will be compromised.

So, keeping that in mind, let's look at *sinus bradycardia* in greater detail.

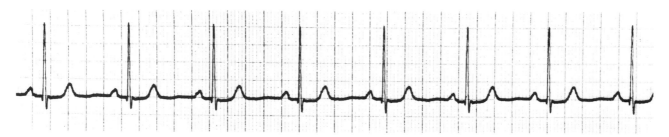

Sinus bradycardia with a heart rate of 62 per minute. This rhythm strip belongs to an eight year old girl. Notice that the P-R interval approaches the upper limit of normal.

Criteria for *sinus bradycardia:*

- Rate—less than 100 in newborns, less than 70 in children.
- Rhythm—regular.
- P waves precede each QRS; P-R interval is constant; the P-P interval regular.
- QRS's are all of normal configuration, R-R interval regular.

Well, *what are some of the more common causes of sinus bradycardia,* you ask. Sinus bradycardia may be *associated* with:

- apnea in the healthy premature infant
- increased vagal tone (due to increased intracranial pressure, hypertension, abdominal distention, etc.)
- adolescent athletes (normal rhythm of *pint-size champions*)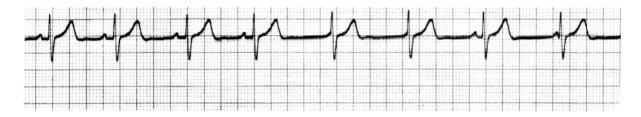
- hypoglycemia (ever feel faint when dieting?)
- following open heart surgery.

Sinus bradycardia is treated when there is evidence of decreased cardiac output (mental confusion, disorientation, lethargy, loss of consciousness, cyanosis). In most cases atropine is the drug of choice. The underlying cause should always be treated and hopefully corrected. Remember, atropine may cause urinary retention!

An exaggerated slow heart rate may allow escape beats or escape rhythms to be initiated from lower, most distal pacemakers. Most commonly, one would see the escape beats originating from the AV junctional tissue. You will recall that escape beats are inscribed late, after the next anticipated normal beat. When escape beats originate in the AV junctional tissue, they are conducted normally through the ventricles. Thus, the QRS is skinny!

Notice that the heart rate slows after beat 4, allowing an AV junctional pacemaker to come through.

SINUS TACHYCARDIA

Tachycardia is a term used to describe a heart rate of greater than 140 in children and greater than 160 in infants. *Sinus tachy* (as those of us who are close call it) is a regular sinus rhythm with an *increased* rate. Usually *sinus tachycardia* will not exceed a rate of 180 in children and 200 in infants. Whew!

Time to be logical. . . . *Sinus tachycardia* has the following characteristics:

- Rate—140–180 in children, 160–200 in infants.
- Rhythm–regular.
- P waves precede each QRS
- P-P interval constant
- P-R interval constant
- A QRS follows each P wave; normal QRS configuration; R-R interval regular.
- Usually has gradual onset; gradual slowing.

Look for yourself!

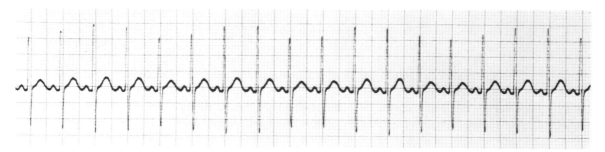

Sinus tachycardia in a three year old with an elevated temperature.

Some *culprits* that may be responsible for sinus tachycardia include anxiety, fever, infection, anemia, CHF, myocarditis, rheumatic fever, decongestants, etc. The treatment for sinus tachycardia consists of *discovering the underlying cause and treating it!* As with all rapid rhythms, ventricular fill time is reduced, thus diminishing cardiac output.

SINUS ARREST

Sinus arrest or *sinus pause* is the result of momentary failure of the SA node to initiate an impulse. Since there is no SA stimulus, no atrial or subsequent ventricular activity occurs. So there's no

_____ and no _____ . (If you said P and QRS, you may go to the head of the class!)

The pause is usually of *short, but undetermined,* duration. Occasionally, an escape beat may interrupt the pause (a built-in safety device of the unit)! Let's take a look.

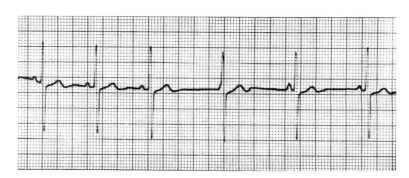

Notice the sinus pause following beat 3. A junctional escape beat interrupts the pause. The normal sinus pacemaker then resumes at a slower rate.

The specifics of *sinus arrest* are as follows:

• Rate usually within normal bounds.
• Rhythm irregular owing to pause(s).
• QRS follows every P wave; P-P interval regular and irregular.
• QRS of normal duration, R-R regular and irregular.

A close cousin of sinus arrest is *sinus block*. Although the sinus pacemaker fires on time, it is blocked somewhere within the sinus mechanism . . . in other words, *it never gets out of the gate!* Usually the pause in sinus block is the duration of two normal sinus impulses.

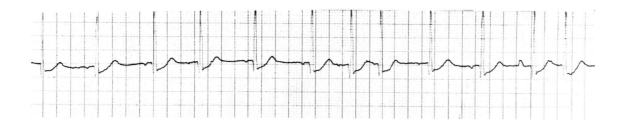

duration of 2 sinus impulses

Sinus pause and sinus arrest are *most commonly caused* by increased vagal tone, hypoxia, and digitalis. Usually treatment is not required unless the pauses are pronounced or of frequent occurrence.

SICK SINUS SYNDROME

Sick sinus syndrome was discussed back on page 62. It is seen when the good ol' SA node fails to function as the dominant pacemaker of the heart. Consequently, one sees a variety of dysrhythmias that are *together* labeled as *sick sinus syndrome*. These dysrhythmias include:

- profound sinus bradycardia
- SA block
- sinus arrest with junctional escape beats
- P.A.T. (remember paroxysmal atrial tachycardia?)
- slow or fast ectopic atrial or junctional rhythms

Sick sinus syndrome may be found in children who have undergone extensive cardiac surgery. This is especially true when the surgery involves the atria and atrial septum.

Oftentimes these children develop frequent episodes of tachycardia requiring propranolol. Usually the tachycardia episodes decrease as the child grows older. If bradycardia is pronounced, pacemaker therapy may be required.

The above strip demonstrates a sick sinus syndrome, though the rate falls within normal limits.

Practice Exercise 2

1. The easiest way to determine rhythm irregularity is to measure the P-P interval or the _____ interval.

2. Analzye this rhythm strip. Bear in mind that the owner of this rhythm is six years old!

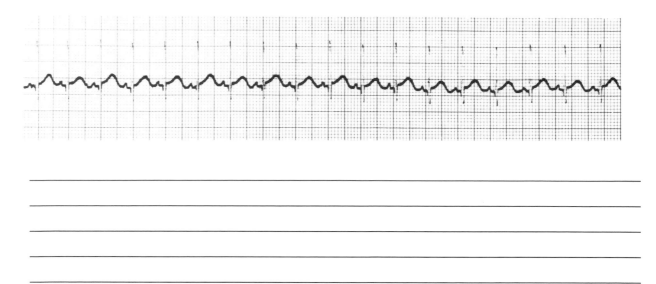

_____

_____

_____

_____

_____

3. Sinus bradycardia in a child is defined as a heart rate (circle the correct answer!)

      less than 90

      less than 70

      less than 80

      less than 60

For **Feedback 2,** refer to page 360.

Input 3: Atrial Dysrhythmias

With no further ado, we are going to begin exploring ectopic activity in children. You will remember from page 53 that we are talking about pacemaker impulses that are generated in abnormal areas of the atria (outside the normal conduction system).

We will start with ectopic rhythms that are generated in the atria. Atrial dysrhythmias give themselves away in that *they have P waves or atrial deflections occurring prior to the QRS's.* The P waves may be premature and may vary in appearance from normal sinus P waves . . . or there may be multiple atrial deflections per QRS (one to a customer please!).

Let's get off to a running start with atrial tachycardia.

ATRIAL TACHYCARDIA

Let's test your short-term memory. . . . (panic!!). Do you remember what the *minimum* and *maximum* inherent rates of SA node discharge are? Well, time's up . . . !

Age	Rate
0–1 month	100–180
1 year	80–180
5 years	70–150
10 years	60–125

In *atrial tachycardia,* the heart rate is usually in excess of 180 beats per minute, considerably *faster* than the inherent firing rate of the SA node (aren't you glad we reviewed those rate limits!). You will recall from Section II that atrial tachycardia often occurs secondary to a reentry phenomenon. In other words, a P.A.C. with a prolonged P-R interval is able to conduct normally as well as backward through the bundle of His to the atria. This *retrograde* or backward conduction reactivates the atria. If this reentry phenomenon continues, atrial tachycardia will result. *Whew!*

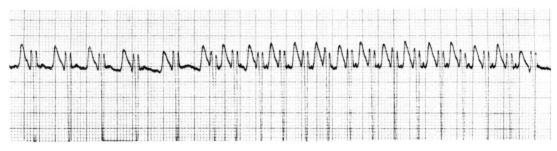

This rhythm strip demonstrates a newborn sinus rhythm. The rhythm slows slightly after beat 4. Beat 6 initiates a burst of atrial tachycardia at a rate of approximately 200 per minute! Since there are definite P waves, we know the rhythm is atrial in origin!

Let's get analytical. . . . *Atrial tachycardia* will have the following features:

- Rate—greater than 180 beats/minute.
- Rhythm—extremely regular.
- P wave—obvious before each QRS.
- P-R may be prolonged owing to tissue refractoriness (the tissue must have sufficient recovery time if the next impulse is to conduct normally).
- QRS—usually of normal duration.

The onset of atrial tachycardia may be gradual, but more often is abrupt, as above. When the onset is abrupt, the rhythm is called *PAROXYSMAL ATRIAL TACHYCARDIA*—P.A.T. to *close* friends.

Atrial tachycardia can exist for a few minutes or go on for days.

As *stimulating* as it may be to feel like you have a machine gun firing in your chest, long bouts of atrial tachycardia will cause decreased cardiac output which may result in congestive heart failure!

Both dobees and don't bees are subject to bouts of atrial tachycardia. Atrial tachycardia, or P.A.T., is found in (1) healthy children (roughly 50 percent of the cases), (2) children with congenital heart disease, and (3) children with Wolff-Parkinson-White Syndrome.

Remember the toilet example on page 58? You will recall that a rapid heart rate reduces cardiac output. (If you flush your toilet 180 times per minute . . . it's all coming back to you . . . I knew the toilet would do it!) So, treatment is aimed at *slowing the heart rate* and *restoring the sinus pacemaker.*

For children with no failure or mild congestive heart failure (CHF), digitalis is the treatment of choice. In more serious cases where CHF is pronounced, or where the rapid rate is poorly tolerated, digitalis is too slow-acting to restore hemodynamic equilibrium quickly. Thus, cardioversion may be the first line of treatment. Verapamil, a relatively new calcium-blocker drug, may also be effective in treating atrial tachycardia. Verapamil, like digitalis, slows AV conduction!

Older children with short bursts of atrial tachycardia may respond well to measures that increase vagal tone (carotid sinus massage, gagging, application of cold or ice water to the face, Valsalva manuever, etc.). Infants, however, may not respond well to these tactics owing to the immaturity of the nervous system. Following restoration of a sinus rhythm, these children usually will be placed on digoxin for six months to prevent further recurrence.

Very *tachy* stuff, huh?

Well, sometimes the ectopic atrial pacemaker becomes impatient, interrupting the underlying, normal rhythm.

PREMATURE ATRIAL CONTRACTION (P.A.C.)

As the name implies, the P.A.C. is premature in its relationship to the sinus rhythm. As rude as that may be, there is also another clue—the premature P wave is different in configuration from the "normal" P wave.

Lets look at an example!

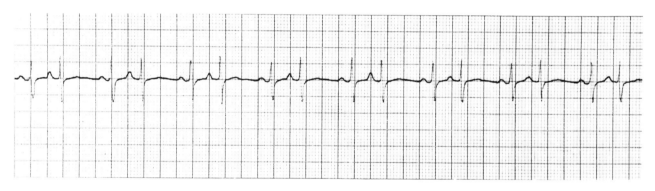

Look closely! Every other beat is a P.A.C. (Bigeminy P.A.C.'s). Notice that the P waves of the P.A.C.'s look distinctly different from the sinus P waves.

Get out the old check list. . . .   rhythms with P.A.C.'s have the following features:

- Rate—normal sinus rate . . . remember . . . the rate varies with age!
- Rhythm—irregular due to premature beats.
- P wave—of the P.A.C. is of different size and/or shape from normal P; P-R interval of normal beats is within normal limits; P-R of ectopic beats may vary from normal.
- QRS—normal duration; R-R interval irregular.
- Pause following the P.A.C. (allowing the sinus mechanism to reset the rhythm). An infant will have a complete compensatory pause (twice the R-R interval), while older children will demonstrate an incomplete compensatory pause (less than twice the R-R interval).

P.A.C.'s may be seen in children with:

- atrial enlargement
- electrolyte imbalances
- hypoxia
- hypoglycemia
- following atrial surgery

. . . and *surprise,* P.A.C.'s are *common* in HEALTHY CHILDREN AND NEWBORNS.

The treatment of P.A.C.'s depends on the underlying cause. If the cardiovascular system is normal, no treatment is usually necessary. If the premature beats are frequent, multifocal, or seen in couplets (two or more together), continuous monitoring should be provided and a physician notified. Usually, digitalis or propranolol are the drugs of choice if treatment is deemed necessary. On to the *romantic sounding* atrial ectopies . . . flutter, fib, wandering. . . .

ATRIAL FLUTTER

Remember the movie "Jaws"? Well, for those of you who are too young, or who have better taste in movies, sharks have a *sawtooth* type fin that protrudes above the water. Atrial flutter resembles a *convention of all Pacific coast great white sharks*—multiple sawtooth waves (sawteeth) with QRS's interspersed.

A Convention of Great White Sharks

Do not color sharks . . . →   ←Water (Pacific Ocean)
they are white   Color this blue

P S   We must humor the author . . .

Atrial flutter arises from an excitable ectopic site within the atria. You will recall that atrial flutter is thought to occur through a reentry mechanism. The atrial flutter rate is *usually* 240–360 beats per minute! However, not all of those impulses are passed through the AV junction. Commonly, one sees a 2:1, 3:1, or 4:1 conduction i.e., one QRS per four sawtooth waves). The sawtooth waves are "F" or flutter waves. (If I had some say, they would be called "S" waves for shark!)

Logic time: Atrial flutter has the following characteristics:

- Atrial rate 240–360 . . . therefore, the ventricular rate is usually ½, ⅓, or ¼ of 240–360.
- Rhythm—usually regular.
- P waves—rather than P waves, there are continuous "F" waves.   ∧∧∧∧∧∧∧∧
- QRS is of normal duration; R-R interval may be regular or irregular depending upon the degree of block in the AV junction.
- Atrial and ventricular activity are related because the interval between a conducted flutter wave and its QRS is always constant.

335

Atrial flutter is seen *rarely* in children, but may be associated with:

• chronic, severe rheumatic fever
• sick sinus syndrome
• hypoxia
• hypoglycemia
• following intra-atrial surgery

The following strip demonstrates a 2:1 atrial flutter . . . sometimes it's difficult to identify flutter waves!

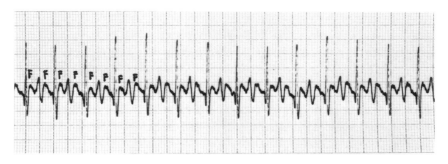

The atrial rhythm is regular at a rate of 300 per minute. Note the "SHARK" waves!

The object of treatment is to reduce the rapid ventricular rate and restore the normal sinus mechanism. (A rapid ventricular rate reduces cardiac output owing to the reduced ventricular fill time.) Digitalis is the first drug of choice. It serves to increase AV block, thus slowing the ventricular rate. In more serious situations (when the rapid rate is poorly tolerated), cardioversion may be the initial treatment of choice.

ATRIAL FIBRILLATION

In *atrial fibrillation* there are no waves, just bizarre, irregular, rapid deflections called "f" waves which distort the baseline. (The baseline *undulates* . . . remember?) The atrial activity has no rhythmic pattern. See for yourself!

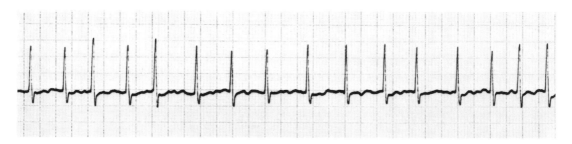

Note the varying R–R interval of atrial fibrillation.

You will notice that there is no coordinated effort in the atria. To quote "the" author,

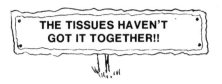

THE TISSUES HAVEN'T
GOT IT TOGETHER!!

"Some parts of the atria are in a state of excitation and some are in a state of refraction."

Let's look at the specifics of atrial fibrillation.

- Atrial rate—400–600 per minute (but who's counting—who could count that!).
- Rhythm—irregularly irregular (everything is irregular).
- P waves—none present; instead, irregular f waves.
- QRS duration normal, but the R-R interval varies continuously.
- Ventricular rate—usually rapid in uncontrolled atrial flutter.

In children, you may see atrial fibrillation associated with:

- electrolyte imbalance
- hypoglycemia
- hyperthyroidism
- intra-atrial surgery
- structural heart defects

As with the adult, treatment is aimed at *reducing the rapid ventricular rate* and restoring sinus rhythm. When the ventricular rate is rapid, there is a reduced cardiac output owing to the decreased ventricular fill time. Similar to other rapid atrial dysrhythmias, digitalis or cardioversion may be the first line of treatment, depending upon how well the child is tolerating the dysrhythmia!

WANDERING ATRIAL PACEMAKER (W.A.P.)

The name says it all . . . the atrial pacemaker wanders! There is a gradual shifting between the SA node and other ectopic atrial foci to be the "big cheese" (site of impulse formation). A wandering atrial pacemaker may result when there is a slight slowing of the SA node impulse formation or when various sites within the atria have similar impulse formation rates.

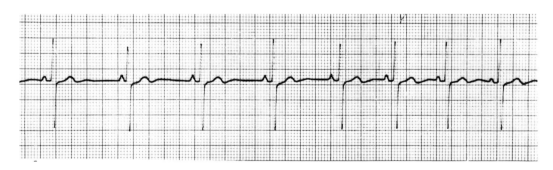

Notice the changing appearance of the P waves and the slight variation in the P-R interval.

337

The following are criteria which help in identifying W.A.P.
- Rate—within normal limits.
- Rhythm—slightly irregular.
- P wave—constantly changing, may be SA, atrial, or junctional in origin (if the pacemaker wanders out of the atria), or may not be visible. P-P interval irregular.
- P-R interval—varies continuously (though the variation is seldom marked).
- QRS's—are related to all P waves; QRS duration within normal limits.

Usually W.A.P. is a benign dysrhythmia and frequently is seen in *otherwise* healthy children.

It may also be seen in conditions such as these:
- acute rheumatic fever
- increased vagal tone (i.e., increased intracranial pressure, hypertension, etc.)
- drugs—digitalis, propranolol

No treatment is required when a wandering atrial pacemaker is found in a healthy child. When associated with other clinical conditions, it is the underlying clinical problem that may require treatment.

Practice Exercise 3

1. The aims of treatment for any rapid atrial dysrhythmia (i.e., P.A.T.) are:

   a. _____

   _____

   b. _____

   _____

2. What are the identifying characteristics of a premature atrial contraction?

   a. _____

   b. _____

   c. _____

3. Analyze this strip:

   _____

   _____

   _____

4. Describe the identifying features of a wandering atrial pacemaker.

   _____

   _____

   _____

For **Feedback 3,** refer to page 360.

A little *junctional escape rhythm lore*—

The heart has many potential pacemakers: the SA node, the atria, the AV junctional tissues, and the ventricles. Only the dominant or fastest pacemaker will normally control the heart. If the sinus pacemaker fails to fire, *or* if the impulse fails to be conducted, *or* if the sinus node discharges impulses so slowly that the heart rate becomes inadequate, a lower, more distal pacemaker will assume the role of pacemaker. Whew! (Remember that!)

JUNCTIONAL ESCAPE RHYTHM

If a rhythm originates in the AV junctional tissue, it is known as a *junctional escape rhythm* or an *idiojunctional rhythm*.

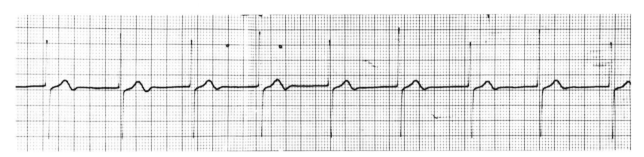

This strip demonstrates a junctional escape rhythm in a five year old female. The heart rate is approximately 64 per minute. Notice that there are no visible P waves occurring before or after the QRS. In this example, the atria and ventricles are being activated at approximately the same time . . . thus, the P wave is hiding within the QRS.

Checklist time . . . otherwise known as "the specifics of junctional escape rhythms":

• Ventricular rate—usually 50–90 in infants and 50–70 in children, though rates may vary.
• Rhythm—regular . . . (escape rhythms are almost always regular).
• P—may be observed before or after the QRS . . . or may be hiding within the QRS. If visible, P waves will be inverted in leads II, III, and aVF.
• QRS—duration normal.

How could this happen, you ask??? A junctional escape rhythm may be associated with the following conditions:

• children who have an otherwise normal heart
• sick sinus syndrome
• increased vagal tone
• following atrial surgery and/or any open heart surgery

If the ventricular rate is adequate, treatment may not be necessary. Remember . . . not only does the slower heart rate compromise the child, so does the loss of *atrial kick*. Therefore, if the patient is symptomatic, atropine or pacing (in exaggerated cases) may be necessary.

JUNCTIONAL ESCAPE BEATS

A *junctional escape beat* is an impulse arising from the junctional tissue due to a brief interruption of the sinus pacemaker. Junctional escape beats will come later than anticipated normal beats (better late than never!). As before, the P wave of the junctional escape beat will occur before or after the QRS . . . or be buried in the QRS. In leads II, III, and aVF the P wave will be inverted. Additionally, the P-R interval of the junctional escape beat will be shorter than the lower limits of normal.

The following tracing demonstrates a slowing of the sinus pacemaker which allows two junctional escape beats to come through. Remember . . . escape beats will always come later in the cardiac cycle than anticipated normal beats.

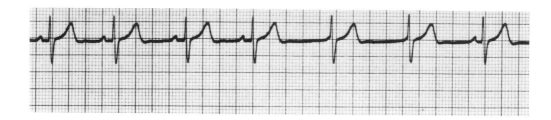

Single, infrequent junctional escape beats have no real significance. If the SA node persistently fires slowly or the impulse fails to conduct, a sustained AV junctional rhythm may be observed. Remember, escape beats or escape rhythms are *never* a primary phenomenon . . . they are *always* secondary to another event. They occur because of failure or disruption of the sinus apparatus. So, you would never want to eradicate escape beats or escape rhythms. It's the proverbial "you don't bite the hand that feeds you."

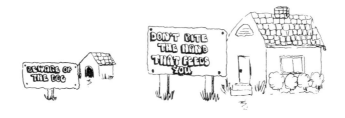

PREMATURE JUNCTIONAL CONTRACTIONS (P.J.C.'s)

Like P.A.C.'s, *premature junctional beats* arise from an excitable focus. The P.J.C. arises within the AV junction, outside the normal conduction system, interrupting the underlying rhythm. The premature beats cause the rhythm to appear irregular. You will recall that a P.J.C. may have a P wave before or after the QRS . . . or the P wave may be "hiding" within the QRS. If visible, the P waves will be inverted in leads II, III, and aVF. Additionally, if a P wave comes before the QRS, the P-R interval will be less than the lower limits of normal. That's a mouthful! The location of the P wave varies depending upon the timing of antegrade and retrograde conduction.

Single, infrequent P.J.C.'s in otherwise healthy children have no clinical significance. They may also be present:

- following surgery near AV junction
- in hypoxic conditions
- in hypoglycemia

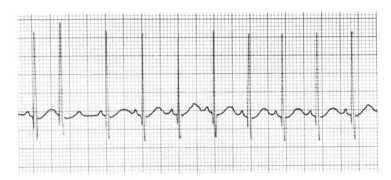

Look closely! Beat 2 is a P.J.C. that interrupts the otherwise normal rhythm. In this instance, the P wave of the P.J.C. is "hiding" in the QRS.

Usually P.J.C.'s require no treatment, though it is important to note their presence and frequency. If the patient shows signs of diminished cardiac output, treatment may be started with digitalis or propranolol (Inderal). (Don't you wish you had stock in companies that make digitalis!)

JUNCTIONAL TACHYCARDIA

In *junctional tachycardia,* a hyperirritable ectopic focus within the AV junction assumes control of the rhythm owing to its rapid rate of discharge . . . usually 160–200 discharges per minute. Junctional tachycardia may result after surgery near the AV node, with digitalis toxicity or with myocarditis. You will remember that the patient with junctional tachycardia experiences a reduced cardiac output from both the rapid ventricular rate and the loss of atrial kick. Atrial activation must be synchronized with ventricular activation to maximize cardiac output!

Let's look at an example of junctional tachycardia.

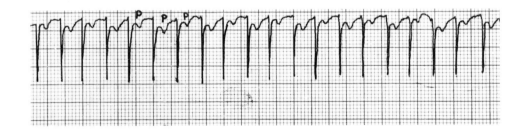

You will notice in this strip, retrograde P waves follow the QRS's indicating that ventricular activation precedes atrial activation. This is a junctional tachycardia with a rate of approximately 200 per minute.

Analysis time. Junctional tachycardia will have the following characteristics:

- Rate—160–220.
- Rhythm—regular (usually).
- P waves—may not be visible (buried in the QRS), or are inverted occurring before or after the QRS. Often because it is difficult to establish definitive P waves, these rhythms are called supraventricular tachycardias.
- P-R interval—if an inverted P wave occurs before the QRS, the P-R will be shorter than the lower limits of normal.
- QRS is usually of normal duration.

Treatment is aimed at decreasing the rapid ventricular heart rate and restoring the sinus pacemaker. Usually a drug combination of digitalis and quinidine is utilized. If rapid treatment is required due to a deteriorating clinical condition, synchronized cardioversion is the treatment of choice (two watt/seconds per kg. of body weight).

PAROXYSMAL SUPRAVENTRICULAR TACHYCARDIA (P.S.V.T.)

P.S.V.T. is the most common dysrhythmia of clinical significance encountered in pediatrics. One finds a hyperexcitable ectopic focus within the atria or junctional tissue discharging rapidly or encounters a reentry phenomenon. If you need a "reentry refresher," please review page 58! Basically, P.S.V.T. is a descriptive category. In other words, when a definitive distinction cannot be made between atrial tachycardia and junctional tachycardia, the rhythm is termed *supraventricular tachycardia*. If the rhythm is *paroxysmal* in nature, it is labeled *P.S.V.T.* Oftentimes, supraventricular tachycardia has a sudden onset. And often, owing to the rapid rate, one cannot determine where in the cardiac cycle P waves are occurring (before, during, or after the QRS). Let's look at a strip of P.S.V.T.

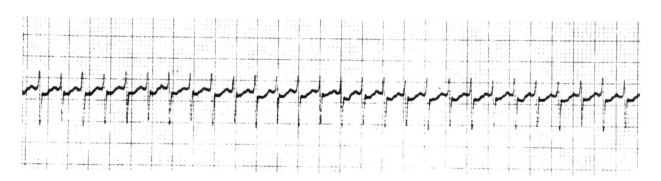

This rhythm strip demonstrates a supraventricular tachycardia at a rate of approximately 250 per minute. It is impossible to tell whether the "bump" between QRS's is a P wave, a T wave, or both. In cases like this, the term supraventricular tachycardia is *most* appropriate! The term implies that the pacemaker is above the level of the ventricles. If the rhythm were ventricular in origin, the QRS would appear widened.

P.S.V.T. has the following identifying features:

- Ventricular rate—250–300 in infants; 160–200 in children.
- P waves—difficult to distinguish owing to the rapid rate.
- QRS—normal duration (the initiating pacemaker is somewhere above the ventricles).

P.S.V.T. is *most often seen* in infants one to three months of age, but there are some *little ones* who like to begin life in the *fast lane* by demonstrating P.S.V.T. in utero. (Definitely type A personality babies!) P.S.V.T. may also be associated with:

- congenital heart disease
- infections
- following cardiac surgery
- adolescents—fatigue, stress, caffeine, tobacco
- no known reason—*unfortunately,* the greatest percentage!

The problem with P.S.V.T. is one we have already encountered *numerous* times—as demonstrated with the toilet flushing on page 58. The rapid ventricular rate causes decreased ventricular filling and thus, decreased cardiac output.

The treatment for P.S.V.T. depends on the severity of the episode. Sometimes the rhythm will spontaneously convert. If of a brief duration, vagal stimulation (such as carotid massage, gagging, application of cold or ice water to the face, or ice water in the stomach) may convert the P.S.V.T. to a sinus rhythm. When associated with congestive heart failure, more definitive treatment is required! Either digoxin or verapamil (drugs which increase AV block) is useful if the child can tolerate the rhythm until the drug takes effect. If the situation is more acute, cardioversion may be used (*two watt/seconds per kg. of body weight*).

Remember, patients receiving digitalis require a downward adjustment of the cardioversion current setting. Infants who have recurrent bouts of P.S.V.T. are usually maintained on digitalis therapy for six months.

Are you tired yet?

Practice Exercise 4

1. What is the difference between a junctional tachycardia and an atrial tachycardia? _____

_____

_____

2. What is happening in this strip, and why?

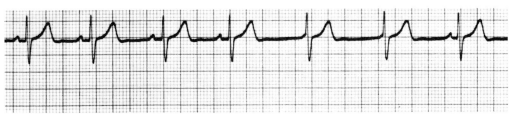

_____

_____

_____

_____

3. What is the treatment for paroxysmal supraventricular tachycardia? _____

_____

_____

_____

For **Feedback 4,** refer to page 361.

Input 5: Ventricular Dysrhythmias

Well, you're still with us, and I believe the worst—meaning the most confusing—may be behind us.

PREMATURE VENTRICULAR CONTRACTIONS (P.V.C.'s)

P.V.C.'s are extra beats arising in an excitable focus or site somewhere in either ventricle (outside the normal conduction system). There is no failure of the normal rhythm, merely additional beats from an irritable focus.

The rundown of rhythms displaying P.V.C.'s:

- Rate—within normal limits for age group.
- Rhythm—underlying rhythm regular, interrupted by premature beats.
- P waves—no P wave prior to the abnormal QRS; may be a P wave following the abnormal QRS. Do you remember why? For a thorough explanation, see page 101.
- QRS—the QRS of the P.V.C. is wide and *bizarre* in relation to the other QRS complexes. You will remember that the QRS is wide because the premature impulse orginates and travels outside the normal conduction system. Thus, conduction is slow!
- T wave—the T wave of the P.V.C. usually appears opposite in direction to the T wave of the normal QRS. In addition, there may be a full compensatory pause after the P.V.C.!

Let's look at some P.V.C.'s!

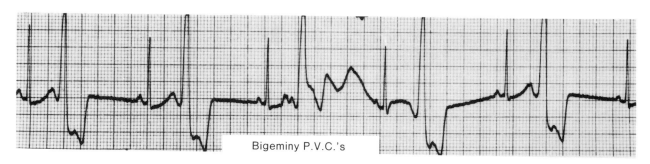

Bigeminy P.V.C.'s

This strip is interesting! Notice the artifact that disrupts the baseline midstrip. Bigeminy P.V.C.'s are the order of the day!

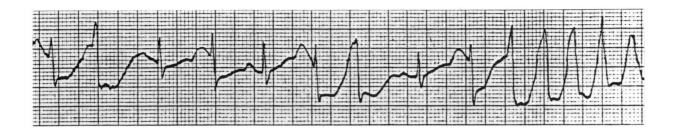

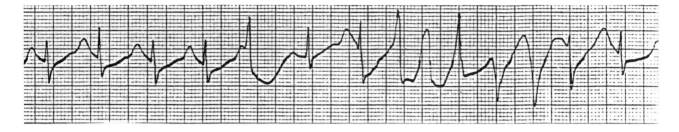

The above two rhythm strips demonstrate frequent P.V.C.'s and short bursts of ventricular tachycardia. These strips were taken from a thirteen year old overdose victim!

One may see P.V.C.'s in children with:

- normal hearts.
- congenital heart disease.
- drug intoxication (e.g., digitalis).
- electrolyte imbalance.
- hypoxia.
- hypoglycemia.

In a healthy child, occasional P.V.C.'s are relatively harmless. When *associated* with an underlying cardiac condition, P.V.C.'s represent *ventricular irritability* and may be the forerunner of ventricular tachycardia or ventricular fibrillation. *Not a good way to go!!* Additionally, multifocal, coupled, and frequent P.V.C.'s and P.V.C.'s precipitated by activity are usually significant.

P.V.C.'s are usually treated with propranolol or lidocaine. Lidocaine therapy involves an initial loading dose—usually **1 mg/kg body weight,** followed by a continuous drip (**20 μg/kg/minute**). If the P.V.C.'s are related to drug or chemical imbalance, the treatment should be directed at the cause. Likewise, P.V.C.'s related to hypoxia may be eliminated with the stabilizing of blood gases! You're asking, "What else does the ventricle do?" I'm so glad you asked. . . .

VENTRICULAR TACHYCARDIA

The following strip demonstrates ventricular tachycardia with an approximate rate of 200 beats per minute.

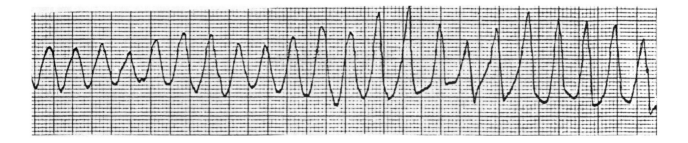

We will not dwell on *ventricular tachycardia* long, not because it isn't important, but because it is a *rare* finding in children.

Let's first look at facts:

- Ventricular rate—slower than P.S.V.T., usually 120–180.
- Rhythm—basically regular.
- P waves—usually not visible. (If visible, they bear no relationship to QRS's.)
- Wide slurred QRS's.

Lidocaine is the drug of choice. A bolus should be given first, followed by a continuous lidocaine infusion.

If lidocaine therapy is ineffective, synchronized cardioversion should be instituted.

You will remember that the usual current setting for cardioversion is *two watt/seconds per kg. of body weight*. You may find ventricular tachycardia associated with:

- severe digitalis toxicity
- myocarditis
- severe electrolyte imbalance
- anesthesia
- following cardiac surgery

What could be worse?

VENTRICULAR FLUTTER

Ventricular flutter is most commonly a *transition rhythm* from ventricular tachycardia to ventricular fibrillation. In ventricular flutter, cardiac output is minimal owing to the rapid, feeble ventricular contractions!

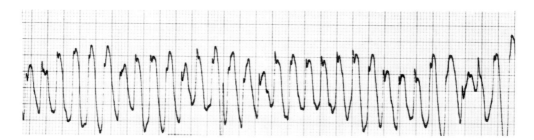

Ventricular flutter, rate 300 per minute.

Usually, the ventricular flutter rate is greater than 200 per minute. Ventricular flutter represents a *true* medical emergency. The treatment is the same as for ventricular fibrillation.

VENTRICULAR FIBRILLATION

Well, you ask, *what could be worse than ventricular flutter*? The answer, *ventricular fibrillation*! *Ventricular fibrillation* represents chaotic, uncoordinated ventricular depolarization (Karen gets all the good lines, page 118). There is *no* effective cardiac output. In effect, the fibrillating heart muscle quivers, but there is *no coordinated* ventricular activity. Death can occur in minutes!

One usually sees P.V.C's or some evidence of myocardial irritability prior to ventricular fibrillation. (See why one cannot ignore P.V.C.'s!)

Ventricular fibrillation may be associated with:

- hypoxia
- digitalis or quinidine intoxication
- anesthesia
- chest trauma
- cardiac catheterization
- hypothermia
- drug overdose

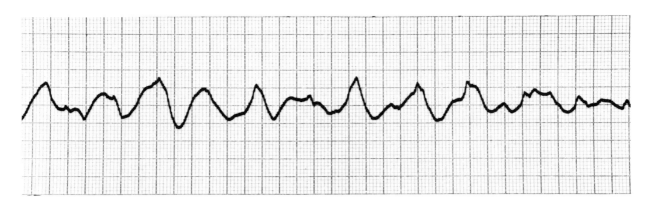

In ventricular fibrillation, one finds:

- Rate—no pulse.
- Rhythm—irregular, fluctuating baseline with no P, QRS, or T waves.

Ventricular fibrillation is a *medical emergency*. The treatment for ventricular fibrillation is electrical defibrillation (**one watt/second per pound**). If a normal sinus rhythm resumes, usually a prophylactic lidocaine drip is initiated and the underlying electrolyte factors corrected. (This is the kind of stuff that will make your heart skip a beat, huh!!)

Last, but not least, it should be noted that ventricular fibrillation is a **rare** finding in children. More commonly, terminal rhythms are bradycardic in nature.

Practice Exercise 5

1. Why is the QRS of a P.V.C. *fat?* _____

   _____

   _____

   _____

2. Lidocaine is the first line of treatment for ventricular tachycardia. What is the usual dosage? _____

   _____

3. Ventricular fibrillation is a common/uncommon finding in children.

4. Draw a strip demonstrating ventricular fibrillation.

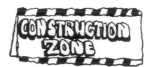

5. If electrical intervention is required for ventricular fibrillation one would use *synchronized cardioversion/defibrillation*? Why? _____

_____

_____

_____

For **Feedback 5,** refer to page 361.

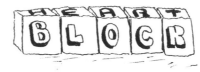

Input 6: Conduction Disturbances

What we're really talking about here is *heart block* (you're saying, it's more like *memory block* to you). We can define *conduction disturbances* as *delays,* or worse still, sometimes *failure* of impulse conduction through the AV junction, through the bundle of His, through the ventricles to the Purkinje fibers. There are three levels of heart block: first degree heart block; second degree heart block; and, third degree heart block. (Clever names.)

FIRST DEGREE HEART BLOCK

The only abnormality in *first degree heart block* is a prolonged P-R interval. Simple enough, huh!!

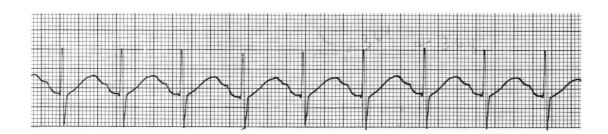

This rhythm strip belongs to a five year old boy taking digitalis. Though it is somewhat difficult to measure here, the P-R measures approximately 0.18 seconds. A normal P-R interval for a five year old is 0.10–0.16 seconds. (If in doubt, check out the Pediatric P-R Interval chart on page 323.) So, for this little guy, we have a first degree AV block!

Analysis please! With a first degree AV block, one finds the following:
- Rate—normal for age group.
- Rhythm—usually regular.
- P waves—normal in appearance and duration; P-R interval prolonged (remember, the duration of the normal P-R interval *varies with age* . . . you may want to refer to page 323).
- QRS—normal duration.

First degree heart block may be associated with

- increased vagal tone (e.g., increased intracranial pressure, hypertension, gastric dilitation).
- rheumatic fever.
- atrial septal defect
- structural heart disease
- following myocardia surgery
- digitalis toxicity

Treatment is usually not required for first degree AV block. In infants, digitalis may be held if prolongation of the P-R interval is seen on the digitalis *predose* rhythm strip, or if, during the administration of digitalis, the P-R continues to increase in duration.

Well, that wasn't too complicated. Let's try second degree heart block. . . .

SECOND DEGREE HEART BLOCK

MOBITZ TYPE I SECOND DEGREE HEART BLOCK

(It's getting worse. . . .)

In *Mobitz type I,* or *Wenckebach,* there is a progressive prolongation of the P-R interval until a P wave is finally blocked (not conducted). In Wenckebach, as the P-R lengthens, the R-R shortens! Wenckebach may be observed in otherwise normal hearts or may be associated with underlying heart disease. You will remember that Wenckebach occurs because of progressive fatigue in the AV junction. (If you would like an in-depth review, turn back to page 140.)

The following are some of the *more frequent* causes of Wenckebach or Mobitz type I second degree heart block in children:

- increased vagal tone
- myocarditis
- structural congenital disease
- cardiac surgery near the AV junction
- digitalis toxicity

Let's have a look! This is a strip of a four year old following recent atrial surgery.

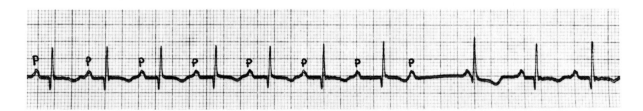

Notice that the P-R interval lengthens until a P wave is finally blocked or not conducted.

Let's analyze the above strip:

1. The heart rate is within normal limits, which is common.
2. The rhythm is irregular. If you look closely, you will notice that the nonconducted P wave principally accounts for the irregularity.
3. The P-R interval progressively lengthens until the eighth P wave fails to conduct.
4. The duration of the QRS's is normal since there is no interference with ventricular activation.

Usually Wenckebach, or Mobitz type I, requires no treatment per se. Treatment is directed at the underlying cause.

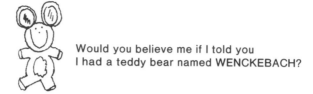

Would you believe me if I told you
I had a teddy bear named WENCKEBACH?

2:1 AV CONDUCTION

Occasionally, a 2:1 (two P waves to one QRS) AV conduction pattern will be observed in children. Since *only* every other P wave is conducted, one cannot determine whether the P-R is constant or whether it becomes progressively longer (as in Wenckebach).

Generally, the causes of 2:1 conduction are the same as for Wenckebach. As a matter of fact, when a 2:1 conduction pattern has QRS's of normal duration, the rhythm is usually a manifestation of Wenckebach. In other words, if one watched a rhythm long enough, eventually two *consecutive* beats would be conducted . . . and one would note that the P-R of the second beat was longer than the first.

Let's look at a strip!

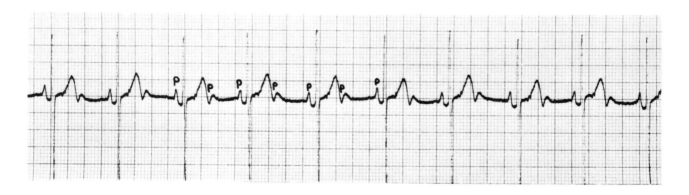

This rhythm strip belongs to a ten day old infant, two days post cardiac surgery to correct a structural anomaly. Notice that the atrial rhythm is regular at a rate of approximately 150 per minute. There are two P waves for every QRS . . . a 2:1 conduction pattern. The P-R of the conducted beats is constant.

Perhaps the most important reason for including this rhythm is to draw a distinction between 2:1 AV conduction and third degree (complete) heart block.

In a 2:1 conduction pattern, *the P-R interval of the conducted beats will always be constant.* In contrast, in a third degree heart block, the interval between the P and the QRS will always *vary,* since there is no relationship between atrial and ventricular activity.

MOBITZ TYPE II SECOND DEGREE HEART BLOCK

Mobitz type II is a *rare* finding in children. For that reason, we will not address the subject here. However, the *finer* identifying features of Mobitz type II (adult version), are discussed on page 142. Should Mobitz type II be observed in children, it is usually related to surgery on or near the bundle of His or the bifurcation of the bundle branches.

THIRD DEGREE HEART BLOCK (*AKA COMPLETE HEART BLOCK)

(Think the *third one is the charm*? . . . I doubt it too!) In *third degree heart block,* all atrial impulses are blocked from reaching and activating the ventricular system. None of the atrial impulses are conducted through to the ventricles to initiate ventricular depolarization. Though the sinus mechanism fires at a normal regular rate and activates the atria normally, none of the impulses reach the ventricular conduction system. Lower pacemakers sense the absence of sinus impulses, so . . . as a self-protection mechanism, a lower pacemaker takes control of the heart (*self-preservation* you might say).

This is, in effect, an escape rhythm mechanism . . . with the *exception* that there is no failure of the sinus node—the sinus impulses are simply blocked from reaching and activating the ventricles. The lower (escape) pacemaker may be initiated from the junctional or ventricular tissue.

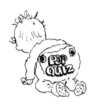 Circle the correct answer!

1. If an escape rhythm is initiated in the AV junction, the QRS complexes will usually be (fat/skinny).

2. If the escape rhythm is initiated in the ventricles, the resulting QRS complexes will be (fat/skinny).

If you answered *skinny* to question number 1, go to the head of the class (I guess you could walk across whatever room you're in)! If you answered *fat,* go to page 148 for some *quick* review. If you answered *fat* to question number 2, take a bow . . . but if you answered *skinny,* again turn to page 148!

All right, down to facts. We have a regular sinus P wave representing atrial depolarization, but then going nowhere . . .

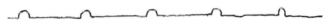

and a "survival" induced QRS either junctional . . .

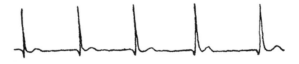

or ventricular . . .

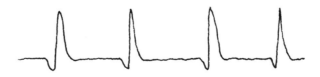

*AKA = *Also known as*

When the atrial activity is combined with the escape mechanism, you will see evidence of the *two independent pacemakers*—the atrial pacemaker and the junctional, or ventricular, pacemaker. These two pacemakers are totally independent of one another . . . and are said to be dissociated (hence, the term *AV dissociation*).

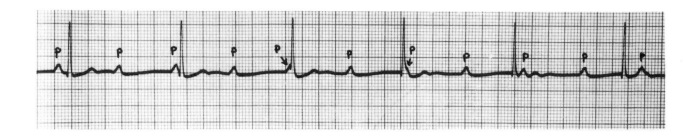

In this strip, you will notice that the atria and the ventricles are functioning independently. The atrial activity is regular at a rate of 83 per minute. The ventricular activity is regular, but slower at a rate of 44 per minute. Atrial activity is not related to ventricular activity . . . *how do I know,* you ask. Look at the P-R interval . . . it *always* varies. *This variation implies AV dissociation.* (AV dissociation is a descriptive term meaning that the atrial and ventricular activity occur independent of one another!)

Let's summarize the characteristics of third degree heart block.

• Both the atrial and ventricular activity is regular.
• Atrial and ventricular rates are different, the atrial rate being faster than the ventricular rate (the atrial rate is usually normal for the age category).
• Atrial and ventricular activation are independent of one another . . . the P-R interval is never constant.
• The ventricular rate is slow and regular.
• The QRS may be skinny (junctional) or fat (ventricular).

Complete heart block may be associated with the following conditions:
• congenital cardiac disease
• following cardiac surgery
• myocarditis
• digitalis toxicity

The aim treatment is to restore an adequate ventricular rate. If ventricular activation is initiated by a junctional pacemaker, atropine may be the treatment of choice. Atropine inhibits vagal effect and, therefore, may speed up the junctional rate. Atropine *will not* eliminate the heart block . . . it may simply increase the rate of the junctional escape pacemaker! If the ventricles are activated by a ventricular pacemaker (fat QRS), isuprel may be administered or ventricular pacing may be initiated.

Occasionally, third degree heart block presents as a congenital anomaly, often associated with transposition of the great arteries. Though certain infants develop congestive heart failure, others adjust to the slow ventricular rate through compensatory mechanisms (such as chamber hypertrophy and increased stroke volume).

BUNDLE BRANCH BLOCK

Our section on blocks would be incomplete if we did not discuss bundle branch blocks. You will remember that the conduction system consists of three fascicles. For a quick review of right and left bundle branch conduction defects, turn back to page 153.

RIGHT BUNDLE BRANCH BLOCK

Right bundle branch block is the most common form of ventricular conduction disturbance seen in children. Commonly, however, the right bundle branch is intact. The delayed right ventricular activation is often due to *congenital problems* that result in right ventricular volume overload (e.g., atrial septal defect). This volume overload and subsequent stretching of the right ventricle results in slower right ventricular activation!

In other cases, right bundle branch block patterns result secondary to right ventricular surgery, such as the repair of a ventricular septal defect or tetralogy of Fallot. In most instances, there is interruption of the Purkinje system rather than the right bundle branch. Just thought you might want to know that!

Unlike the adult patient, the rsR′ or "M" pattern is a common finding in a *healthy juvenile EKG specimen,* though the QRS is within normal limits! If you have forgotten the normal pediatric QRS durations, you may want to review page 324. So, in a right bundle branch block, you can expect to see:

- rsR′ in lead V_1
- QRS duration greater than the upper limits of normal for age
- wide, slurred S wave in lead I, V_5, and V_6

Let's take a look!

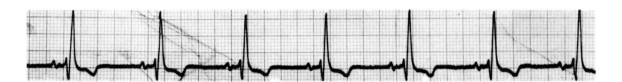

This is a sixteen year old female with right ventricular hypertrophy. The rhythm demonstrates a right bundle branch block with a heart rate of 62 per minute. P.S. This is a lead V_1 monitor tracing.

LEFT BUNDLE BRANCH BLOCK

Left bundle branch block is extremely rare in children . . . in fact, so rare that we could not find a single one! We are told, however, that should *you* come across a *true* left bundle branch block, you can expect to see:

- wide S waves in leads V_1 and V_2
- QRS duration greater than the upper limits of normal for age
- slurred and wide R waves in V_5 and V_6

So much for bundle branch blocks . . . right? Carry on!

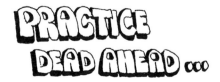

PRACTICE DEAD AHEAD ∞

Practice Exercise 6

1. Describe the abnormality in this strip and the probable treatment. This is a five year old female with congestive failure.

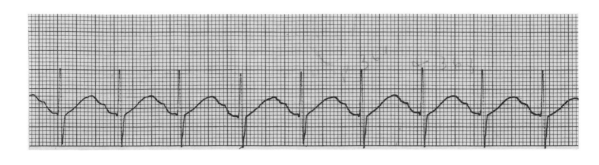

_____

_____

_____

_____

2. Draw a picture of Mobitz type I (Wenckebach).

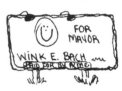

3. This is a tough question! Analyze and distinguish between the following two strips:

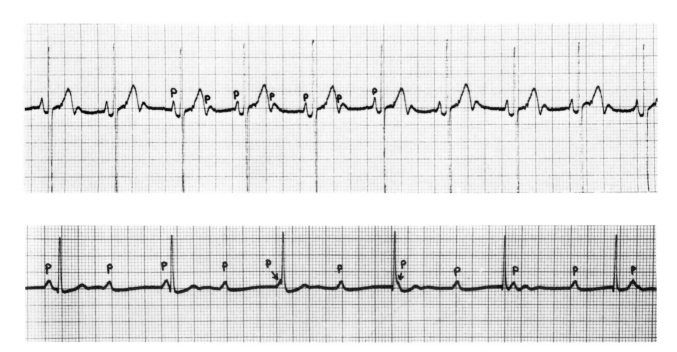

For **Feedback 6,** refer to page 362.

Potassium (K^+) norms, according to Hughes and Griffith (*Synopsis of Pediatrics,* 6th Edition, 1984, Mosby) are as follows:

SERUM POTASSIUM VALUES	
Age	**Potassium Level Norms**
Premie	4.5–7.2 mEq. per liter
Full term	5.0–7.5 mEq. per liter
2 days–3 mos.	4.0–6.2 mEq. per liter
3 mos.–1 year	3.7–5.6 mEq. per liter
1–16 years	3.5–5.0 mEq. per liter

You will remember from earlier sections, potassium (K^+) ions play an important role in the repolarization activities of the myocardial cells. Since the T wave represents repolarization, look for changes in the EKG near the T wave.

HYPOKALEMIA

Hypokalemia is the term used for potassium levels below the suggested low norm. On the EKG, hypokalemia may produce *depressed ST segments* and *prominent U waves.*

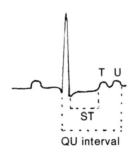

You will remember that the U wave is thought to represent late repolarization of the Purkinje fibers. Because of this *add-on* feature (the U wave), the QT interval appears prolonged. In reality, there is now a QU interval! Whew!

Hypokalemia is most commonly caused by vomiting, diarrhea, or diuretic therapy. It is important to remember that *hypokalemia causes electrical instability* and may produce any of the following dysrhythmias:

- P.V.C.'s
- atrial tachycardia or P.A.T.
- junctional tachycardia
- supraventricular tachycardia or P.S.V.T.
- ventricular tachycardia
- ventricular fibrillation

Unfortunately, U waves are *difficult* to spot . . . and we did not spot any!  Usually, when an extreme hypokalemia is confirmed by lab values, one may be able to go back to a 12 lead EKG and discern U waves . . . though the U waves are not evident in all leads.

Treatment for hypokalemia involves the administration of potassium supplement, oral or intravenous, depending upon the severity of the hypokalemia.

HYPERKALEMIA

Hyperkalemia is the term used for potassium levels that exceed the upper limits of the suggested norms (refer back to the table, p. 355).

In mild hyperkalemia, tall, peaked T waves can be observed.

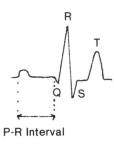

As potassium levels increase, the P-R interval prolongs and the QRS widens.

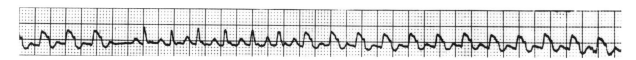

P-R Interval

In pronounced cases of hyperkalemia (K^+ levels *greater* than 9.0 mEq. per liter), the P wave may be absent and the widened QRS's may become diphasic. Look at this example!

Neonate showing EKG manifestations of hyperkalemia (10.9 K^+).

Hyperkalemia may be associated with kidney damage or infusions of *excessive amounts of potassium replacements*. Hyperkalemia *depresses* the normal electrical activity of the myocardial cells. So, the child with hyperkalemia is at risk for *sinus bradycardia, first degree heart block, escape rhythms, ventricular fibrillation, etc.*

Treatment for severe hyperkalemia (*greater than 7.0 mEq. per liter*) is aimed at reducing the serum potassium levels. Drug treatment may include calcium gluconate (counteracts effects on the neuromuscular system), sodium bicarb (shifts serum K^+ into the cells), or concentrated glucose (increases cellular uptake of K^+). *These drug solutions do not remove K^+ from the body!* Rather, they shift serum K^+ into the cell. In addition, dialysis may be used. For mild cases of hyperkalemia, Kayexalate (orally or rectally) is administered.

THIS IS MOSTLY A REVIEW . . . RIGHT?!

DIGITALIS TOXICITY

High serum levels of digitalis may provoke characteristic EKG pattern changes and dysrhythmias. We will look at specific dysrhythmias momentarily. *Please remember,* there are certain factors that pre-dispose the child to digitalis toxicity, such as the following:

- renal impairment
- elevated serum calcium (Ca^{++})
- acute hypoxia
- decreased serum potassium (K^+)

Digitalis toxicity usually involves disturbances in the formation and conduction of impulses. As you remember from page 306, digitalis in excessive amounts retards AV conduction, producing various forms of heart block—*sinus block, first degree AV block, second degree AV block, blocked P.A.C.'s, paroxysmal atria tachycardia with block, escape beats,* etc. Additionally, one may find supraventricular tachy-arrthymias, premature atrial and junctional beats, and P.V.C.'s (the multifocal variety) associated with digitalis toxicity.

Here is a rhythm strip demonstrating digitalis toxicity.

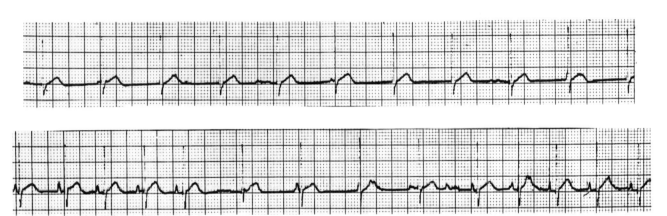

In the top strip, observe the junctional escape rhythm. In the second strip, the sinus pacemaker is evident for several beats, then gives way to the junctional escape rhythm. Finally, the sinus pacemaker resumes control. Remember . . . an escape rhythm will only be observed when there is failure or disruption of a higher pacemaker.

Ths most common EKG changes associated with *therapeutic* levels of digitalis are:

- shortened QT interval
- slowed heart rate
- slight prolongation of the P-R interval
- changes in the ST segment

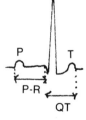

You should also remember, a child "isn't only a heart"—a digitalis toxic child may have anorexia, nausea, vomiting, or diarrhea. Usually digitalis is held if the P-R interval is increasing, new dysrthymias are occurring, or the pulse is below 100 in infants or 70–80 in children.

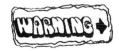 If a child is on digitalis, any new dysrthymia should be considered "suspect" for digitalis toxicity until ruled otherwise (by official "digitalis toxicity rulers" . . . otherwise known as physicians).

Practice Exercise 7

1. Abnormalities associated with potassium imbalance will be observed in the _____ segment of the EKG.

2. Construct an EKG complex demonstrating mild hyperkalemia.

3. Check all the dysrhythmias that may be related to digitalis toxicity:

   ☐ sinus bradycardia
   ☐ first degree heart block
   ☐ blocked P.A.C.'s
   ☐ P.V.C.'s
   ☐ P.A.C.'s
   ☐ junctional tachycardia
   ☐ Wenckebach

For **Feedback 7,** refer to page 362. For **Feedback 7,** refer to page 362.

Input 8: Kids' Artifact

Last, but not least, we need to acknowledge that children's monitors, like adult's monitors, occasionally display *artifact.* You may find it helpful to review Section VI (beginning on page 169). *Artifact,* you will recall, is an electrical signal which appears on the monitor that originates from sources other than the heart! Sound familiar?

Owing to their high activity levels, children are prone to "creating" motion artifact. That means that special attention should be given to skin preparation. It is also helpful to secure the monitor cable and wires in a manner that reduces motion. (Tough job, right?)

Since Section VI is comprehensive, we will not belabor the point.

Look at this rhythm strip (lead II) from a premie. Can you find the artifact? . . . And better yet, can you guess what is causing it?

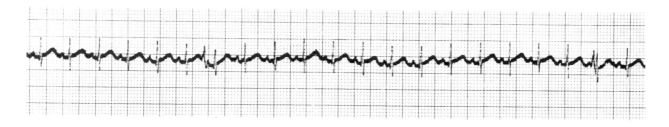

See the peculiar spiked waves occurring before complex 7 and before complex 20? These are hiccoughs! Neat, huh. Baby hiccoughs!

358

I thought about asking you to draw a baby hiccough . . . but, I reconsidered since this is the *last* input section!

. . . And, here's one more baby rhythm strip to ponder. This one belongs to an eleven month old "*little lamb.*" See what you think!

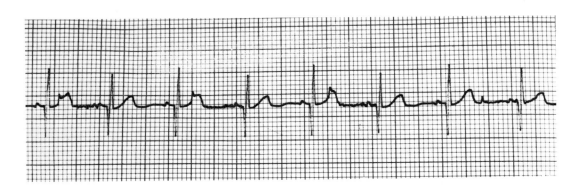

Notice that the T waves of beats 1, 3, and 5 are distorted. Grounds for blocked P.A.C.'s, right?! Well, *not* exactly, because there will *always be* pauses following P.A.C.'s (conducted or blocked P.A.C.'s). This is just one more example of baby artifact that may be confused with certain dysrhythmias!

There is no practice exercise associated with Input 8 . . . just be on the LOOKOUT for artifact!

NOW LEAVING

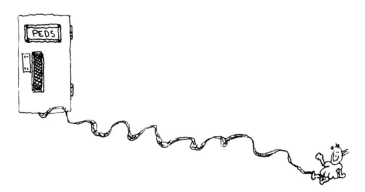

Feedback 1

1. The heart rate, the duration of P-R, QRS, and QT intervals all vary with _____AGE_____!

Circle the correct answer:

2. The heart rate increases/(decreases) with increasing age.

3. The P-R interval (lengthens)/shortens with increasing age.

4. The duration of the QRS is (longer)/shorter with increasing age.

5. The duration of the QT interval increases/(decreases) with increasing age.

6. What does this picture represent?

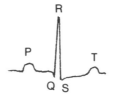

This is a normal cardiac complex with the exception that there is ST segment depression. Commonly, ST segment depression is associated with hypokalemia or digitalis administration.

Feedback 2

GOOD WORK!

1. The easiest way to determine rhythm irregularity is to measure the P-P interval or the _____R-R_____ interval.

2. This rhythm is a sinus tachycardia. For a normal six year old, a heart rate should be approximately 100 per minute. One would need to *investigate* and treat the underlying cause!

3. Sinus bradycardia in a child is defined as a heart rate of (less than 70) per minute. (Remembering heart rates is the most difficult part of this whole process!)

Feedback 3

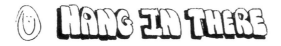

HANG IN THERE

1. The aims of treatment for any rapid atrial dysrhythmia are:
   a. Reduce the rapid ventricular rate.
   b. Restore hemodynamic equilibrium—restore a sinus rhythm!

2. The identifying characteristics of a premature atrial contraction are:
   a. The beat is premature, interrupting the underlying rhythm.
   b. There is a P wave before the premature beat and characteristically, the premature P wave is of a different configuration.
   c. There is a pause following the premature beat, allowing the sinus pacemaker to reset itself.

3. This strip demonstrates an atrial flutter with a variable ventricular response. You will remember from page 64 that the ventricular response will be irregular if there is variable AV block. The identification of atrial flutter is confirmed by the rate and the regularity of the F (shark) waves. The atrial rhythm is regular at a rate of 300 per minute!

4. In a wandering atrial pacemaker, one finds:
   • a normal rate
   • a slightly irregular rhythm
   • P waves that constantly change in appearance since the pacemaker wanders around in the atria
   • a varying P-R interval
   • the QRS duration usually within normal limits

Feedback 4

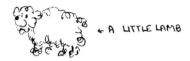

← A LITTLE LAMB

1. The difference between a junctional tachycardia and an atrial tachycardia is slight when it comes to heart rate! However, cardiac output will be more significantly reduced in a junctional tachycardia owing to the loss of atrial kick.

2. The underlying rhythm here is sinus rhythm at a rate of 75 per minute. (If this strip belongs to a newborn, it is a sinus bradycardia!) When the sinus pacemaker slows, a junctional escape pacemaker takes over for two beats. Then, back to sinus rhythm.

3. The treatment for paroxysmal supraventricular tachycardia consists of using measures to slow the ventricular rate and restore the sinus pacemaker. Vagotonic maneuvers (carotid massage, gagging, ice water applied to the face) may *break* the rhythm. If these measures are ineffective, digoxin or verapamil may be used to increase AV block. In acute situations, cardioversion may be used. Cardioversion is usually applied using a current setting of two watt/seconds per kg. of body weight.

Feedback 5

1. The QRS of a P.V.C. is wide and bizarre because the beat originates in the ventricular myocardium outside the normal conduction system. Because the impulse travels a retrograde (backward) pathway outside the normal conduction route, ventricular depolarization takes more time . . . therefore, the QRS is *fat*!

2. Lidocaine is usually administered one mg. per kg. of body weight initially, followed by a continuous drip at a rate of 20 μg per kg. per minute.

3. Ventricular fibrillation is a common/(uncommon) finding in children.

4. Your drawing of ventricular fibrillation should look something like this!

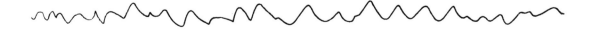

5. If electrical intervention is required for ventricular fibrillation, *defibrillation* is utilized because there is no effective cardiac activity. Synchronized cardioversion is only used when there is an effective underlying rhythm. (R waves are required to synchronize the patient's rhythm with the defibrillator unit).

If you need a quick review, see page 194.  The usual current setting for pediatric defibrillation is one watt/second per pound.

Feedback 6

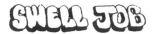

1. Since this is a rhythm strip from a five year old, the rhythm is a borderline sinus bradycardia. Normally the heart rate of a five year old would approach 100 per minute. In this example, the heart rate is approximately 94 per minute. Additionally, the P-R interval measures 0.18 seconds. The upper limits of normal for a five year old is 0.16 seconds. Thus, this is a borderline sinus bradycardia with a first degree AV block. Treatment probably is not warranted.

2. Hope your Wink E. Bach looks something like mine! Note the increasing P-R interval until finally, a P wave is not conducted.

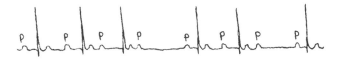

3. You will notice that there are more P waves than QRS's in each strip! The critical thing to observe is that in strip 1, the P-R interval of the conducted beats is constant. In strip 2, the P-R always varies, thus indicating AV dissociation. Strip 1 represents a 2:1 conduction pattern (a form of second degree AV block). Strip 2 represents third degree or complete AV block.

Feedback 7

1. Abnormalities associated with potassium (K⁺) imbalance will be observed in the <u>ST</u> segment of the EKG.

2. Hope you were in compliance with all construction codes! Your EKG complex should look *something* like mine!

3. *All* of the following dysrhythmias may be related to digitalis toxicity!
   - ☑ sinus bradycardia
   - ☑ first degree heart block
   - ☑ blocked P.A.C.'s
   - ☑ P.V.C.'s
   - ☑ P.A.C.'s
   - ☑ junctional tachycardia
   - ☑ Wenckebach

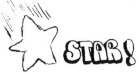 STAR!

NOTES

Section XIV
Test Your Skill

If you would like to test your newly acquired abilities, find a comfortable chair and complete this review exercise. And remember, *it's okay to use the book to answer the questions* . . . that's why the book is attached to the review exercise!

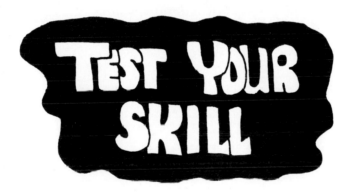

REVIEW EXERCISE

This is an exercise to tie all the loose ends together. Try to answer each question on your own. If you get stuck, CHEAT! (That's why the book is attached to the review exercise!)

1. Label the parts of the myocardial conduction system.

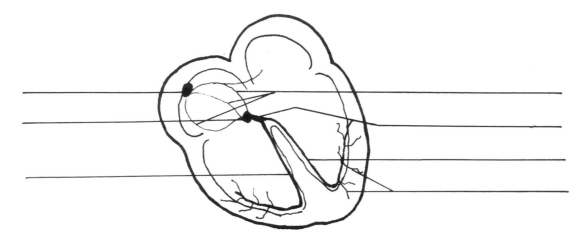

2. On EKG, the P wave represents _____ .

The normal P-R interval measures _____ to _____

small boxes wide, or _____ seconds. The QRS represents

_____ and should be *less* than

_____ small squares or less than _____ seconds.

The _____ represents recovery of the ventricles following contraction.

3. Name three methods of calculating heart rate.
   a.
   b.
   c.

4. The treatment for sinus tachycardia consists of _____

_____

_____ .

5. The patient with atrial fibrillation has a/an _____ pulse.

The irregularity of the ventricular response is a result of _____

_____

_____ .

6. In the normal heart, the AV junction is generally unable to conduct greater than _____ impulses per _____ . The AV junction will _____ impulses over this rate. This is referred to as a _____ block.

7. "Saw-toothed" F waves are characteristic of _____ . In this rhythm, there are actually two rates to calculate. The atrial or flutter rate may be between _____ per minute. Characteristically, the ventricular rate will vary between _____ beats per minute. Usually atrial flutter is a (regular/irregular) rhythm.

   What effect would digitalis have on atrial flutter? _____

   _____

   _____

   _____ .

   If the heart rate (ventricular rate) is between _____ and _____ , one should always *consider* atrial flutter.

8. What is an escape rhythm? When would one see an escape rhythm? What is the probable treatment?

   _____

   _____

   _____

   _____

   _____

   _____

9. In order to qualify as a junctional beat, the P R interval must be _____

   _____ .

10. Describe the criteria that must be met in order to identify a beat as a P.V.C. _____

    _____

    _____

    _____

    _____

11. P.V.C.'s are harmful in patients with coronary disease; P.V.C.'s indicate _____

    _____ , and may forewarn of _____ .

    The drug of choice to suppress ventricular ectopic activity is _____ .

12. Describe what is meant by "R on T" pattern when referring to P.V.C.'s. _____

    _____

    _____

    _____

    _____

13. What are the identifying features of ventricular tachycardia—and how should it be treated?

_____

_____

_____

_____

14. Describe myocardial activity and the EKG picture associated with ventricular fibrillation. What is the appropriate treatment? _____

_____

_____

_____

_____

_____

AND NOW, THE FUN PART

15. For each of the following rhythms, write one descriptive sentence that would help a new learner identify the rhythm. Then, draw a picture from what you have described!

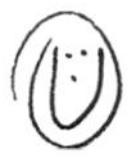

a. Mobitz type I (Wenckebach): _____

_____

_____

b. Mobitz type II: _____

_____

_____

_____

c. Complete (third degree) heart block: _____

_____

_____

_____

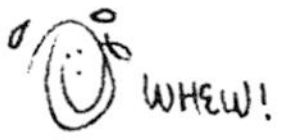

WHEW!

16. When looking at a 12 lead EKG, which chest lead is most helpful in identifying bundle branch

blocks? _____

17. Mild hyperkalemia may be suspected if _____

_____ T waves appear on the EKG. Digitalis effect

causes a _____

of the ST segment.

18. With myocardial ischemia, the ST segment will appear _____

_____ .

ST elevation represents _____ . The hallmark

finding on EKG indicative of myocardial infarction (tissue death) is the _____ wave in

upright leads and the _____ wave in downwardly directed leads.

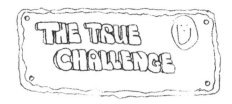

Describe the following EKG rhythm strips, including rate, regularity, etc. *If you feel comfortable,* apply a name. If you need help getting started, look back to page 33 for some tips on interpretation of abnormal rhythm patterns!

19.

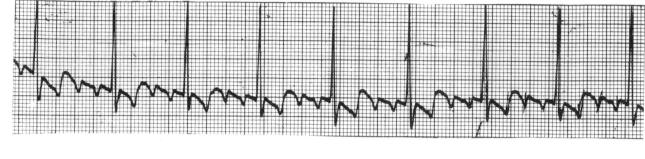

_____

_____

_____

_____

20.

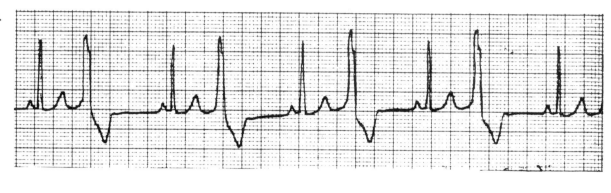

_____

_____

_____

_____

21.

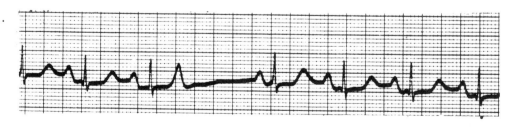

_____

_____

_____

_____

22.

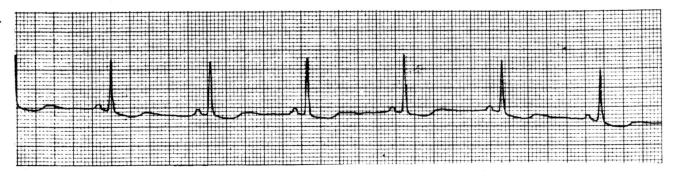

_____
_____
_____
_____

23.

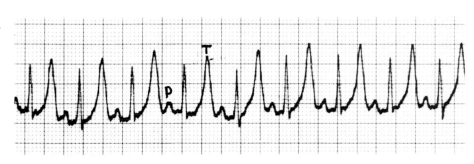

_____
_____
_____
_____

24.

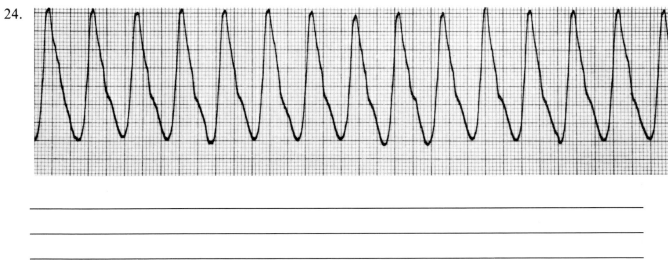

_____
_____
_____
_____

25.

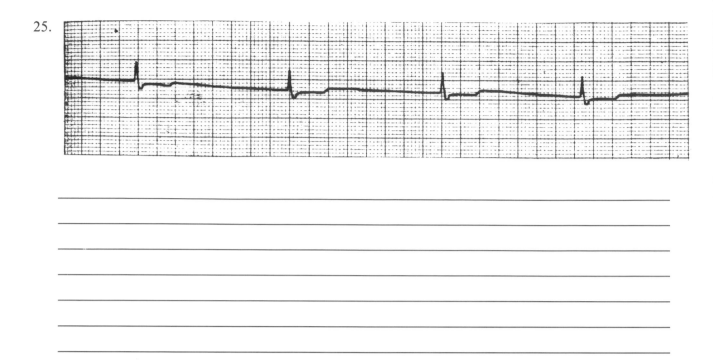

_____
_____
_____
_____
_____
_____
_____

ARE WE HAVING FUN YET ? ☺

26.

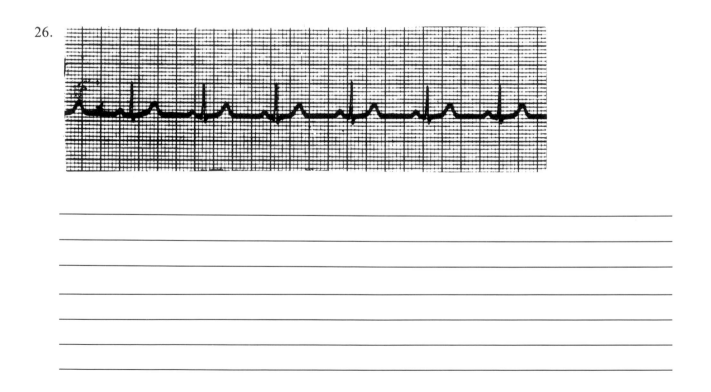

_____
_____
_____
_____
_____
_____
_____

27.

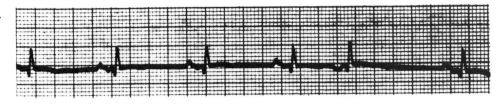

_____

_____

_____

_____

28.

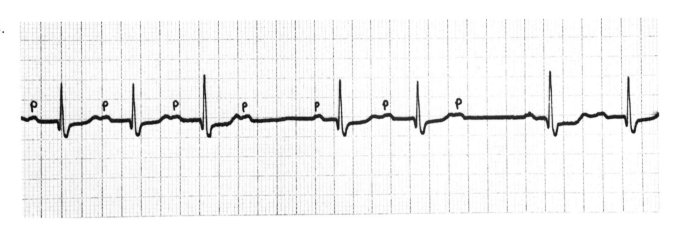

_____

_____

_____

_____

29.

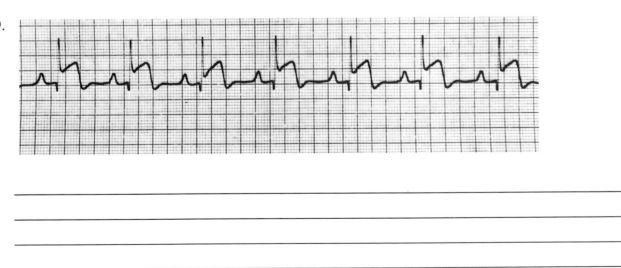

_____

_____

_____

_____

30.

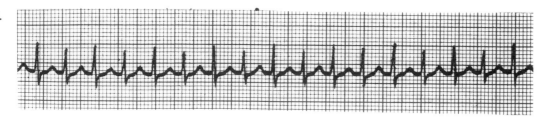

31.

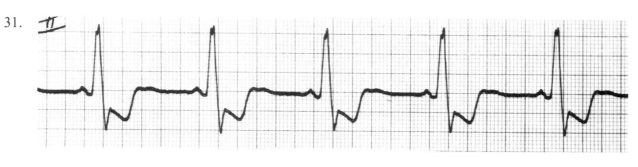

32.

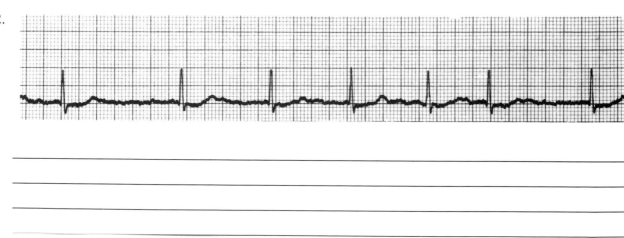

33.

V_1

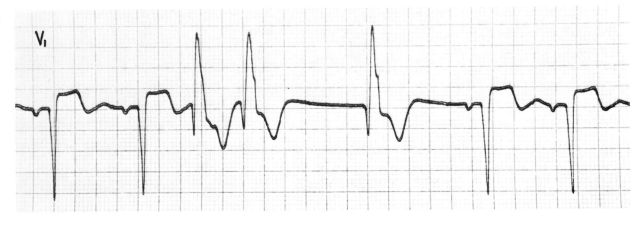

_____
_____
_____
_____
_____

34.

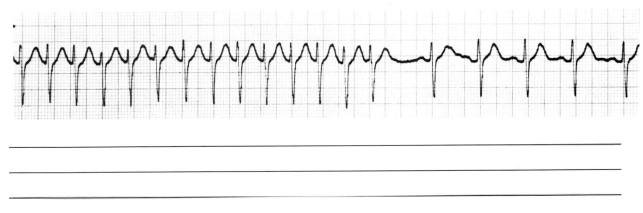

_____
_____
_____
_____
_____

35.

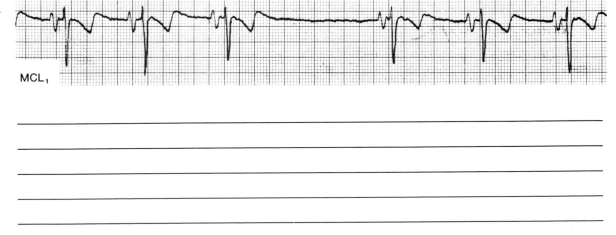

MCL_1

_____
_____
_____
_____
_____

36.

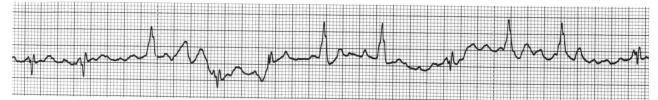

This is an example of motion artifact that masks the underlying rhythm. Describe actions that you would take to determine the significance of the rhythm disturbance. Then, describe methods for correcting the problem.

_____

_____

_____

_____

_____

37. What are these two rhythms? Which dysrhythmia has the greater significance, and why?

A.

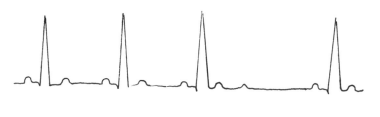

P-R = 0.14
QRS = 0.08
Heart Rate = 75

B.

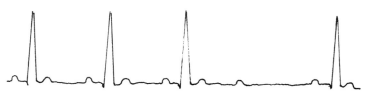

P-R = 0.14
QRS = 0.08
Heart Rate = 75

_____

_____

_____

_____

_____

_____

_____

_____

38. 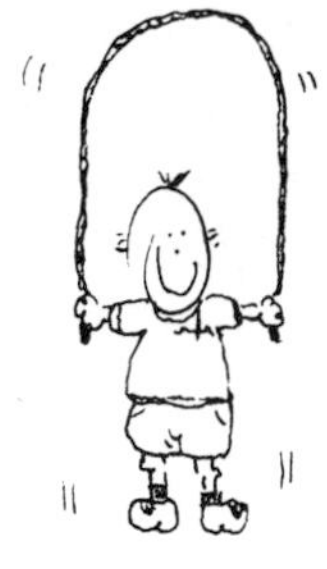   This is a _____ . The major distinctions between a pediatric and an adult rhythm are:

a. _____ rate

b. duration of the _____ interval

c. duration of the _____ .

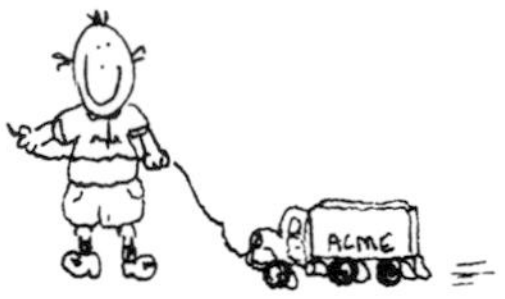

39. Correctly match the following Class I antiarrhythmic drugs with their appropriate actions.

Class IA (Quinidine, Pronestyl, Norpace)   Little effect on conduction
Class IB (Lidocaine, Dilantin)   Conduction slowed significantly
Class IC (Enkaid, Rhythmol)   Moderate slowing of conduction

40. List three reasons or three conditions warranting the insertion of a temporary pacemaker.

a. _____

b. _____

c. _____

41. Pacemaker non-capture means that _____

_____

_____

Draw a picture of ventricular non-capture.

42. Correctly match the following diagnostic abbreviations with the appropriate hemodynamic measurements.

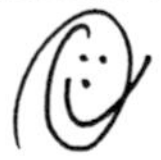

CVP   left ventricular function
PCWP   myocardial contractile force
LVEDP   right heart preload
CO   left heart preload

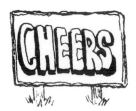

CHEERS HERE'S HOPING YOU DID WELL !

Remember, the major objective of this book was to assist you in describing EKG events . . . if you have learned some JARGON along the way, that's a *BONUS!* Just keep in mind that people have a great tendency to disagree over terminology!

ANSWERS FOR THE REVIEW EXERCISE BEGIN ON THE NEXT PAGE.

REVIEW EXERCISE ANSWERS

The answers to questions 1 through 18 are strategically placed throughout the book . . . very clever, right? ☺ Since those questions have "concrete" answers, I will refer to you to the appropriate page in the text. Then I will discuss the interpretations of the rhythm strips in detail!

1. Refer to page 14 to verify your answer.

2. Answers can be found on pages 15–20. If you had difficulty remembering any of these facts, you may want to reread Section I in its entirety.

3. Calculating heart rate (three methods) is discussed beginning on page 27.

4. The treatment of sinus tachycardia is discussed on page 51.

5. If you had difficulty with this question, refer to page 68.

6. Look back to the discussion on physiologic block, page 63.

7. Atrial flutter is discussed on pages 64 and 66. Reread the entire section if necessary.

8. Escape rhythms are reviewed on pages 80 and 121.

9. Double check your answers on page 82.

10. How did you do with this one? P.V.C.'s are wide and bizzare in appearance interrupting the underlying rhythm; the QRS measures a minimum of 0.12 seconds; there is no P wave preceding the QRS. Review page 102 if you had difficulty!

11. Verify your answers on pages 102–103.

12. This one was easy! If you experienced a memory lapse, see pages 103–104.

13. Ventricular tachycardia is always difficult to "definitely" identify. You may want to reread page 113.

14. The chaotic, uncoordinated ventricular depolarization of ventricular fibrillation is discussed on pages 118–119.

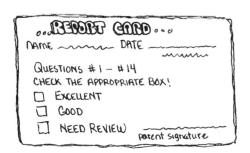

My favorite part of this review exercise is questions 15 a, b, and c! Everyone always laughs at the way I draw. . . . so I have my fun on these questions! ☺

15a. Refer to page 140 for a textbook example and description of Wenckebach.

15b. Page 144 clearly depicts Mobitz type II.

15c. Complete heart block is discussed on page 149.

16. V_1 is the lead that most clearly identifies bundle branch block. See pages 154 and 157.

17. Potassium and digitalis effects can be found on pages 218 and 305.

18. ST segment depression connotes myocardial ischemia. ST elevation represents current injury. And, the development of a pathologic Q wave in upright leads and the loss of R wave in negative leads represents myocardial necrosis. For a quick review see Section X, pages 231–238.

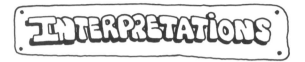

Before we begin to discuss the various rhythm strips, I need to repeat myself. The important aspect of dysrhythmia interpretation is accurately describing the electrical events. Do not compare how *I've written the interpretation* with how *you've written it*! Rather, make certain you have described what I have described! And remember, it is possible that you and I may see the same electrical events differently!

19. The rhythm appears regular. There is more atrial activity than ventricular activity. Atrial waves are "saw-toothed" in appearance and occur at a rate of 300 per minute. The QRS's are "skinny" and occur regularly at a rate of 75 per minute. Atrial waves (F waves) march through the rhythm. This is atrial flutter with 4:1 conduction (four flutter waves for every QRS). The fourth flutter wave is buried in the QRS—I know it is there however, because flutter waves are continuous, never stopping. If you need review, turn to page 64.

20. This one is easy! A normal sinus beat is followed by a P.V.C., then the whole cycle repeats. This is ventricular bigeminy. The heart rate should be determined by counting the patient's pulse for one full minute. It is helpful to count both apical and radial pulses because not all abnormal beats will be adequately perfused. The P-R interval of normally conducted beats is approximately 0.08 seconds. For review, see page 103.

21. The rhythm is irregular. There is a pause noted after the third beat. The underlying rhythm is a sinus rhythm with an approximate rate of 80 beats per minute—however, when a rhythm is irregular, it is important to count the rate over one full minute! The P-R interval is constant and measures 0.20 seconds; the QRS is constant and measures slightly less than 0.08 seconds. Looking closely at the pause, you will notice the preceding T wave is abnormally peaked. AH-HA! There must be a P wave sitting on top of the T wave! This is a P.A.C. that does not conduct. And as always, when a P.A.C. occurs, there is a pause allowing the sinus mechanism to reset itself. If you need review, turn to pages 55–56.

22. The rhythm is regular with a ventricular rate of slightly less than 60 per minute. The P-R is constant measuring approximately 0.14 seconds; the QRS is constant measuring approximately 0.08 seconds. There is slight scooping or depression of the ST segment. This is a sinus bradycardia with a slightly depressed ST segment. The ST depression may represent digitalis effect.

23. The rhythm is rapid and regular. The ventricular rate is approximately 120 per minute. The P-R is constant measuring 0.16 seconds; the QRS is constant measuring approximately 0.08 seconds. Giant, peaked, "tentlike" T waves are evident throughout. This is a sinus tachycardia with tall, peaked T waves (suggestive of hyperkalemia). If you need review, turn to page 218.

24. The rhythm is rapid and fairly regular with a ventricular rate of approximately 125 per minute. There is no obvious atrial activity; the QRS's are wide and bizarre. Though there are no fusion or capture beats to confirm the "diagnosis," this is most likely ventricular tachycardia and should be treated as such. If you need review, turn to page 113.

25. The rhythm is slow and fairly regular with a ventricular rate of approximately 40 per minute. There is no obvious atrial activity preceding the QRS. The QRS complexes are narrow measuring slightly greater than 0.08 seconds. This is a junctional escape or idiojunctional rhythm. If you need review, look back to page 80.

26. You guessed it!!! Normal sinus rhythm. The ventricular rate is approximately 80 beats per minute. The P-R is constant measuring approximately 0.14 seconds; the QRS is constant measuring approximately 0.06 seconds. *I hope you don't need review!*

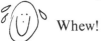 Whew!

27. The rhythm is not regular; therefore, one would need to count the pulse for one full minute. The underlying rhythm appears to be sinus rhythm. The P waves of the sinus beats appear jagged. The P-R of the sinus beats is constant measuring 0.16 seconds. The QRS of the sinus beats is constant measuring 0.08 seconds. The rhythm is interrupted by a premature beat. The premature beat is preceded by an inverted P wave; the P-R measures slightly greater than 0.12 seconds! To be a premature junctional beat the P-R would need to be *less* than 0.12. So, about the best I can say is that this is a sinus rhythm interrupted by a premature beat of supraventricular origin (I know it's not of ventricular origin because the QRS is "skinny").

28. The rhythm is irregular, so to determine the rate, I would need to count the pulse for one full minute. The P waves all appear uniform in appearance but the P-R interval gets progressively longer until a P wave fails to conduct. Then, the cycle repeats, though irregularly. This is good ol' Wenckebach (Mobitz type I second degree heart block). If you need review, turn to page 140.

29. The rhythm is regular with a ventricular rate of approximately 60 per minute. The P waves are uniform in appearance. The P-R is constant measuring 0.28 seconds. The QRS is narrow followed by ST elevation. So, this is a sinus rhythm with a first degree heart block and ST elevation. One would need to do a 12 lead EKG to determine in which leads the ST elevation is present. ST elevation is suggestive of current injury, and appears in the leads overlooking the area of injury. If you need a quick review, turn to pages 236–237.

30. The rhythm is regular and rapid with a ventricular rate of approximately 185 beats per minute. (I used the cheat guide on page 39.) It is difficult to identify any clear P waves, but the QRS is constant measuring 0.08 seconds. Therefore, I know the rhythm is not of a ventricular origin. Since I am uncertain of P waves, I'm simply going to describe this strip as "supraventricular tachycardia, rate 185, Q.R.S. = 0.08 seconds."

31. The underlying rhythm here is sinus bradycardia with a rate of 50 per minute. The QRS's are wide and bizarre, *but* there is a P wave preceding each QRS. The P-R interval measures 0.16 seconds. The QRS's measure almost 0.20 seconds in duration! This is a bundle branch block. To know whether this is right or left bundle branch block, I would need to inspect lead V_1. So, in summary, this is a sinus bradycardia with bundle branch block! For review, see page 153.

32. Everything about this rhythm is *IRREGULAR*! There is lots of atrial activity, but no definitive atrial wave forms. The QRS complexes are uniform in appearance, occur irregularly, and measure 0.08 seconds. This is our *old friend* atrial fibrillation. For a refresher, see page 68.

33. *OOOOOh!* Well, the underlying rhythm is a sinus rhythm with a rate of 70 per minute. The P-R interval is of normal duration. The R waves are absent and there is marked ST segment elevation suggesting anterior wall infarction! Beats 3 and 4 are P.V.C.'s and beat 5 is a ventricular escape beat. A strip like this presents a *true* treatment dilemma. Refer back to page 238 for a review of R waves in lead V$_1$.

34. The beginning of this rhythm strip shows a supraventricular tachycardia at a rate of 166 per minute. I am calling it a supraventricular tachycardia because there is no clear evidence of P waves and the QRS duration is within normal limits. The rhythm then converts *spontaneously* to a sinus tachycardia with a rate of slightly greater than 100 per minute. The P-R interval of the sinus beats measures approximately 0.16 seconds. The QRS of the sinus beats measures approximately 0.08 seconds.

35. This strip demonstrates a sinus rhythm with *flipped* or inverted T waves. The P waves are biphasic in appearance and the P-R interval measures approximately 0.20 seconds. There is a 2.2 second pause between beats 3 and 4. This is a sinus pause since the *next anticipated event* during the pause is a P wave. For a quick review, see page 130.

36. The significance of the disturbance can be determined by comparing the patient's pulse with the rhythm strip. When artifact is present, the pulse (rate and sequence) will assist one in locating QRS complexes. Motion artifact can often be eliminated or reduced by correct skin preparation and an ample quantity of gel on the electrode patches. To prevent cable wire movement, the cable may be clipped to the patient's clothing. If motion artifact relates to respiration, reposition the lead away from the diaphragm. For review, see Section VI, page 169.
NOTE: ATTACHING THE ELECTRODES OVER BONY AREAS WILL REDUCE MOTION ARTIFACT!

37. A *toughie!* Diagram A is a sinus rhythm with a blocked P.A.C. (notice that the unaccompanied P wave occurs *early* or prematurely in the cycle). There is a pause following the blocked P.A.C. The significance of P.A.C.'s is the significance of the underlying disorder. Frequently, blocked P.A.C.'s are observed in digitalis toxicity. Diagram B represents a Mobitz type II second degree AV block! In Mobitz type II, a P wave is suddenly blocked without warning. The blocked P wave is neither early nor late . . . it occurs *right on time*. Mobitz type II occurs because of intermittent bilateral bundle branch block and is almost always associated with *extensive* myocardial damage. Oftentimes, a pacemaker is prophylactically inserted when Mobitz type II is observed. *ALWAYS DETERMINE IF UNACCOMPANIED P WAVES OCCUR EARLY, LATE, OR RIGHT ON TIME!* For review, see pages 56 and 143.

38. This is a kid. The major distinctions between a pediatric and an adult rhythm are:

    a. <u>heart</u> rate
    b. duration of the <u>P-R</u> interval
    c. duration of the <u>QRS</u>

39. Class IA (Quinidine, Pronestyl, Norpace) → Little effect on conduction
    Class IB (Lidocaine, Dilantin) → Conduction slowed significantly
    Class IC (Enkaid, Rhythmol) → Moderate slowing of conduction

    For a quick review of Class I drug actions, turn to page 302.

40. A temporary pacemaker may be inserted to treat any of the following conditions:

    a. second degree AV blocks associated with acute myocardial infarction
    b. drug-induced bradyarrhythmias
    c. third degree heart block
    d. symptomatic bradycardia

41. Pacemaker non-capture means that <u>a pacemaker generated impulse fails to produce the desired effect</u> <u>(atrial depolarization or ventricular depolarization)</u>. See page 209 for a quicker review of non-capture!

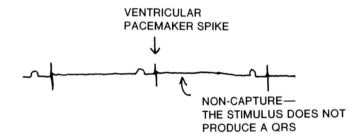

VENTRICULAR
PACEMAKER SPIKE

NON-CAPTURE—
THE STIMULUS DOES NOT
PRODUCE A QRS

42.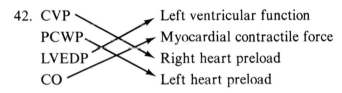

CVP → Left ventricular function
PCWP → Myocardial contractile force
LVEDP → Right heart preload
CO → Left heart preload

For a refresher, review section XI!

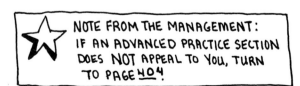

NOTE FROM THE MANAGEMENT:
IF AN ADVANCED PRACTICE SECTION
DOES NOT APPEAL TO YOU, TURN
TO PAGE 404.

NOTES

Section XV
The Final Analysis: *Advanced* Arrhythmia Interpretation Practice

The purpose of this text has been to aid learners in gaining basic EKG interpretation competence. However, complicating rhythm strip interpretation is the fact that few "live" strips resemble their "textbook" cousins. Frequently, multiple anomalies can be found in one tracing. For example, ectopic activity may complicate conduction disturbances, or multifocused excitability may obliterate an underlying rhythm.

TEXTBOOK COUSINS

NON-TEXTBOOK COUSINS

The analysis and interpretation of complex or "difficult" rhythms is aided by:

- knowledge of a patient's physical findings and overall sense of well being.
- review of the patient's underlying pathology, including current drug therapy, electrolyte, and cardiac enzyme lab values
- observing the rhythm pattern over time (a six second strip is often too short to distinguish patterns)
- "tete to tete" consultation with a colleague

REMEMBER:
In *all* instances, the naming of rhythm anomalies is far *less* important than an accurate description of electrical events!

The following practice strips are included for their "less than textbook" quality. Use your *best* analysis skills and describe what you see! My analysis follows at the end of this section, page 398.

BLAST OFF!

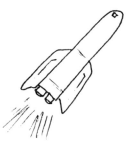

Advanced Practice Exercise

Review each strip carefully. Describe all that you see!

1.

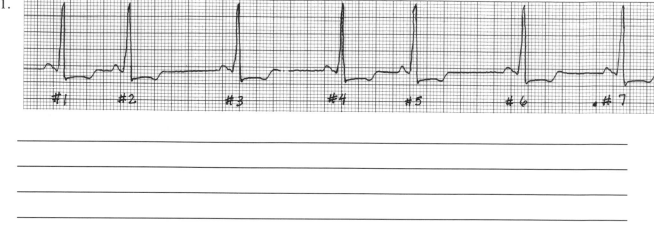

_____

_____

_____

_____

_____

2.

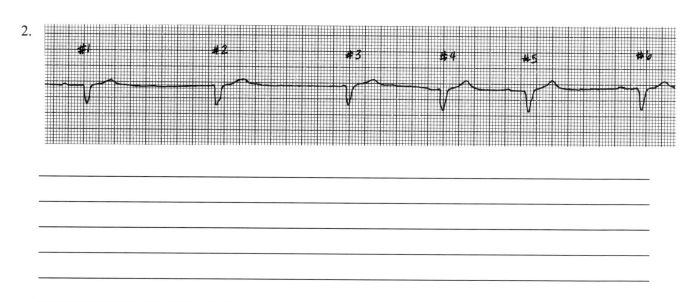

_____

_____

_____

_____

_____

3.

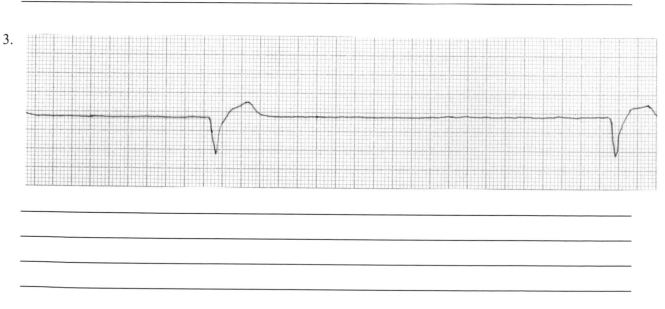

_____

_____

_____

_____

4.

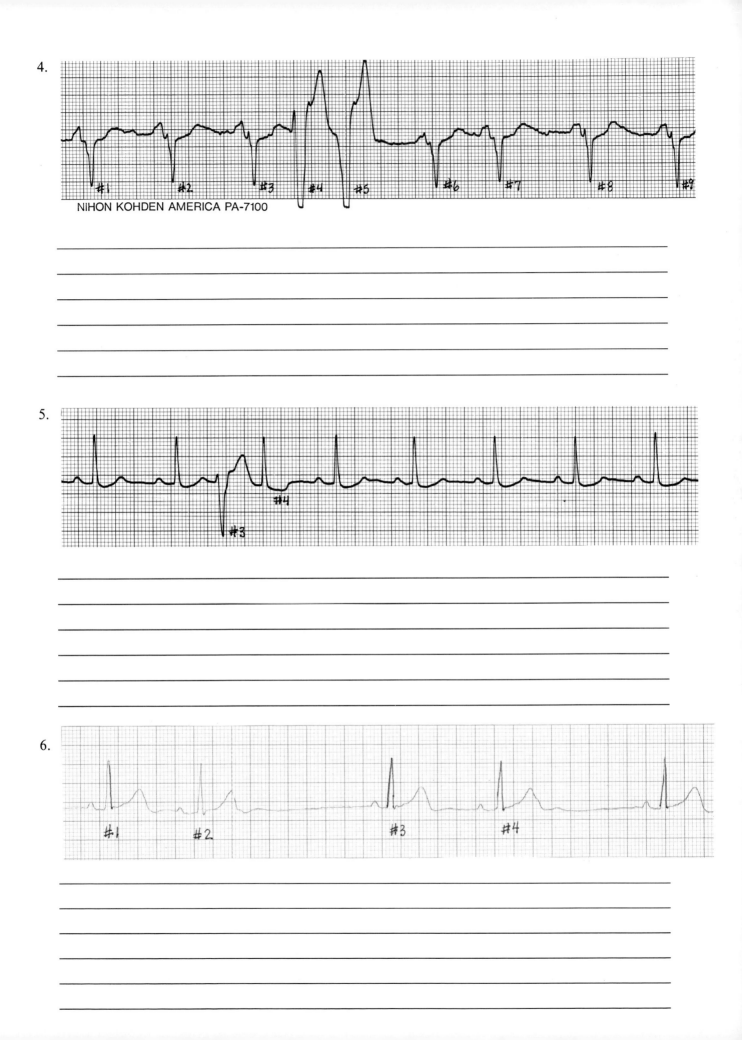

NIHON KOHDEN AMERICA PA-7100

#1   #2   #3   #4   #5   #6   #7   #8   #9

_____
_____
_____
_____
_____
_____

5.

#3   #4

_____
_____
_____
_____
_____
_____

6.

#1   #2   #3   #4

_____
_____
_____
_____
_____
_____

7.

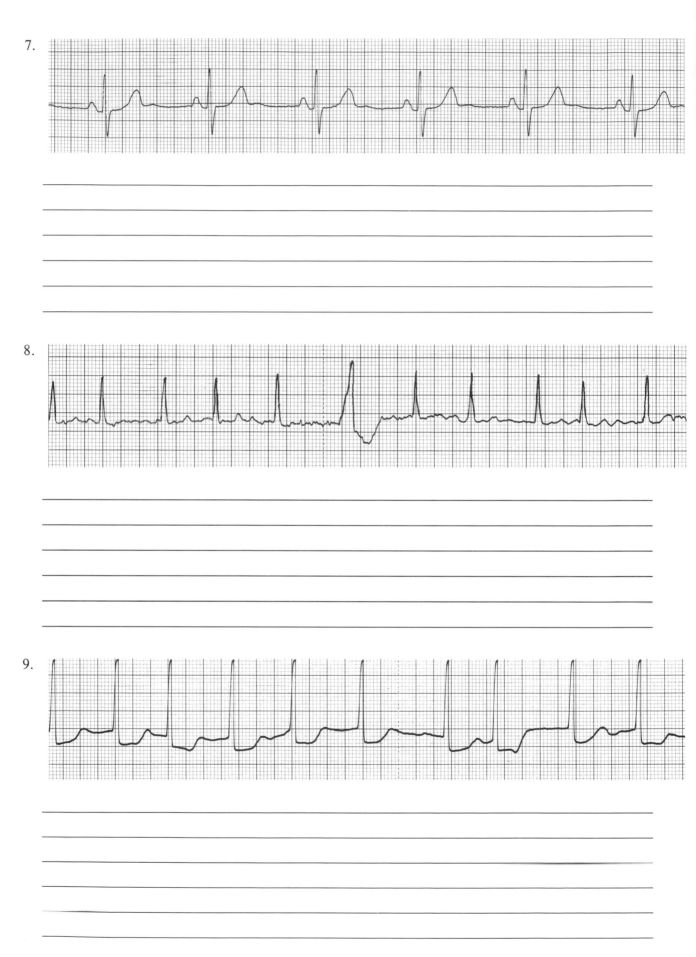

_____
_____
_____
_____
_____
_____

8.

_____
_____
_____
_____
_____
_____

9.

_____
_____
_____
_____
_____
_____

10.

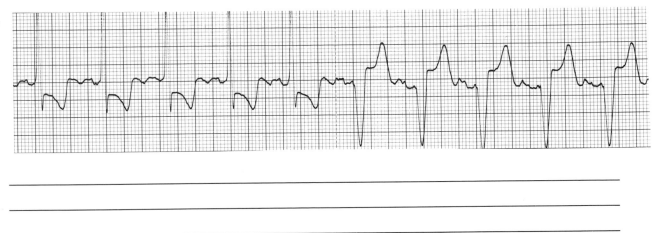

_____

_____

_____

_____

_____

_____

11.

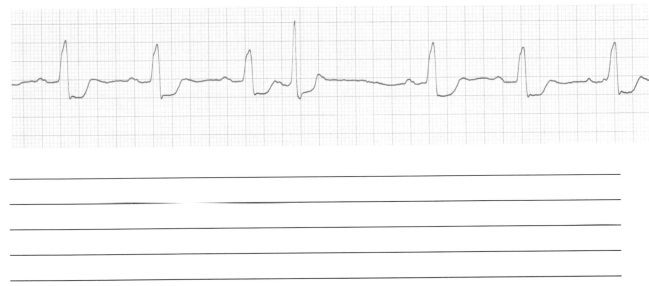

_____

_____

_____

_____

_____

_____

12.

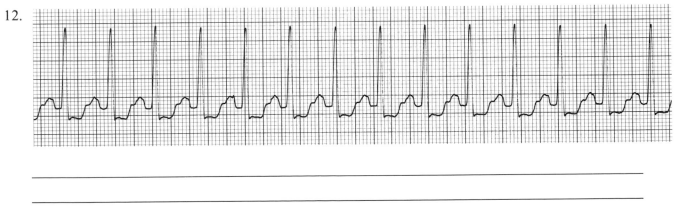

_____

_____

_____

13.

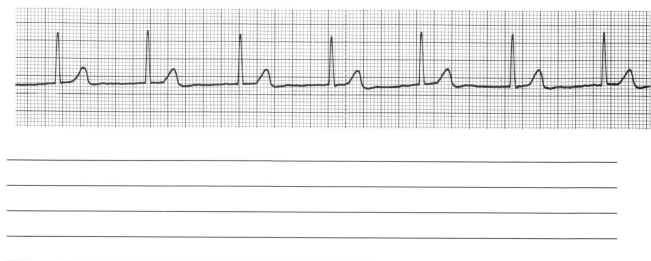

14. A.

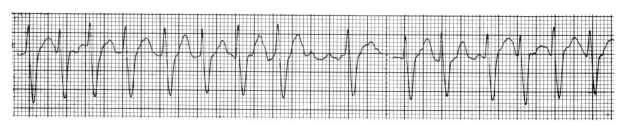

B.

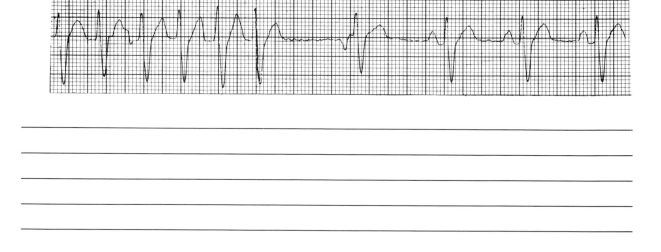

15.

A.

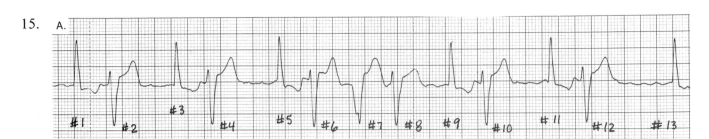

#1   #2   #3   #4   #5   #6   #7   #8   #9   #10   #11   #12   #13

B.

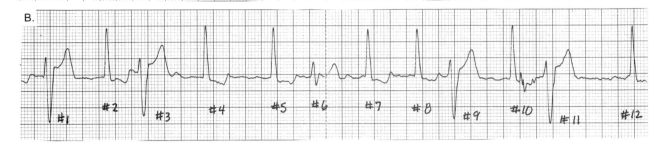

#1   #2   #3   #4   #5   #6   #7   #8   #9   #10   #11   #12

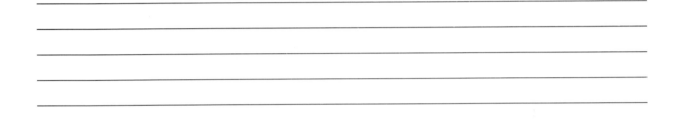

_____

_____

_____

_____

_____

_____

16.

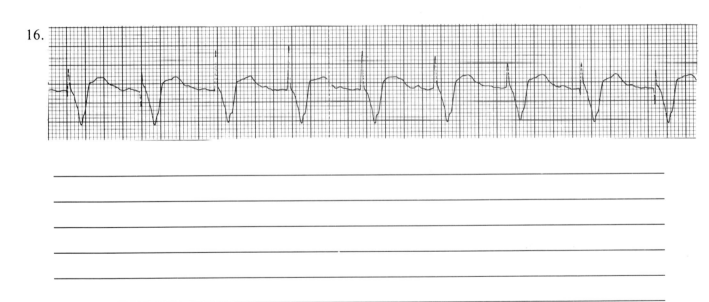

_____

_____

_____

_____

_____

_____

17.

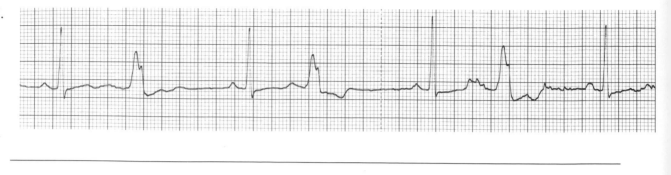

_____
_____
_____
_____
_____
_____

18.

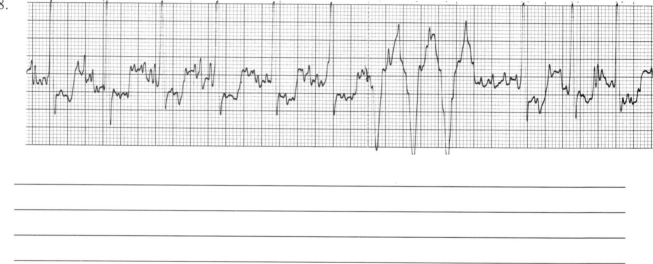

_____
_____
_____
_____
_____
_____

19.

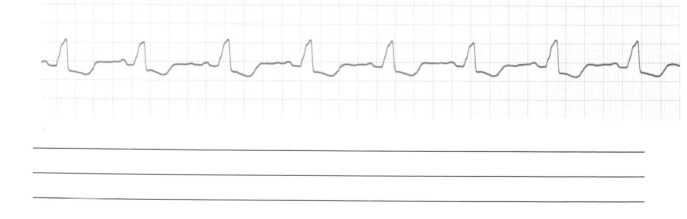

_____
_____
_____
_____

20.

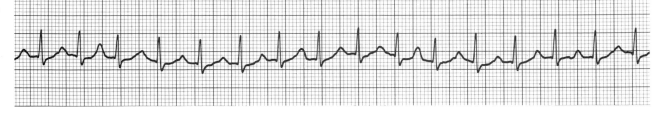

21.

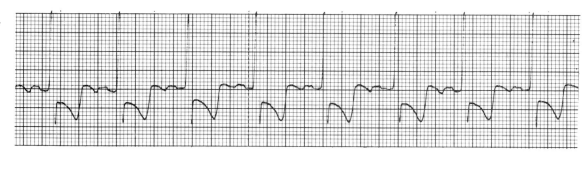

22.

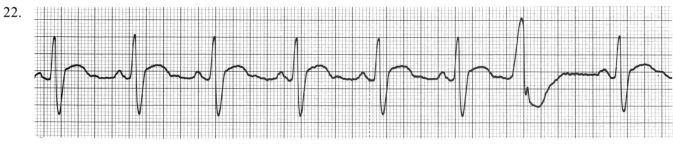

23.

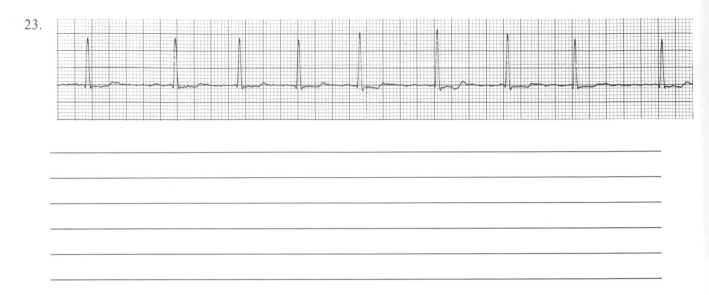

24.

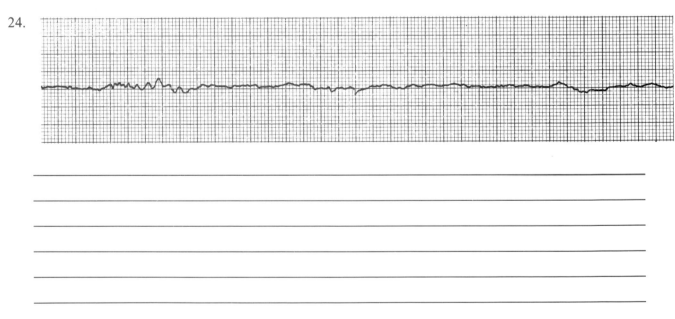

25.

A.

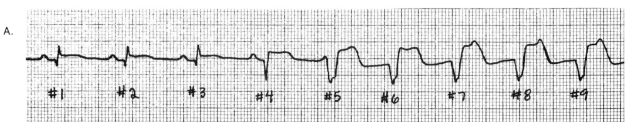

#1   #2   #3   #4   #5   #6   #7   #8   #9

B.

_____

_____

_____

_____

_____

_____

26.

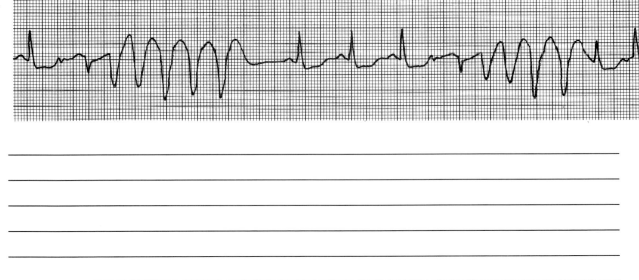

_____

_____

_____

_____

_____

_____

27.

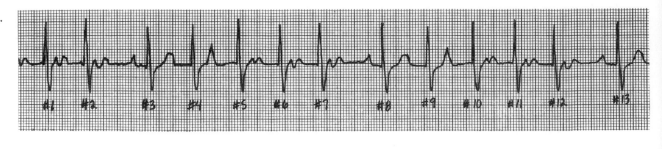

#1 #2 #3 #4 #5 #6 #7 #8 #9 #10 #11 #12 #13

_____
_____
_____
_____
_____
_____

28.

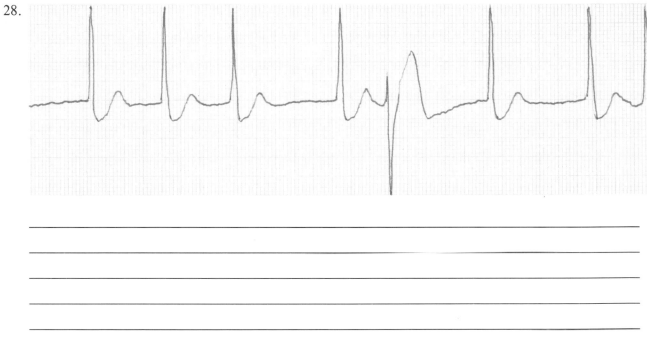

_____
_____
_____
_____
_____
_____

29.

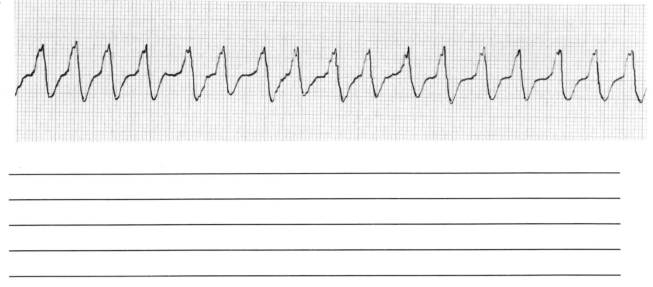

_____

_____

_____

_____

_____

_____

30.

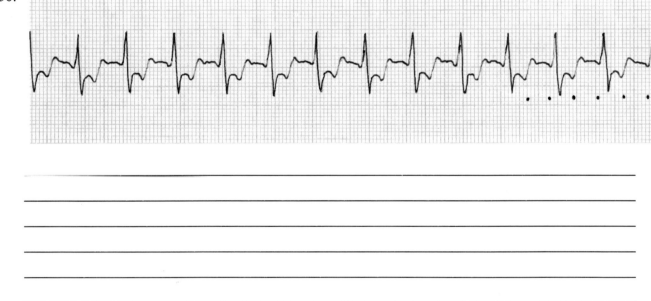

_____

_____

_____

_____

_____

_____

INTERPRETATIONS

No two individuals analyze rhythm strips in the same manner so, I do not expect your verbage to match mine!! Be certain, however, that your descriptions contain the "fundamentals."

1. By eyeball analysis, this rhythm is irregular. Every QRS is preceded by a P wave. Certain P waves appear different in configuration. My tendency is to identify something familiar and work backwards. Beats #3 and #4 appear similar—slow sinus beats. Beats #3 and #4 have identical upright P waves and the P-R interval of those two beats measures 0.16 seconds. The QRS complexes measure slightly less than 0.12 seconds. The ST segments are significantly depressed and the T waves are inverted. Beat #5 occurs earlier than expected in the cycle, the P wave is of a different configuration, and the P-R interval is shorter in duration. This is a P.A.C. Following the P.A.C. is the normal anticipated pause allowing the sinus mechanism to reset itself. Beats #6 and #7 appear to be sinus beats. Now back to the beginning of the strip. Beat #1 is a sinus beat. (Note the constant P-R interval of beats #1, #3, #4, #6, and #7.) Beat #2 is a P.A.C., coming earlier than anticipated, and followed by a pause. Viola! The underlying rhythm is a sinus rhythm interrupted by P.A.C.'s (beats #2 and #5). The ST depression and inverted T waves noted throughout are suggestive of ischemia. How did you do?

2. This rhythm is slow and irregular. Beats #1, #5, and #6 all look alike in that they have clearly iden- tifiable P waves appearing before the following QRS's. The P-R interval measures approximately 0.28 seconds—grounds for first degree AV block. The QRS complexes throughout measure a "hair less" than 0.12 seconds. Beats #5 and #6 represent the underlying rhythm, a pronounced sinus bradycardia (rate approximately 40) with first degree AV block. Measure the interval between beats #5 and #6 and compare that to the interval between beats #1 and #2. You will notice that beat #2 is inscribed later than expected. Beats #2 and #3 represent an escape rhythm generated from the AV junctional tissues (the QRS's are not preceded by a P wave and the QRS duration is within normal limits). Beat #4 may have a P wave, though the P-R interval is shorter than beats #5 and #6. (Limb leads would better display atrial activity.) Note the slight ST elevation throughout. In summary, the underlying rhythm is a *slow* sinus bradycardia with first degree AV block. There is a period of sinus arrest (a failure) and a resulting idiojunctional response. The sinus pacemaker resumes near the end of the strip. This patient was in the recovery phase of an acute M.I.

3. S L O W, irregular, ineffective ventricular rhythm. This is known as an agonal or dying heart rhythm. This rhythm strip followed an unsuccessful code arrest.

4. First, I have scanned the strip to determine that beats #1, #2, #3, #7, #8, and #9 appear identical. The P-R interval of those beats measures approximately 0.18 seconds. There is obvious artifact throughout the strip. Though somewhat difficult to measure precisely, the QRS appears to be 0.12 seconds in duration (normal duration is *less* than 0.12 seconds). The underlying rhythm is sinus rhythm (rate somewhere in the mid-sixties) with slightly delayed ventricular conduction. I would need to view lead V_1 for a better analysis and to distinguish right v.s. left bundle branch block. Beats #4 and #5 are coupled P.V.C.'s with the first P.V.C. falling near the vulnerable T wave of beat #3. Coupled P.V.C.'s signify major ventricular irritability. Beat #6 is a "funny-looking beat" (FLB), but it is atrial in origin. In summary, this is a sinus rhythm with bundle branch block with coupled P.V.C.'s.

5. The underlying rhythm is slightly irregular, probably secondary to a slight sinus arrhythmia (related to respiration). The approximate rate is 70 beats per minute. With the exception of beats #3 and #4, all P waves and QRS complexes appear identical. There is a "slight" first degree AV block present since the P-R interval measures approximately 0.21 seconds. Beat #3 is a P.V.C. though it does not interrupt the rhythm of the underlying pacemaker. This is an interpolated P.V.C. with the same sig- nificance of any other P.V.C. (you may wish to refer back to page 107 for review). Beat #4 is probably a sinus beat. Interpolated P.V.C.'s typically cause a prolongation of the P-R interval of the next beat.

I suspect a P wave is hidden in the recovery phase of the interpolated P.V.C. In any event, this is a sinus rhythm with borderline first degree AV block interrupted by a P.V.C. (interpolated). Generalized ST scooping is present throughout. *Note:* Frequently a prolonged P-R interval and ST scooping is found with digitalis administration!

D IGITALIS

6. This rhythm is slow and irregular. It would be necessary to count the rhythm for a full minute to determine the heart rate. Each QRS in the strip is preceded by a P wave. The P-R interval is inconsistent. Beat #1 has a P-R interval measuring 0.18 seconds. The P-R interval of beat #2 measures approximately 0.23. Then comes a pause. Interestingly, the same relationships exist with beats #3 and #4! Wait a minute! Look closely. There is a bump at the finale of the "beat #2 T wave" and another more obvious bump after the "beat #4 T wave." These bumps are no doubt P waves! This is Mobitz type I or a Wenckebach rhythm. The P-R gets progressively longer until a P wave fails to conduct. Then, the cycle starts over again. Generally, Wenckebach is considered a benign dysrhythmia!

7. This rhythm is slow and regular with a rate near 50 beats per minute. Identically appearing P waves precede each QRS. The P-R interval is constant and measures 0.18 seconds. The QRS's are uniform in appearance and measure 0.11 seconds. There is slight sagging of the ST segment. This is a sinus bradycardia.

8. Here we find an irregularly irregular rhythm. There are no clear P waves. The baseline appears to undulate. A lone P.V.C. breaks the ranks. This rhythm is atrial fibrillation with a P.V.C. One would need to count the rate for one full minute to accurately determine heart rate.

9. This strip presents another irregularly irregular rhythm with fairly marked ST depression. Though T waves are pronounced following the ST depression, there are no definitive P waves preceding the QRS complexes. QRS complexes measure within normal limits. For a better view of atrial activity, I would monitor on leads II, III, or aVF. This rhythm strip is fine atrial fibrillation with pronounced ST depression. If you think rhythm interpretation is tedious and frustrating, you are correct!

10. **NEVER PANIC!** Always made the monitor believe *you* are in control! My first eyeball analysis reveals that P waves come before every beat! Thus, I can relax. This is *not* a ventricular anything. I am going to begin my analysis at the beginning of the strip. The first five beats occur regularly with an approximate rate of 85 per minute. Though some notching exists, the P waves appear uniform and the constant P-R interval measures 0.20 seconds. (Notching of the P wave may represent atrial hypertrophy.) The QRS complexes measure 0.12 seconds in duration, grounds for bundle branch block. An analysis of the second half of the strip reveals an approximate rate of 85 beats per minute. The P-R interval measures 0.22 seconds. The QRS complexes measure 0.12 seconds in duration. The second half of the strip also reveals a bundle branch block. My best guess is that this rhythm represents alternating right and left bundle branch blocks—no doubt a function of severe myocardial ischemia/damage. Both the right and left bundle branch blocks produce ST-T wave distortion. To be certain, more information is warranted and a 12-lead EKG is in order!

11. Another strange rhythm strip! The rhythm is regular (approximate rate 62) with a premature beat appearing midstream. A P wave presents before each QRS of the underlying rhythm. The P-R interval is prolonged, measuring 0.24 seconds. Thus, a first degree AV block is present. The QRS complexes of the underlying rhythm measure approximately 0.14 seconds, signifying bundle branch block. To determine right v.s. left bundle branch block, one would need to view lead V_1. The underlying rhythm is a sinus rhythm with both first degree AV block and bundle branch block. The premature beat interrupting the rhythm has a QRS measuring 0.14 seconds. Is it ventricular or supraventricular in

origin? I believe it is a P.A.C. with delayed ventricular conduction (prolonged QRS duration). There is a probable P wave resting on the downstroke of the previous T wave. I did not describe ST depression because, in the face of bundle branch block, repolarization occurs in a distorted manner.

12. The rhythm is regular with a rate of 125 beats per minute. P waves are present before each QRS and begin on the downstroke of the preceding T wave. The P-R interval is constant and measures slightly less than 0.20 seconds. The QRS duration is constant and measures slightly greater than 0.08 seconds. This rhythm is a sinus tachycardia with marked ST depression.

13. Here is a nice, pretty, regular rhythm with an approximate rate of 58 beats per minute. The QRS duration is within normal limits and the T waves are peaked in appearance. No P waves are obvious prior to, or following, the QRS. This rhythm is a junctional (escape) rhythm. A potassium level may be in order since prominent peaked T waves are a primary feature of hyperkalemia. Also, hyperkalemia depresses normal electrical activity and may precipitate conduction disturbances such as junctional rhythms!

14. This is a tough one, so I thought two consecutive rhythm strips (A and B) might be helpful! I always look for something "known" when I begin analysis. The last three beats of the second strip (B) demonstrate a sinus rhythm with an approximate rate of 75 per minute. The P-R interval measures 0.18 seconds and the QRS is greater than the normal limits, measuring 0.14 seconds. So, the last three beats represent a sinus rhythm with bundle branch block. One would need to view lead V_1 to determine right v.s. left bundle branch block. Now back to the beginning, Strip A. At first glance, the rhythm resembles a ventricular tachycardia. The rhythm is fairly regular, the QRS's are widened, and there are no clearly distinguishable P waves. However, in the middle of Strip A there appears to be two consecutive P waves. Presumably the second P wave conducts through to the ventricles (a sinus beat). The QRS's of the rapid rhythm are similar in appearance to those at the end of the second strip. If the rapid rhythm was ventricular in origin, the QRS's would be wide, but they would be configured *differently* from the sinus beats, secondary to retrograde or backward conduction. So, what is the rapid rhythm? I'm not certain either! It might be a "masked" atrial flutter given the two consecutive P waves (rate 300) in the middle of the top strip. Rather than risk confusion, I would simply describe this strip as a rapid rhythm (rate 150) of supraventricular origin. The rapid rhythm breaks spontaneously in the bottom strip. There is a pause, followed by a beat with an inverted P wave, then on to sinus rhythm. Treatment would be aimed at preventing a recurrence of the earlier rapid rhythm. WHEW!!

15. Another difficult strip for consideration! I hope having two consecutive rhythm strips helped. To be certain, this is a chaotic rhythm. In beginning my analysis, I look for beats similar in appearance! In the second strip (B), beats #2, #4, #5, #7, #8, #10, and #12 look reasonably similar, as do beats #1, #3, #9, and #11.

First, I'll consider beats #2, #4, #5, #7, #8, #10, and #12 (B). No clear (obvious) P waves precede these beats, but the baseline undulates. The QRS complexes are within normal limits, measuring 0.10 seconds. Note the ST segment depression and biphasic T wave following those QRS's. The underlying rhythm here is atrial fibrillation with ST segment depression.

Now back to beats #1, #3, #9, and #11 in Strip B. One can easily be misled believing these are sinus beats with a bundle branch block configuration! However, there are *no* P waves preceding these prolonged QRS complexes (QRS measures 0.16 seconds)! Look back at the ST segment and T waves of beats #4, #5, and #7 of Strip B. What appears to be P waves preceding the widened QRS's are in fact the biphasic T waves of the previous beat. *Ugh!* These wide beats are most likely P.V.C.'s Beat #6 (Strip B) is also a P.V.C. but of a different configuration (signifying irritability of different ventricular focus).

Now back to Strip A. Beats #2, #4, #6, #7, #8, #10, and #12 are likely P.V.C.'s! This rhythm is an atrial fibrillation with *extreme* ventricular irritability as is evidenced by frequent P.V.C.'s, multifocused ventricular excitability, and consecutive P.V.C.'s. Clearly, lidocaine therapy would be in order.

PRESS BUTTON . . .

(electronic stripreader activator)

. . . IF YOU WISH TO CONTINUE!

---

16. This strip demonstrates a pacemaker generated ventricular rhythm. No doubt the pacemaker was inserted to correct failure or ineffectiveness of a higher pacemaker. Note the pacemaker spikes initiating each QRS. The ventricular pacemaker rate is approximately 75 per minute.

17. The underlying rhythm is a sinus rhythm with an estimated rate of 70 beats per minute. The P-R interval of the sinus beats measures 0.18 seconds and the QRS measures less than 0.12 seconds in duration. The rhythm is interrupted by unifocal P.V.C.'s occurring in a bigeminal pattern. Note the artifact at the end of the rhythm strip.

18. This strip demonstrates a regular underlying rhythm, rate 88 beats per minute. The atrial activity is masked by a major artifact evident throughout the tracing. The QRS's of the underlying rhythm measure 0.12 seconds. Though distorted, there is evidence of significant ST depression. There is a probable run of P.V.C.'s in the second half of the strip. As a first course of action, I would treat the "assumed" P.V.C.'s (lidocaine) and then attempt to diminish the artifact (antiartifact tips can be found on page 180). This rhythm was a sinus rhythm with bundle branch block interrupted by a short burst of ventricular tachycardia!

19. This strip seems simple compared to some of the previous examples! The rhythm is regular at an approximate rate of 66 beats per minute. The P-R interval is constant and measures 0.16 seconds. The QRS is abnormally wide, measuring almost 0.16 seconds. This is a sinus rhythm with a bundle branch block. One would need to review lead V_1 to accurately distinguish right from left bundle branch block.

20. The rhythm is regular with a rate of 136 beats per minute. When P waves cannot clearly be distinguished, I tend to use the term *supraventricular*. There may be P waves occurring on top of the T waves, but I am uncertain. Because the QRS is within normal limits (0.08 seconds), I know the rhythm cannot be of ventricular origin. Thus we have a supraventricular tachycardia with a rate of 136 beats per minute. In all probability, this is a sinus tachycardia. P waves can be seen more distinctly when monitoring on leads II, III, or aVF. The ST segment sags throughout.

21. UGH! The rhythm is regular, occurring at an approximate rate of 80 beats per minutes. A widened P wave precedes each QRS (suggested atrial hypertrophy) and the constant P-R interval measures 0.20 seconds. The QRS measures 0.10 seconds. There is marked ST depression which suggests ischemia. (It is important to view all leads to determine the location and extent of ST depression.) This is a sinus rhythm!

22. Here we have a sinus rhythm with a rate of 75 beats per minute. The rhythm is interrupted by a lone P.V.C. (note the retrograde P wave following the widened QRS). The P-R interval measures 0.20 seconds and the QRS of the sinus beats measures 0.20 seconds (major conduction delay). There is evidence of ST elevation; however, abnormal ventricular depolarization causes abnormal ventricular repolarization. One would need to view a 12-lead EKG for further analysis. This is a sinus rhythm with a bundle branch block and ST elevation interrupted by a P.V.C. How are you doing? I'm stopping for dinner!

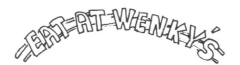

23. The rhythm is irregularly irregular with an undulating baseline. This is an atrial fibrillation. The QRS measures 0.08 seconds.

24. This rhythm strip demonstrates an undulating baseline with no evidence of effective ventricular activation. With no patient to observe, one would assume this is ventricular fibrillation and grounds for immediate resuscitation. However, the truth of the matter is that this patient lost his electrodes! In fact, the patient had a normal sinus rhythm once the leads were reattached!

25. Two continuous rhythm strips were presented to assist in rhythm interpretation. The first three beats in Strip A demonstrate a sinus rhythm with a rate of 75 beats per minute and ST elevation. The P-R interval measures 0.20 seconds and the QRS measures approximately 0.08 seconds. The P wave of beat #4 occurs on time, though the P wave is slightly more pronounced than in the previous three beats. The QRS of this beat is configured differently, but measures less than 0.12 seconds in duration. The pacemaker for this beat is located within the atria, but obviously travels a different pathway, resulting in a QRS with a different configuration. Looking ahead to the next series of ventricular beats, I suspect that beat #4 is a fusion beat—partly formed by a sinus impulse and partly formed by an ectopic ventricular impulse. The remainder of Strip A demonstrates a ventricular rhythm, rate of 79 beats per minute. Given that the ventricular rate is faster than the earlier sinus rate, this rhythm is presumed to be ectopic in nature. Some practitioners would call this a "slow ventricular tachycardia." Fortunately, near the end of Strip B, the sinus pacemaker resumes pacemaker control! This type of rhythm presents somewhat of a treatment dilemma. Aggressive clinicians will elect to administer lidocaine based on the premise that, if the faster ventricular rhythm is abolished, a slower sinus rhythm will prevail. Conservative clinicians may refrain from aggressive therapy if the patient tolerates the rhythm. The rationale behind conservative treatment is the concern that this may be a ventricular escape mechanism, and, if abolished, there may be no underlying sustaining rhythm. To me, the strongest clue supporting an ectopic v.s. escape origin is beat #4, the fusion beat. It is helpful to know that this patient had an acute inferior wall myocardial infarction in progress. WHEW!!

26. The underlying rhythm is sinus rhythm (see mid-strip) with a rate of 80 beats per minute. The P-R interval and QRS measure 0.16 seconds and 0.11 seconds, respectively. Note the ST segment depression suggesting myocardial ischemia. The sinus rhythm is interrupted by bursts of ventricular tachycardia, rate approximately 160 per minute. You will note each "run" of ventricular tachycardia begins with a "funny-looking beat" that has a P wave, and a QRS less wide than those of the ventricular tachycardia. These funny-looking beats are fusion beats and strongly support a ventricular tachycardia classification. Clearly, there is pronounced ventricular irritability!

27. This strip is a killer! Note that the rhythm is irregular. Three slight pauses are evident in the tracing. At first glance, the atrial activity appears to be "a mess." QRS complexes measure approximately 0.14 seconds in duration, demonstrating delayed ventricular conduction (bundle branch block). To begin my analysis, I look at the last beat in the strip (#13) because it appears reasonably normal. I will use it as my guidepost as I examine other complexes. The trick is to determine what mechanism is causing the varying P waves and the irregular ventricular response. Beat #8 resembles beat #13, so I'll begin there. Beat #8 looks like a sinus beat with a P-R interval measuring 0.24 seconds. Beat #9 has no obvious P wave, but the T wave is exceptionally fat. There may be a P wave occurring on the downstroke of the T wave. If so, the P-R interval would be longer than the P-R interval of the preceding complex. The same thing goes for beat #10. There is no obvious P wave, but the T wave is distorted, and appears different. If a P wave is occurring on top of the T wave, this P-R interval would be even greater than in the previous beat. In beats #11 and #12, it is somewhat easier to measure the increasing P-R interval. Following beat #12, there is a pause. Then the cycle appears to begin again. The same pattern exists in beats #3 through #7, with a pause following beat #7. This is a second degree AV block—type I, Wenckebach, accompanied by a bundle branch block. (A conduction system filled with delays!) As is typical of Wenckebach, the P-R gets progressively longer and the R-R interval becomes increasingly shorter until an atrial impulse fails to conduct. This conduction failure relates to refractoriness of the AV junction and is usually caused by ischemia!

28. This rhythm is irregularly irregular and is interrupted by a P.V.C. This is a "fine" atrial fibrillation. The QRS measures 0.12 seconds. This ventricular conduction delay probably accounts for the early distortion (ST segment depression) of ventricular repolzarization.

29. This is one of those "treat now and ask questions later" strips. This looks like a ventricular tachycardia at a rate of 166 per minute. See page 113 for a quick review

30. This strip demonstrates a rapid rhythm with a rate of approximately 120 beats per minute. The QRS duration is 0.12 seconds. This *may* be a sinus tachycardia with a first degree AV block (P-R measures almost 0.24 seconds) and a bundle branch block. However, I am a suspicious character by nature. Any time I see a "sing-song" rapid, regular rhythm, it makes me suspect an atrial flutter. (Sometimes, turning the strip upside down assists me in detecting atrial flutter waves.) I would want to see a rhythm strip of leads II, III, or aVF where atrial activity is more pronounced. I have drawn dots on the strip where I suspect flutter waves. If I am correct, this is a 2:1 atrial flutter. If I am wrong, this is a sinus tachycardia as described above. Beyond looking at other leads, one might have the patient perform a Valsalva maneuver. The Valsalva maneuver momentarily increases the degree of AV block and may make flutter waves more obvious.

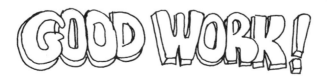

DIPLOMA ☆

LET IT BE RECOGNIZED THAT

NAME : _____

HAS SUCCESSFULLY COMPLETED

THE ART OF EKG INTERPRETATION

ON THIS DAY OF _____, 19___.

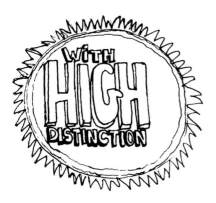

WITH HIGH DISTINCTION

Karen Ehrat

KAREN S. EHRAT, Ph.D.
PROFESSOR IN ABSTENTIA

Index

Atrial
SR — 32
S arrythmias — 72
SB 72
ST 73
PACs 74
a-tach 74
aflutter 75
a bib 76

junctional escape 94
PJC 96
junctional tach 96

Ventricular

PVCs
shells labs 21, 22, 21
67, 68, 69, 70